Manual of Neonatal Respiratory Care

Second Edition

Steven M. Donn, M.D.

Professor of Pediatrics
Director, Division of Neonatal-Perinatal Medicine
C.S. Mott Children's Hospital
University of Michigan Health System
Ann Arbor, Michigan, USA

Sunil K. Sinha, M.D., Ph.D.

Professor of Paediatrics
University of Durham
Consultant in Paediatrics and Neonatal Medicine
The James Cook University Hospital
Middlesbrough, UK

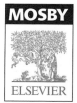

MOSBY

ELSEVIER

MOSBY
ELSEVIER

1600 John F. Kennedy Blvd.
Ste 1800
Philadelphia, PA 19103-2899

MANUAL OF NEONATAL RESPIRATORY CARE
Copyright © 2006, Mosby Inc.

ISBN-13: 978-0-323-03176-9
ISBN-10: 0-323-03176-5

Notice

Knowledge and best practice in this field are constantly changing. As new research and experience broaden our knowledge, changes in practice, treatment, and drug therapy may become necessary or appropriate. Readers are advised to check the most current information provided (i) on procedures featured or (ii) by the manufacturer of each product to be administered, to verify the recommended dose or formula, the method and duration of administration, and contraindications. It is the responsibility of the practitioners, relying on their own experience and knowledge of the patient, to make diagnoses, to determine dosages and the best treatment for each individual patient, and to take all appropriate safety precautions. To the fullest extent of the law, neither the Publisher nor the Editors assumes any liability for any injury and/or damage to persons or property arising out of/or related to any use of the material contained in this book.

Library of Congress Cataloging-in-Publication Data
Manual of neonatal respiratory care/edited by Steven M. Donn and Sunil K. Sinha.—2nd ed.
   p. ; cm.
  Includes bibliographical references and index.
  ISBN 0-323-03176-5
    1. Respiratory therapy for newborn infants—Handbooks, manuals, etc. I. Donn, Steven M. II. Sinha, Sunil K., M.D., Ph.D.
  [DNLM: 1. Respiration Disorders—therapy—Infant, Newborn. 2. Intensive Care, Neonatal—methods. 3. Respiratory Therapy—Infants, Newborn. 4. Ventilators, Mechanical. WS 280 M294 2006]
  RJ312.M36 2006
  618.92′206—dc22   2005049578

Acquisitions Editor: Todd Hummel
Editorial Assistant: Martha Limbach
Publishing Services Manager: Frank Polizzano
Project Manager: Joan Nikelsky
Design Direction: Steve Stave

Working together to grow
libraries in developing countries
www.elsevier.com | www.bookaid.org | www.sabre.org
ELSEVIER BOOK AID International Sabre Foundation

Printed in the United States of America
Last digit is the print number: 9 8 7 6 5 4 3 2 1

Dedication

To my teachers and mentors, who helped shape and guide my career, with special recognition to the late Harry Shirkey, who first exposed me to clinical research and taught me about child advocacy; Jerry Lucey, who supported and encouraged me in my earliest research endeavors; Alistair Philip, who could not have been a better role model, friend, and mentor; and Dieter Roloff, who gave me the opportunity to develop professionally; to my late parents—Elaine, who developed my organizational skills and study habits (almost before I could walk), and Richard, from whom I inherited my love of writing; to my late grandfather, Phil, for always pushing me to do my best; and to my wife, Paula, from whom I learned what true courage is.

—SMD

To my network of colleagues and friends across the world, whose support and encouragement have always been very valuable; and my wife, Lalita, and son, Ian, with gratitude for bearing with the sacrifices imposed and the time taken from them while completing this task. Nonetheless, they will unanimously join me in dedicating this book to my elder son, Akashdeep, who died too young to see this world but who made me a better and complete person. If only an occasional child benefits from this work, we will all consider this some recompense.

—SKS

Contributors

Namasivayam Ambalavanan, M.D.
Assistant Professor of Pediatrics
Division of Neonatology
University of Alabama at Birmingham
  Medical Center
Birmingham, Alabama, USA

Jeanette M. Asselin, M.S., R.R.T.
Manager, Neonatal & Pediatric
  Critical Care Research Group
Children's Hospital & Research
  Center at Oakland
Oakland, California, USA

Mohammad A. Attar, M.D.
Clinical Instructor of Pediatrics
Division of Neonatal-Perinatal
  Medicine
C.S. Mott Children's Hospital
University of Michigan Health System
Ann Arbor, Michigan, USA

C. Fred Baker, M.D.
Fellow in Neonatology
Department of Pediatrics
C.S. Mott Children's Hospital
University of Michigan Health System
Ann Arbor, Michigan, USA

Eduardo Bancalari, M.D.
Professor of Pediatrics
Director, Division of Newborn
  Medicine
University of Miami, School of
  Medicine
Miami, Florida, USA

Kenneth P. Bandy, R.R.T.
Technical Director
Department of Critical Care Support
  Services
University of Michigan Health System
Ann Arbor, Michigan, USA

Keith J. Barrington, M.D.
Associate Professor
Departments of Paediatrics and
  Obstetrics and Gynaecology
McGill University
Director, NICU
Royal Victoria Hospital
Montreal, Quebec, Canada

Daniel G. Batton, M.D.
Medical Director of Newborn
  Medicine
William Beaumont Hospital
Royal Oak, Michigan, USA

**J. Harry Baumer, F.R.C.P.,
F.R.C.P.C.H.**
Consultant Paediatrician
Derriford Hospital
Plymouth, Devon, UK

Michael A. Becker, R.R.T.
Clinical Specialist
Department of Critical Care Support
  Services
C.S. Mott Children's Hospital
University of Michigan Health
  System
Ann Arbor, Michigan, USA

Vinod K. Bhutani, M.D.
Professor of Pediatrics
Division of Neonatology
Lucile Packard Children's Hospital
Stanford University Medical Center
Palo Alto, California, USA

**Elaine Boyle M.B., Ch.B., M.Sc.(Dist.),
M.D., M.R.C.P., M.R.C.P.C.H.**
Specialist Registrar
Lothian Universities Hospital Trust
Edinburgh, Scotland, UK

J. Bert Bunnell, Sc.D.
Chairman and Chief Executive Officer
Bunnell Incorporated
Assistant Adjunct Professor
Department of Bioengineering
University of Utah
Salt Lake City, Utah, USA

Mary K. Buschell, R.R.T.
Clinical Specialist
Department of Critical Care Support
 Services
C.S. Mott Children's Hospital
University of Michigan Health System
Ann Arbor, Michigan, USA

Waldemar A. Carlo, M.D.
Professor of Pediatrics
Director of Neonatology
University of Alabama at Birmingham
 Medical Center
Birmingham, Alabama, USA

Robert L. Chatburn, R.R.T.
Associate Professor of Pediatrics
Case Western Reserve University
Director of Respiratory Care
University Hospitals of Cleveland
Cleveland, Ohio, USA

*Malcolm L. Chiswick, M.D., F.R.C.P.,
F.R.C.P.C.H., D.C.H.*
Professor of Paediatrics and Child
 Health
University of Manchester
Consultant Paediatrician, Neonatal
 Medical Unit
St. Mary's Hospital for Women and
 Children
Manchester, UK

Reese H. Clark, M.D.
Director of Research
Pediatrix Medical Group
Sunrise, Florida, USA

Jonathan M. Davis, M.D.
Professor of Pediatrics
Director of Neonatology
Winthrop-University Hospital
Mineola, New York, USA

Eugene M. Dempsey, M.D.
Fellow in Neonatology
McGill University
Montreal, Quebec, Canada

Steven M. Donn, M.D.
Professor of Pediatrics
Director, Division of Neonatal-
 Perinatal Medicine
C.S. Mott Children's Hospital
University of Michigan Health System
Ann Arbor, Michigan, USA

David J. Durand, M.D.
Division of Neonatology
Children's Hospital & Research
 Center at Oakland
Oakland, California, USA

*Avroy A. Fanaroff, M.D., F.R.C.P.,
F.R.C.P.C.H., F.R.C.P.E.*
Professor and Chair, Department of
 Pediatrics
Case Western Reserve University
 School of Medicine
Eliza Henry Barnes Chair of
 Neonatology
Physician-in-Chief
Rainbow Babies & Children's Hospital
Cleveland, Ohio, USA

Jonathan M. Fanaroff, M.D., J.D.
Senior Fellow in Neonatology
Department of Pediatrics
Rainbow Babies & Children's Hospital
Case Western Reserve University
Cleveland, Ohio, USA

*S. David Ferguson, M.A., F.R.C.P.,
F.R.C.P.C.H.*
Consultant Paediatrician
Royal Gwent Hospital
Gwent, Wales, UK

*David J. Field, F.R.C.P.C.H., F.R.C.P.
(Ed.), D.M.*
Professor of Neonatal Medicine
University of Leicester
Leicester, UK

Alistair R. Fielder, F.R.C.P., F.R.C.S., F.R.C.Ophth.
Professor of Ophthalmology
Imperial College School of Medicine
Academic Unit of Ophthalmology
The Western Eye Hospital
London, UK

Neil N. Finer, M.D.
Professor of Pediatrics
Director, Division of Neonatology
Unversity of California, San Diego
    Medical Center
San Diego, California, USA

David S. Foley, M.D.
Assistant Professor of Surgery
Division of Pediatric Surgery
University of Louisville
Louisville, Kentucky, USA

Molly R. Gates, M.S., R.N.C.
Neonatal Outreach Coordinator
Department of Nursing
C.S. Mott Children's Hospital
University of Michigan Health
    System
Ann Arbor, Michigan, USA

Linda Genen, M.D.
Associate Medical Director, NICU
Winthrop-University Hospital
Assistant Professor of Pediatrics
SUNY Stony Brook School of
    Medicine
Mineola, New York, USA

Dale R. Gerstmann, M.D.
Staff Neonatologist
Utah Valley Regional Medical
    Center
Provo, Utah, USA

Jay P. Goldsmith, M.D.
Chairman Emeritus
Department of Pediatrics
Ochsner Clinic Foundation
Clinical Professor of Pediatrics
Tulane University
New Orleans, Louisiana, USA

Anne Greenough, M.D., F.R.C.P., F.R.C.P.C.H., D.C.H.
Professor of Clinical Respiratory
    Physiology
Department of Paediatrics
Guy's, King's, and St. Thomas' School
    of Medicine
King's College Hospital
London, UK

Samir Gupta, M.D., M.R.C.P.I., F.R.C.P.C.H.
Senior Clinical Fellow
Department of Neonatal Medicine
The James Cook University Hospital
Middlesbrough, UK

Ronald B. Hirschl, M.D.
Associate Professor of Surgery
Division of Pediatric Surgery
C.S. Mott Children's Hospital
University of Michigan Health System
Ann Arbor, Michigan, USA

Martin Keszler, M.D.
Professor of Pediatrics
Division of Neonatology
Georgetown University Medical Center
Washington, D.C., USA

John P. Kinsella, M.D.
Professor of Pediatrics
Medical Director: Newborn Emergency
    Medical Transport Service
Medical Director: ECMO Service
The Children's Hospital/University of
    Colorado School of Medicine
Denver, Colorado, USA

Lawrence R. Kuhns, M.D.
Professor of Radiology
Division of Pediatric Radiology
C.S. Mott Children's Hospital
University of Michigan Health System
Ann Arbor, Michigan, USA

Thierry Lacaze-Masmonteil, M.D., Ph.D.
Professor of Pediatrics
Department of Paediatrics
University of Alberta
Edmonton, Alberta, Canada

Kimberly LaMar, N.D., R.N.C., C.N.N.P.
Director, Professional Practice, Development, and Research
Banner Desert Medical Center
Mesa, Arizona, USA

M. Jeffrey Maisels, M.D.
Chairman of Pediatrics
William Beaumont Hospital
Royal Oak, Michigan, USA
Clinical Professor of Pediatrics
University of Michigan Medical School
Ann Arbor, Michigan, USA
Clinical Professor of Pediatrics
Wayne State University
Detroit, Michigan, USA

Neil McIntosh, D.Sc.(Med.), F.R.C.P., F.R.C.P.E., F.R.C.P.C.H.
Professor of Paediatrics
Department of Child Life and Health
University of Edinburgh
Edinburgh, Scotland, UK

Anthony D. Milner, M.D., F.R.C.P., F.R.C.P.C.H., D.C.H.
Professor of Neonatology
Department of Paediatrics
Guy's, King's, and St. Thomas' School of Medicine
St. Thomas' Hospital
London, UK

Colin J. Morley, M.A., D.C.H., M.D., F.R.C.P., F.R.C.P.C.H.
Professor of Paediatrics
Director of Neonatal Medicine
Royal Women's Hospital
Melbourne, Victoria, Australia

Joanne J. Nicks, R.R.T.
Clinical Specialist
Department of Critical Care Support Services
C.S. Mott Children's Hospital
University of Michigan Health System
Ann Arbor, Michigan, USA

Donald M. Null, Jr., M.D.
Medical Director NBICU Primary Children's Medical Center
Professor of Pediatrics
University of Utah School of Medicine
Salt Lake City, Utah, USA

Elvira Parravicini, M.D.
Assistant Attending, Division of Neonatology
Children's Hospital of New York–Presbyterian
Assistant Professor of Clinical Pediatrics
Columbia University College of Physicians and Surgeons
New York, New York, USA

Gilberto R Pereira, M.D.
Neonatologist, Children's Hospital of Philadelphia
Professor of Pediatrics
University of Pennsylvania School of Medicine
Philadelphia, Pennsylvania, USA

Jeffrey M. Perlman, M.B.
Professor of Pediatrics
Director, Division of Neonatology
Weill Cornell University Medical Center
New York, New York, USA

Christian F. Poets, M.D.
Professor of Pediatrics
Director of Neonatology
University Children's Hospital
Tuebingen, Germany

Richard A. Polin, M.D.
Director, Division of Neonatology
Children's Hospital of New York–Presbyterian
Professor of Pediatrics
Columbia University College of Physicians and Surgeons
New York, New York, USA

Tonse N. K. Raju, M.D., D.C.H.
Medical Officer/Program Scientist
Pregnancy and Perinatology Branch
Center for Developmental Biology
 and Perinatal Medicine
National Institute of Child Health and
 Human Development
National Institutes of Health
Bethesda, Maryland, USA

*Janet M. Rennie, M.A., M.D., F.R.C.P,
F.R.C.P.C.H, D.C.H.*
Consultant and Senior Lecturer in
 Neonatal Medicine
Elizabeth Garret Anderson Obstetric
 Hospital
University College London Hospitals
London, UK

*Sam W. J. Richmond, F.R.C.P,
F.R.C.P.C.H.*
Consultant in Paediatrics
Neonatal Unit
Sunderland Royal Infirmary
Sunderland, UK

Gauravi K. Sabharwal, M.D.
Clinical Lecturer
Division of Pediatric Radiology
C.S. Mott Children's Hospital
University of Michigan Health System
Ann Arbor, Michigan, USA

Saroj Saigal, M.D., F.R.C.P. (C.)
Senior Scientist, Canadian Institute
 for Health Research
Professor of Pediatrics
McMaster University
Hamilton, Ontario, Canada

Subrata Sarkar, M.D.
Clinical Assistant Professor of
 Pediatrics
Division of Neonatal-Perinatal
 Medicine
C.S. Mott Children's Hospital
University of Michigan Health System
Ann Arbor, Michigan, USA

Andreas Schulze, M.D.
Associate Professor of Pediatrics
Director, Division of Neonatology
Department of Obstetrics and
 Gynecology
Klinikum Grosshadern and The
 Dr. von Hauer Children's Hospital
University of Munich
Munich, Germany

Robert E. Schumacher, M.D.
Associate Professor of Pediatrics
Division of Neonatal-Perinatal
 Medicine
Medical Director, Holden Neonatal
 Intensive Care Unit
C.S. Mott Children's Hospital
University of Michigan Health System
Ann Arbor, Michigan, USA

Rupa Seetharamaiah, M.D.
Research Fellow
Section of Pediatric Surgery
C.S. Mott Children's Hospital
Department of Surgery
University of Michigan Health System
Ann Arbor, Michigan, USA

*Sunil K. Sinha, M.D., Ph.D., F.R.C.P,
F.R.C.P.C.H.*
Professor of Paediatrics
University of Durham
Consultant in Paediatrics and
 Neonatal Medicine
The James Cook University Hospital
Middlesbrough, UK

Emidio M. Sivieri, M.S.
Section on Newborn Pediatrics
Pennsylvania Hospital
Philadelphia, Pennsylvania, USA

Alan R. Spitzer, M.D.
Senior Vice President and Director
The Center for Research and
 Education
Pediatrix Medical Group
Sunrise, Florida, USA

Barbara S. Steffes, M.D.
Fellow in Neonatology
Department of Pediatrics
C.S. Mott Children's Hospital
University of Michigan Health System
Ann Arbor, Michigan, USA

Win Tin, M.R.C.P., F.R.C.P.C.H.
Consultant in Paediatrics and
    Neonatology
The James Cook University Hospital
Middlesbrough, UK

Stefano Tredici, M.D.
Research Fellow
Department of General Surgery
University of Michigan Health System
Ann Arbor, Michigan, USA

*Unni Wariyar, M.D., F.R.C.P.,
F.R.C.P.C.H.*
Consultant in Paediatrics and
    Neonatology
Royal Victoria Infirmary Hospital
Newcastle-upon-Tyne, UK

Thomas E. Wiswell, M.D.
Staff Neonatologist
The Florida Hospital
Orlando, Florida, USA

*Jonathan P. Wyllie, F.R.C.P.,
F.R.C.P.C.H.*
Consultant in Paediatrics and
    Neonatology
The James Cook University Hospital
Middlesbrough, UK

Foreword

A successful transition from fetal to neonatal life is dependent on the profound cardiorespiratory adaptation occurring at this time. Unfortunately, this unique sequence of events frequently requires medical intervention, especially in preterm infants. Furthermore, the consequences of pathophysiologic changes and resultant therapeutic interventions in such neonates may have long-lasting effects on the developing respiratory system and on neurodevelopmental outcome of this high-risk population.

Recognition of the importance of neonatal respiratory management was an early milestone in the history of neonatology. The role of surfactant deficiency in the etiology of neonatal respiratory distress syndrome was confirmed 45 years ago, and thus the way was paved for the introduction of assisted ventilation for this population in the 1960s. I was privileged to be introduced to the field of neonatal pediatrics in the early 1970s at a time when the advent of continuous positive airway pressure demonstrated how physiologic insight could be translated into effective therapy. The decade of the 1970s offered many other innovations in neonatal respiratory care, including noninvasive blood gas monitoring, xanthine therapy for apnea, the first real understanding of the pathogenesis and management of meconium aspiration syndrome and of three frequently interrelated conditions—group B streptococcal pneumonia and persistent fetal circulation and pulmonary hypertension of the newborn. The decade ended in remarkable fashion with the introduction of exogenous surfactant therapy and recognition that the novel technique of high-frequency ventilation allows effective gas exchange in sick neonates.

The past 25 years have allowed us to build dramatically on the foundation of this earlier period in neonatal respiratory management. The improved survival of low-birth-weight infants has been nothing short of spectacular. However, many key issues in neonatal respiratory care still need to be addressed. For preterm infants the focus is clearly to reduce the unacceptably high incidence of bronchopulmonary dysplasia and chronic neonatal lung disease. What constitutes optimal ventilatory strategy in the delivery room and subsequent goals for gas exchange? What is the risk/benefit ratio of current and future pharmacologic adjuncts to ventilatory support-such as inhaled nitric oxide, xanthine, and antioxidant therapy (to name a few)? For preterm and term infants with malformations of the respiratory system, advances in pre- and postnatal imaging and surgical techniques hold great promise for improved outcomes.

Great strides are being made in our understanding of the molecular basis of normal and abnormal lung development. Furthermore, it is being increasingly recognized that genotypic characteristics may greatly influence the impact of environmental factors on lung development. These scientific advances need to be translated into improved neonatal outcomes. As care providers to neonates, it is our responsibility to encourage clinical trials and other patient-based investigation that will allow the optimization of the outcome of neonatal respiratory care.

This comprehensive manual, with contributions by a distinguished group of physicians/scientists, will contribute to this goal. The editors have assembled leaders in the field of developmental pulmonology, with expertise spanning neonatal physiology, pathogenesis of disease, and unique approaches to management of both simple and complex disorders. The result is a comprehensive text that provides a strongly international insight into neonatal respiratory care in a user-friendly format.

Richard J. Martin, M.B., F.R.A.C.P.
Professor of Pediatrics, Neonatology and
Reproductive Biology, and Biophysics
Case Western Reserve University School of Medicine
Director of Neonatology
Rainbow Babies & Children's Hospital
Cleveland, Ohio, USA

Preface

It has been a little more than 6 years since the publication of the first edition of the *Manual of Neonatal Respiratory Care*. Changes and advances continue to occur at an astonishing rate, with new devices, pharmaceuticals, and therapeutic strategies evolving every day. The milieu of the neonatal intensive care unit has also changed; acuity has increased, care has become more complex, and new, daunting challenges continue to arise. Today's clinicians, especially those in training, are faced with enormous tasks and a myriad of treatment choices that can confuse even the most seasoned professionals.

The purpose of this book is to try to put into perspective the management of neonatal respiratory failure, which is still the most prominent problem in neonatal intensive care. It is our aim to provide an overview of the various facets of respiratory care, including lung development, pulmonary function and pathophysiology, diagnosis, and management of neonatal respiratory disorders. Our contributors were selected from the world's experts, and the list literally spans five continents. We hope that this offers a more global point of view and enables the practitioner to choose strategies to which he might not otherwise be exposed. The equipment we feature in this book was chosen because it is widely used, and the choice should not be misconstrued as a specific preference of the editors or contributors.

This edition of the *Manual of Neonatal Intensive Care* has some notable changes. In addition to updating the original chapters of the first edition, new chapters have been added on lung and airway anomalies, respiratory gas conditioning, oxygen therapy and toxicity, pulse oximetry, noninvasive ventilation, proportional assist ventilation, nutritional support, and outcomes of infants with chronic lung disease. Controversies continue to abound, and some of the chapters were chosen for exactly that reason.

It is our good fortune to have become part of the Elsevier network, and we appreciate all of the help and guidance we received during the production of the book. Special thanks go to Judy Fletcher, who understood the need for a book such as this, to Todd Hummel, our acquisitions editor, to Martha Limbach, his assistant, and to Joan Nikelsky, our project manager. Despite living in the electronic era, manuscripts still need to be typed, corrected, and re-typed. Collating 76 chapters from 70 contributors was not easy, and we would like to acknowledge the outstanding effort, organization, patience, and persistence of Susan Peterson in Ann Arbor and Vicky Hall in Middlesbrough. Their help and contributions in the production of this book are greatly appreciated.

Finally, we would like to acknowledge our colleagues, who support us in so many ways, including letting us bring our new gadgets into the NICU, and our families, who spend many nights alone while we are gadgeteering in the NICU.

Steven M. Donn, M.D.
Ann Arbor, Michigan, USA

Sunil K. Sinha, M.D., Ph.D.
Middlesbrough, UK

Contents

SECTION III. Procedures and Techniques

SECTION IV. Monitoring the Ventilated Patient

SECTION V. Noninvasive and Invasive Ventilatory Techniques

SECTION X. Other Considerations

SECTION XI. Ethical Considerations

SECTION XII. Ventilatory Case Studies

List of Abbreviations

A	alveolar
a	arterial
A-aDO$_2$	alveolar-arterial oxygen gradient
ABG	arterial blood gas
ACD	alveolar capillary dysplasia
ACT	activated clotting time
A/C	assist/control
ADP	adenosine diphosphate
AH	absolute humidity
ALTE	apparent life-threatening event
AMP	adenosine monophosphate
Ao	aortic
AOI	apnea of infancy
AOP	apnea of prematurity
AP	anteroposterior
ARDS	adult (or acute) respiratory distress syndrome
ASD	atrial septal defect
ATP	adenosine triphosphate
ATPS	ambient temperature and pressure, saturated with water vapor
BAER	brainstem audiometric evoked responses
BPD	bronchopulmonary dysplasia
BPM	beats per minute
BR	breath rate
BTPS	body temperature and pressure, saturated with water vapor
C	compliance
°C	degrees Celsius
C$_{20}$	compliance over last 20% of inflation
C$_D$ (or C$_{DYN}$)	dynamic compliance
C$_L$	compliance
C$_{ST}$	static compliance
CAHS	central alveolar hypoventilation syndrome
cAMP	cyclic adenosine monophosphate
CAP	constant airway pressure
CaO$_2$	oxygen content of arterial blood
CBC	complete blood cell count
CBF	cerebral blood flow
CBG	capillary blood gas
cc	cubic centimeter
CCAM	congenital cystic adenomatoid malformation
CDH	congenital diaphragmatic hernia

CDP	constant or continuous distending pressure
cGMP	cyclic guanosine monophosphate
CHAOS	congenital high-airway obstruction syndrome
CHD	congenital heart disease
CLD	chronic lung disease
CLE	congenital lobar emphysema
cm	centimeter
CMV	conventional mechanical ventilation
CMV	cytomegalovirus
CNS	central nervous system
CO	cardiac output
CO_2	carbon dioxide
COHb	carboxyhemoglobin
CPAP	continuous positive airway pressure
CPL	congenital pulmonary lymphangiectasis
CPR	cardiopulmonary resuscitation
CPT	chest physiotherapy
CRP	C-reactive protein
CSF	cerebrospinal fluid
CT	computed tomography
CV	conventional ventilator or ventilation
CVP	central venous pressure
CXR	chest x-ray (radiograph)
D	diastole
2D Echo	2-dimensional echocardiogram
DIC	disseminated intravascular coagulation
dL	deciliter
2,3-DPG	2,3-diphosphoglycerate
DPPC	dipalmitoylphosphatidylcholine
DR	delivery room
D_5W	dextrose 5% in water
E	elastance
ECG	electrocardiogram
ECMO	extracorporeal membrane oxygenation
EDRF	endothelial-derived relaxing factor
EEG	electroencephalogram
EF	ejection fraction
ELBW	extremely low birth weight
EMG	electromyogram
EMLA	eutectic mixture of lidocaine and prilocaine
ERV	expiratory reserve volume
ET	endotracheal
$ETCO_2$	end-tidal carbon dioxide
ETCPAP	endotracheal continuous positive airway pressure
ETT	endotracheal tube
EXIT	ex utero intrapartum treatment

F or f	frequency
°F	degrees Fahrenheit
FDA	Food and Drug Administration [U.S.]
FEV_1	forced expiratory volume in one second
FiO_2	fraction of inspired oxygen
FOE	fractional oxygen extraction
Fr	French
FRC	functional residual capacity
FSP	fibrin split products
FTA	fluorescent treponemal antibody
G	gravida
g	gram
GA	gestational age
GER	gastroesophageal reflux
GERD	gastroesophageal reflux disease
GMP	guanosine monophosphate
GTP	guanosine triphosphate
GUIs	graphical user interfaces
hr	hour
Hb	hemoglobin
HCH	hygroscopic condenser humidifier
HFJV	high-frequency jet ventilation
HFO	high-frequency oscillation
HFOV	high-frequency oscillatory ventilation
HFV	high-frequency ventilation
Hg	mercury
HME	heat and moisture exchanger
HR	heart rate
HSV	herpes simplex virus
Hz	Hertz
H_2O	water
I	inertance
IC	inspiratory capacity
ID	internal diameter
I:E	inspiratory:expiratory ratio
Ig	immunoglobulin
IL	interleukin
IMV	intermittent mandatory ventilation
iNO	inhaled nitric oxide
I/O	input/output
IP	inspiratory pressure
IPPV	intermittent positive pressure ventilation
IRV	inspiratory reserve volume
I/T	immature-to-total neutrophil ratio
IUGR	intrauterine growth retardation or restriction

IV	intravenous
IVH	intraventricular hemorrhage
IVS	interventricular septum
°K	degrees Kelvin
K	constant
kDa	kilodalton
kg	kilogram
kPa	kilopascal
L	liter
LA	left atrium
LBW	low birth weight
LCD	liquid crystalline display
LED	light-emitting diode
LOS	length of stay
L/min	liters per minute
LVEDD	left ventricular end-diastolic dimension
LVID	left ventricular internal diameter
LVIDD	left ventricular internal diameter at diastole
LVIDS	left ventricular internal diameter at systole
µg	microgram
m	meter
MAP	mean arterial pressure
MAS	meconium aspiration syndrome
mcg	See µg.
MD	minute distance
mEq	milliequivalent
MetHb	methemoglobin
mg	milligram
MIC	mean inhibitory concentration
min	minute
mL	milliliter
mm	millimeter
MMV	mandatory minute ventilation
mo	month
mOsm	milliosmoles
MRI	magnetic resonance imaging
MSAF	meconium-stained amniotic fluid
msec	millisecond
MCT	medium-chain triglyeride
MV	minute ventilation
NEC	necrotizing enterocolitis
NICU	neonatal intensive care unit
NO	nitric oxide
NO_2	nitrogen dioxide
NOS	nitric oxide synthase

O_2	oxygen
O_2 Sat	blood oxygen saturation
OI	oxygenation index
P	para
P_{50}	point of 50% saturation of hemoglobin with oxygen
Paw	airway pressure
$P\bar{a}w$	mean airway pressure
P_E	elastic pressure
P_I	inertial pressure
P_I	inspiratory pressure
P_{IP}	intrapleural pressure
P_R	resistive pressure
P_{ST}	static pressure
P_{TP}	transpulmonary pressure
PvO_2	partial pressure of oxygen, venous
P_ACO_2	partial pressure of carbon dioxide, alveolar
P_aCO_2	partial pressure of carbon dioxide, arterial
P_AO_2	partial pressure of oxygen, alveolar
P_aO_2	partial pressure of oxygen, arterial
PAV	proportional assist ventilation
PB	periodic breathing
PC	pressure control
PCA	postconceptional age
PCO_2	partial pressure of carbon dioxide
PDA	patent ductus arteriosus
PEEP	positive end-expiratory pressure
PFC	persistent fetal circulation
PG	prostaglandin
PH_2O	partial pressure of water vapor
PIE	pulmonary interstitial emphysema
PiO_2	partial pressure of oxygen in humidified air
PIP	peak inspiratory pressure
PL	pressure limit
PLV	partial liquid ventilation
PMA	postmenstrual age
PN_2	partial pressure of nitrogen
PMA	pre-market approval [U.S.]
PO_2	partial pressure of oxygen in dry air
PPHN	persistent pulmonary hypertension of the newborn
ppm	parts per million
PRBCs	packed red blood cells
prn	as needed
PRVC	pressure-regulated volume control
PS_{max}	pressure support, maximum
psig	pounds per square inch, gauge
PSV	pressure support ventilation
PT	prothrombin time
PTT	partial thromboplastin time

PTV	patient-triggered ventilation
PUFA	polyunsaturated fatty acid
PV-IVH	periventricular-intraventricular hemorrhage
PVL	periventricular leukomalacia
P_VO_2	mixed venous PO_2
PVR	pulmonary vascular resistance
Q	perfusion
q	every
R	resistance
r	radius
R_{AW}	airway resistance
R_E	expiratory resistance
R_I	inspiratory resistance
R_{ST}	static resistance
RBCs	red blood cells
RDS	respiratory distress syndrome
REM	rapid eye movement
RH	relative humidity
RhSOD	recombinant human superoxide dismutase
ROP	retinopathy of prematurity
ROS	reactive oxygen species
RR	respiratory rate
RSV	respiratory syncytial virus
RV	reserve volume
S	end-systole
$S_{1\ (2,3,4)}$	first (second, third, fourth) heart sound
SAHS	sleep apnea hypopnea syndrome
SaO_2	arterial oxygen saturation
SpO_2	pulse oximetry saturation
SvO_2	venous oxygen saturation
sec	second
sGC	soluble guanylate cyclase
SIDS	sudden infant death syndrome
SIMV	synchronized intermittent mandatory ventilation
SNIPPV	synchronized nasal intermittent positive pressure ventilation
SOD	superoxide dismutase
SP	surfactant protein
sq	square
STPD	standard temperature and pressure, dry
T	temperature
T_E	expiratory time
T_I	inspiratory time
$TcPCO_2$	transcutaneous carbon dioxide level
$TcPO_2$	transcutaneous oxygen level
TBW	total body water

TCPL(V)	time-cycled, pressure-limited (ventilation)
TCT	total cycle time
TEF	tracheoesophageal fistula
TGV	thoracic gas volume
THAM	tris-hydroxyaminomethane
TLC	total lung capacity
TLV	total liquid ventilation
TNF	tumor necrosis factor
TPN	total parenteral nutrition
TRH	thyroid-releasing hormone
TTN, TTNB	transient tachypnea of the newborn

U	unit(s)
UAC	umbilical artery catheter

V	volume
$\dot{V}$	flow
$\ddot{V}$	rate of change of flow
V_A	alveolar volume
$\dot{V}_A$	alveolar ventilation
$\dot{V}_{CO_2}$	carbon dioxide elimination
V_D	deadspace volume
V_T	tidal volume
V_{TE}	expiratory tidal volume
V_{TI}	inspiratory tidal volume
VA	venoarterial
VACTERL	vertebral abnormalities, anal atresia, cardiac abnormalities, tracheoesophageal fistula and/or esophageal atresia, renal agenesis and dysplasia, and limb defects
VAPS	volume-assured pressure support
VC	vital capacity
VCF	velocity of circumferential fiber shortening
VCV	volume controlled ventilation
VDRL	venereal disease research laboratory
VLBW	very low birth weight
V/Q	ventilation-perfusion
VS	volume support
VSD	ventricular septal defect
VTI	velocity time interval
VV	venovenous

WBCs	white blood cells
wk	week(s)

yr	year(s)

Lung Development and Maldevelopment

Development of the Respiratory System

Vinod K. Bhutani

I. Introduction
   A. Prenatal development of the respiratory system is not complete until sufficient gas exchange surface has formed to support the newborn at birth.
   B. Pulmonary vasculature must also achieve sufficient capacity to transport carbon dioxide and oxygen through the lungs.
   C. Gas exchange surface must be structurally stable, functional, and elastic to require minimal effort for ventilation and to be responsive to the metabolic needs of the infant.
   D. Structural maturation of the airways, chest wall, and respiratory muscles and neural maturation of respiratory control are integral to the optimal function of the gas exchange "unit."
   E. Respiratory system development continues after birth and well into childhood (Table 1-1).
   F. Fundamental processes that impact on respiratory function:
      1. Ventilation and distribution of gas volumes
      2. Gas exchange and transport
      3. Pulmonary circulation

TABLE 1-1. Magnitude of Lung Development from Fetal Age to Adulthood

	30 wk	Term	Adult	Increase*
Surface area (m²)	0.3	4.0	100	23
Lung volume (mL)	25	200	5000	23
Lung weight (g)	25	50	800	16
Alveoli (no.)	Few	50 m	300 m	6
Alveolar diameter (μ)	32*	150	300	10
Airway branching (no.)	24	24	24	03

*Two-Fold increase after term postconceptional age.
m, million.

4. Mechanical forces that initiate breathing and those that impede airflow
5. Organization and control of breathing
II. Lung Development
   A. Background: The lung's developmental design is based on the functional goal of allowing air and blood to interface over a vast surface area and an extremely thin yet intricately organized tissue barrier. The developmental maturation is such that growth (a quantitative phenomenon) progresses separately from maturation (a qualitative phenomenon). A tension skeleton composed of connective tissue fibers determines the mechanical properties of the lungs: axial, peripheral, and alveolar septal.
      1. Axial connective tissue fibers have a centrifugal distribution from the hilum to the branching airways.
      2. Peripheral fibers have a centripetal distribution from the pleura to within the lungs.
      3. Alveolar septal fibers connect the axial and peripheral fibers.
   B. Functional anatomy (Table 1-2)
      1. Fetal lung development takes place in seven phases (see Table 1-2).
      2. Demarcations are not exact but arbitrary, with transition and progression occurring between each.
      3. Little is known about the effects of antenatal steroids on the transition and maturation of fetal lung development.

TABLE 1-2. Stages of Prenatal and Postnatal Structural Lung Development

Phase	Postconceptional Age	Length: Terminal Bronchiole to Pleura	Structure
Embryonic	0-7 wk	<0.1 mm	Budding from the foregut
Pseudoglandular	8-16 wk	0.1 mm	Airway division commences and terminal bronchioles formed
Canalicular	17-27 wk	0.2 mm	3 generations of respiratory bronchioles; primitive saccule formation with type I and type II epithelial cells; capillarization
Saccular	28-35 wk	0.6 mm	Transitional saccules formed; true alveoli appear
Alveolar	>36 wk	11 mm	Terminal saccules formed; true alveoli appear
Postnatal	2 mo	175 mm	5 generations of alveolar ducts; alveoli form with septation
Early childhood	6-7 yr	400 mm	Airways remodeled; alveolar sac budding occurs

TABLE 1-3. Factors That Influence Fetal Lung Maturation

Physical	Hormonal	Local
Fetal respiration	Glucocorticoids	cAMP
Fetal lung fluid	Prolactin	Methylxanthines
Thoracic volume (FRC)	Insulin	

    C. Factors that impact fetal lung growth:
       1. Physical, hormonal, and local factors play a significant role (Table 1-3).
       2. The physical factors play a crucial role in structural development and may influence the size and capacity of the lungs.
       3. Hormonal influences may be stimulatory or inhibitory.
    D. Fetal lung fluid and variations in lung development: Production, effluence, and physiology are dependent on physiologic control of fetal lung fluid.
       1. Production: Secretion commences in mid-gestation, during the canalicular phase, and composition distinctly differs from that of fetal plasma and amniotic fluid (Table 1-4).
       2. Distending pressure: Daily production rate of 250 to 300 mL/24 hr results in distending pressure of 3 to 5 cm H_2O within the respiratory system. This hydrostatic pressure seems to be crucial for fetal lung development, including the progressive bifurcations of the airways and development of terminal saccules.
       3. Fetal breathing: During fetal breathing movements, tracheal egress of lung fluid (up to 15 mL/hr) during expiration (compared to minimal loss during fetal apnea) ensures that lung volume remains at about 30 mL/kg (equivalent to FRC). Excessive egress has been associated with pulmonary hypoplasia (Figure 1-1), whereas tracheal ligation has been associated with pulmonary hyperplasia.
  III. Upper Airway Development
    A. Airways are heterogeneous, conduct airflow, and do not participate in gas exchange. Starting as the upper airways (nose, mouth,

TABLE 1-4. Chemical Features of Fetal Fluids

Fluid	Osmolality (mOsm/L)	Protein (g/dL)	pH	Sodium (mEq/L)	Potassium (mEq/L)	Chloride (mEq/L)	Bicarbonate (mEq/L)
Fetal lung fluid	300	0.03	6.27	140	6.3	144	2.8
Fetal plasma	290	4.1	7.34	140	4.8	107	24
Amniotic fluid	270	0.1-0.7	7.07	110	7.1	94	18

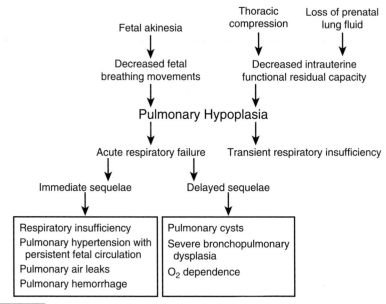

Fetal akinesia → Decreased fetal breathing movements

Thoracic compression, Loss of prenatal lung fluid → Decreased intrauterine functional residual capacity

Pulmonary Hypoplasia

Acute respiratory failure → Immediate sequelae

Transient respiratory insufficiency → Delayed sequelae

Immediate sequelae:
Respiratory insufficiency
Pulmonary hypertension with persistent fetal circulation
Pulmonary air leaks
Pulmonary hemorrhage

Delayed sequelae:
Pulmonary cysts
Severe bronchopulmonary dysplasia
O_2 dependence

FIGURE 1-1. Probable mechanisms and sequelae of pulmonary development during prolonged amniotic leak. (Modified from Bhutani VK, Abbasi S, Weiner S: Neonatal pulmonary manifestations due to prolonged amniotic leak. Am J Perinatol 1986; 3:225, © Thieme Medical Publishers, with permission.)

pharynx, and larynx), they lead to the trachea. From there, the cartilaginous airways taper to the small bronchi and then to the membranous airways and to the last branching, the terminal bronchioles (Table 1-5). The lower airways and the gas exchange area commence with the respiratory bronchioles. The upper airways are not rigid but are distensible, extensible, and compressible. The branching is not symmetric and dichotomous but irregular. The lumen is not circular and is subject to rapid changes in cross-sectional area and diameter because of a variety of extramural, mural, and intramural factors.

B. Anatomy: Includes the nose, oral cavity, palate, pharynx, larynx, hyoid bone, and extrathoracic trachea.

C. Function: Conducts, humidifies, and warms (or cools) to body temperature; filters air into the lungs; helps to separate functions of respiration and feeding; and shares in the process of vocalization.

D. Patency control: Stable pressure balance between collapsing forces (inherent viscoelastic properties of the structures and that of the constricting tone) and the dilator forces of supporting musculature help to maintain upper airway patency. Negative pressure in the airways, neck flexion, and changes in head and neck posture narrow the airways. Intrinsic and extrinsic muscles of the upper airway can generate dilator forces, such as flaring of the ala nasi.

TABLE 1-5. Classification, Branching, and Lumen Size of Adult Human Airways

Branch Order	Name	Number	Diameter (mm)	Cross-sectional Area (cm²)
0	Trachea	1	18	2.54
1	Main bronchi	2	12.2	2.33
2	Lobar bronchi	4	8.3	2.13
3	Segmental bronchi	8	5.6	2.00
4	Subsegmental bronchi	16	4.5	2.48
5-10	Small bronchi	32-1025	3.5-1.3	3.11-13.4
11-14	Bronchioles	2048-8192	1.99-0.74	19.6-69.4
15	Terminal bronchioles	32,768	0.66	113
16-18	Respiratory bronchioles	65,536-262,144	0.54-0.47	180-534
19-23	Alveolar ducts	524,288-8,388,608	0.43	944-11,800
24	Alveoli	300,000,000	0.2	

IV. Lower Airway Development
    A. Anatomy
        1. Conducting airways of the intrathoracic trachea
        2. Respiratory gas exchange in portions of the terminal and respiratory bronchioles and alveolar ducts
    B. Function of airway smooth muscle
        1. Tone is evident early in fetal life and plays a significant role in controlling airway lumen.
        2. In the presence of respiratory barotrauma, there appears to be a propensity for airway reactivity, perhaps as a component of the smooth muscle hyperplasia seen in BPD.
        3. Patency control: Excitatory and inhibitory innervations lead to bronchoconstriction and dilation, respectively.
        4. Narrow airways: Narrowing of the airways leads to increased resistance to airflow, an increased resistive load during breathing, and thereby to increased work of breathing and wasted caloric expenditure. Clinical factors associated with airway narrowing are listed in Table 1-6.
V. Thoracic and Respiratory Muscle Development
    A. Anatomy
        1. Three groups of skeletal muscles are involved in respiratory function:
           a. Diaphragm
           b. Intercostal and accessory muscles
           c. Abdominal muscles

Table 1-6. Clinical Conditions Associated with Narrowing of the Airways

Airway Inflammation
Mucosal edema
Excessive secretions
Inspissation of secretions
Tracheitis
Bronchoconstriction
Reactive airways
Exposure to cold, dry air
Exposure to bronchoconstricting drugs
Bronchomalacia
Prolonged mechanical ventilation
Congenital
Secondary to vascular abnormality
Trauma
Foreign body
Mucosal damage from ventilation, suction catheters
Subglottic stenosis
Congenital
Choanal stenosis
High arched palate
Chemical
Aspiration of gastric contents
Hyper-/hypo-osmolar fluid in the airways

2. These muscles constitute the respiratory pump that helps conduct the air in and out of the lungs.
3. During quiet breathing, the primary muscle for ventilation is the diaphragm.
4. The diaphragm is defined by its attachments to the skeleton:
   a. That part attached to the lumbar vertebral regions is the crural diaphragm.

　　　b. That part attached to the lower six ribs is the costal diaphragm.
　　　c. Both parts converge and form a single tendon of insertion.
　　5. Innervation of the diaphragm is by alpha motor neurons of the third through fifth cervical segments, the phrenic nerve.
　　6. Attached to the circumference of the lower thoracic cage, its contraction pulls the muscle downward, displaces the abdomen outward, and lifts up the thoracic cage.
　　7. In the presence of a compliant thoracic cage, relative to the lungs the thoracic cage is pulled inward (sternal retraction).
　　8. The concomitant pressure changes during inspiration include reduction of intrapleural pressure and an increase in intra-abdominal pressure.
　B. Respiratory contractile function
　　1. Strength, endurance, and the inherent ability to resist fatigue may assess the performance of the respiratory muscles.
　　2. Strength is determined by the intrinsic properties of the muscle (such as its morphologic characteristics and types of fibers).
　　3. Clinically, strength may be measured by the pressures generated at the mouth or across the diaphragm at specific lung volumes during a static inspiratory or expiratory maneuver.
　　4. Endurance capacity of a respiratory muscle depends on the properties of the system as well as the energy availability of the muscles.
　　5. Clinically, endurance is defined as the capacity to maintain either maximal or submaximal levels of ventilation under isocapnic conditions. It may be standardized as maximal ventilation for duration of time, as ventilation maintained against a known resistive load, or as sustained ventilation at a specific lung volume (elastic load). It is also determined with respect to a specific ventilatory target and the time to exhaustion (fatigue).
　　6. Respiratory muscles fatigue when energy consumption exceeds energy supply.
　　7. Fatigue is likely to occur when work of breathing is increased, strength is reduced, or inefficiency results so that energy consumption is affected.
　　8. Hypoxemia, anemia, decreased blood flow to muscles, and depletion of energy reserves alter energy availability.
　　9. Clinical manifestations of respiratory muscle fatigue include progressive hypercapnia and apnea.
　C. Postnatal maturation
　　1. Lung size, surface area, and volume increase in exponential fashion for about 2 months after term gestation.
　　2. Control of breathing (feedback control through chemoreceptors and stretch receptors), and the neural maturation of the respiratory centers also appears to coincide with maturation at about 2 months postnatal age.
　　3. Beyond this age, lung volumes continue to increase during infancy, slowing during childhood but still continuing to grow structurally into early adolescence (Table 1-7).

TABLE 1-7. Postnatal Maturation of the Lung

Age	Number of Alveoli	Surface Area (m²)	Respiratory Rate (breaths/min)
Birth	24,000,000	2.8	45 (35-55)
5-6 mo	112,000,000	8.4	27 (22-31)
~1 yr	129,000,000	12.2	19 (17-23)
~3 yr	257,000,000	22.2	19 (16-25)
~5 yr	280,000,000	32.0	18 (14-23)
Adult	300,000,000	75	15 (12-18)

4. It is this biologic phenomenon that provides a scope of recovery for infants with BPD.
5. In healthy infants, the increasing lung volume and cross-sectional area of the airways are associated with a reduction in the normal respiratory rate.

Suggested Reading

Bancalari E: Pulmonary function testing and other diagnostic laboratory procedures in neonatal pulmonary care. In Thibeault DW, Gary GA (eds): Neonatal Pulmonary Care, 2nd ed. East Norwalk, CT, Appleton-Century Crofts, 1986, pp 195-234.

Bhutani VK, Shaffer TH, Vidyasager D (eds): Neonatal Pulmonary Function Testing: Physiological, Technical and Clinical Considerations. Ithaca, NY, Perinatology Press, 1988.

Bhutani VK, Sivieri EM: Physiological principles for bedside assessment of pulmonary graphics. In Donn SM (ed): Neonatal and Pediatric Pulmonary Graphics. Principles and Clinical Applications. Armonk, NY, Futura Publishing, 1998, pp 57-79.

Bhutani VK, Sivieri EM, Abbasi S: Evaluation of pulmonary function in the neonate. In Polin RA, Fox WW (eds): Fetal and Neonatal Physiology, 2nd ed. Philadelphia, WB Saunders, 1988, pp 1143-1164.

Comroe JH. Physiology of Respiration, 2nd ed. Chicago, Year Book Medical Publishers, 1974.

Comroe JH, Forster RE, Dubois AB, et al: Clinical Physiology and Pulmonary Function Tests, 2nd ed. Chicago, Year Book Medical Publishers, 1971.

Polgar G, Promadhat V: Pulmonary Function Testing in Children. Philadelphia, WB Saunders, 1971.

Rodarte JR, Rehder K: Dynamics of respiration. In Geiger SR (ed): Handbook of Physiology, Section 3: The Respiratory System, vol III. Bethesda, MD, American Physiological Society, 1986, pp 131-144.

Stocks J, Sly PD, Tepper RS, Morgan WJ (eds): Infant Respiratory Function Testing. New York, Wiley-Liss, 1996.

West JB: Respiratory Physiology: The Essentials. Oxford, Blackwell Scientific Publications, 1974.

2

Developmental Lung Anomalies

Mohammad A. Attar and Subrata Sarkar

I. Introduction
   A. Most pulmonary malformations arise during the embryonic and the pseudoglandular stages of lung development.
   B. The spectrum of developmental malformation related to lung bud formation, branching morphogenesis, and separation of the trachea from the esophagus includes laryngeal, tracheal, and esophageal atresia; tracheoesophageal fistula; pulmonary aplasia; and bronchogenic cysts.
   C. Development abnormalities related to the pseudoglandular stage of lung development and failure of the pleuroperitoneal cavity to close properly include intralobar pulmonary sequestration, cystic adenomatoid malformation, tracheomalacia and bronchomalacia, and congenital diaphragmatic hernia.
   D. The spectrum of abnormalities arising at the canalicular and saccular stages of lung development is related to growth and maturation of the respiratory parenchyma and its vasculature and includes acinar dysplasia, alveolar capillary dysplasia, and pulmonary hypoplasia.
   E. Acute lung injury in the neonatal period may alter subsequent alveolar and airways growth and development.
II. Categorization of Lung Anomalies
   A. Lung anomalies can be localized to the lung or may be part of multiple organ involvement.
   B. Lung anomalies may be associated with other congenital anomalies that are part of a syndrome.
   C. Congenital anomalies in the lung can be categorized as malformations in:
      1. The tracheobronchial tree
      2. Distal lung parenchyma
      3. Abnormalities in the pulmonary arterial and venous trees and the lymphatics
III. Pulmonary and Extrapulmonary Malformations: The most common pulmonary and extrapulmonary malformations are congenital diaphragmatic hernia (CDH), cystic adenomatoid malformations (CAMs), tracheoesophageal fistula (TEF), bronchopulmonary sequestration (BPS), and congenital hydrothorax.
   A. Tracheoesophageal fistula (TEF)
      1. TEF occurs in 1 in 3000 to 4500 live births.

2. TEF may result from failure of the process of separation of the primitive foregut into the respiratory and alimentary tracts at 3 to 6 weeks of gestation.

3. TEF usually is found in combination with various forms of esophageal atresia. The most common combination is esophageal atresia with a distal tracheoesophageal fistula (about 85% of cases).

4. Infants often present with respiratory distress secondary to airway obstruction from excess secretions or aspiration of gastric contents into the lung through the fistula.

5. Excessive salivation and vomiting soon after feedings are often the first clue to diagnosis.

6. Esophageal atresia itself is diagnosed when it is not possible to pass a catheter into the stomach. The diagnosis is confirmed by radiographic studies showing a distended, blind upper esophageal pouch filled with air and the presence of the catheter coiled in the pouch.

7. TEF without esophageal atresia (H-type fistula) is extremely rare and usually presents after the neonatal period.

B. Laryngotracheoesophageal cleft
1. There is a long connection between the upper airway and the esophagus caused by failure of dorsal fusion of the cricoid, which is normally completed by the eighth week of gestation. Several subtypes are present.

2. Patients have chronic aspiration, gag during feeding, and develop pneumonia.

3. The diagnosis is made by bronchoscopy.

C. Congenital high-airway obstruction syndrome (CHAOS)
1. CHAOS may be caused by laryngeal atresia, subglottic stenosis, a laryngeal web, or a completely occluding laryngeal cyst.

2. Prenatal diagnosis of upper airway obstruction can be inferred from secondary changes such as enlarged echogenic lung, flattened or inverted diaphragm, fetal ascites, or hydrops.

3. MRI may be helpful in localizing the level of obstruction prenatally.

D. Tracheal agenesis
1. Tracheal agenesis is a rare, but fatal, anomaly caused by displacement of the tracheoesophageal septum.

2. The length of the agenetic segment is variable.

3. At birth, this anomaly is suspected when attempts at intubation are unsuccessful.

4. Tracheal agenesis may be associated with esophageal atresia, and most cases are associated with other anomalies that form a pattern that overlaps but is distinctive from the VACTERL association.

E. Tracheal stenosis
1. Tracheal stenosis is a malformation in which the trachea is narrow, either because of intrinsic abnormality in cartilage formation or because of external compression from abnormal vessel formation or vascular rings.

2. The major cause of intrinsic tracheal stenosis is an abnormality in cartilaginous ring formation, either from posterior fusion of the

normally C-shaped rings or as the result of formation of a complete cartilaginous sleeve, as reported in children with craniosynostosis anomalies, including Crouzon, Apert, and Pfeiffer syndromes.
3. Symptoms include biphasic stridor and expiratory wheezing.
4. Diagnosis is by bronchoscopy.

F. Tracheomalacia and bronchomalacia
   1. Absence or softening in the cartilaginous rings causes the trachea to collapse on expiration. There is a reduction in the cartilage–to–soft tissue ratio.
   2. The anomaly may be segmental or diffuse.
   3. Infants with laryngomalacia present with variable inspiratory stridor that worsens with crying, feeding, and upper respiratory obstruction.
   4. The tracheomalacia may be associated with other congenital anomalies such as vascular rings and TEF.

G. Bronchopulmonary sequestration
   1. Bronchopulmonary sequestration develops as a mass of nonfunctioning lung tissue, not connected to the tracheobronchial tree, which receives its blood supply from one or more anomalous systemic arteries arising from the aorta.
   2. There are two forms of bronchopulmonary sequestration, depending on whether it is within (intralobar) or outside (extralobar) the visceral pleural lining.
   3. Most infants with bronchopulmonary sequestration are asymptomatic in the neonatal period.
   4. If the sequestration is sufficiently large, there may be persistent cyanosis and respiratory distress.
   5. Some cases may present with large unilateral hydrothorax, possibly secondary to lymphatic obstruction, or with congestive heart failure secondary to large left-to-right shunting through the sequestration.
   6. The classic appearance on radiography consists of a triangular or oval-shaped basal lung mass on one side of the chest, usually the left.
   7. Diagnosis is confirmed by CT scan of the chest and MRI.

H. Congenital bronchogenic cysts
   1. These cysts are caused by abnormal budding and branching of the tracheobronchial tree.
   2. Typically the cysts lie in the posterior mediastinum, near the carina, but they also may be found in the anterior space.
   3. The cysts are filled with a clear, serous fluid unless they become infected. Their walls usually contain smooth muscle and cartilage.
   4. The diagnosis may be considered if a space-occupying lesion is detected on a chest radiograph obtained for investigation of respiratory distress.

I. Congenital lobar emphysema (CLE)
   1. CLE can be classified as lobar overinflation or regional or segmental pulmonary overinflation.
   2. CLE may result from malformation in the bronchial cartilage, with absent or incomplete rings; from a cyst in the bronchus; or from

a mucous or meconium plug in the bronchus. It also may result from extrinsic bronchial obstruction caused by dilated vessels or from intrathoracic masses such as bronchogenic cysts, extralobar sequestration, enlarged lymph nodes, and neoplasms.

3. CLE usually affects the upper and middle lobes on the right, and the upper lobe on the left.
4. These lesions cause air trapping, compression of the remaining ipsilateral lung or lobes, and respiratory distress.
5. Age at the time of diagnosis is closely related to the severity of the respiratory distress and the amount of functioning lung.
6. Diagnosis is by radiography, which reveals the lobar distribution of the hyperaeration with compression of adjacent pulmonary parenchyma.

IV. Malformations of the Distal Lung Parenchyma
  A. Pulmonary agenesis and aplasia (see Chapter 53)
    1. These anomalies are forms of arrested lung development that result in the absence of the distal lung parenchyma.
    2. Pulmonary agenesis is complete absence of one or both lungs, including the bronchi, bronchioles, vasculature, and respiratory parenchyma.
    3. Pulmonary aplasia occurs when only rudimentary bronchi are present; each bronchus ends in a blind pouch, with no pulmonary vessels or respiratory parenchyma.
    4. Pulmonary aplasia arises early in lung development, when the respiratory primordium bifurcates into the right and left primitive lung buds.
    5. Developmental arrest at a later stage may result in lobar agenesis or pulmonary dysplasia; some bronchial elements are present, but not alveoli.
    6. Unilateral pulmonary agenesis is more common than the bilateral pulmonary agenesis.
    7. Some infants with pulmonary agenesis may die in the delivery room; others may have severe respiratory distress that does not respond to mechanical ventilation.
    8. Radiography shows homogeneous density in place of the lung; the ribs appear crowded on the involved side, and there is mediastinal shift. A CT scan of the chest confirms the absence of lung tissue on one side.

  B. Pulmonary hypoplasia
    1. This anomaly develops as a result of other anomalies in the developing fetus. Many of these anomalies physically restrict growth or expansion of the peripheral lung.
    2. Pulmonary hypoplasia occurs in infants with renal agenesis or dysplasia, urinary outlet obstruction, loss or reduction of amniotic fluid from premature rupture of membranes, diaphragmatic hernia, large pleural effusions, congenital anomalies of the neuromuscular system, and chromosomal anomalies, including trisomies 13, 18, and 21.

C. Congenital diaphragmatic hernia (CDH) (see Chapter 52)
   1. CDH occurs in one per 2000 to 3000 births.
   2. Fifty percent of these hernias are associated with other malformations, especially neural tube defects, cardiac defects, and malrotation of the gut.
   3. In CDH, the pleuroperitoneal cavity fails to close. This allows the developing abdominal viscera to bulge into the pleural cavity and stunts the growth of the lung.
   4. The most common site is the left hemithorax, with the defect in the diaphragm being posterior (foramen of Bochdalek in 70% of infants).
   5. The left side of the diaphragm is involved more commonly than the right.
   6. The severity of the resulting pulmonary hypoplasia varies, probably depending on the timing of the onset of compression; early, severe compression of the lungs is associated with more severe hypoplasia.
   7. There is a decrease in the number and size of the alveoli and a decrease in the pulmonary vasculature.
   8. Infants with a large CDH present at birth with cyanosis, respiratory distress, a scaphoid abdomen, decreased breath sounds on the side of the hernia, and displacement of heart sounds to the opposite side.
   9. Prenatal diagnosis is often made by ultrasonographic studies, which are carried out because of the presence of polyhydramnios.
   10. Often there is severe pulmonary hypertension, likely because of the increased proportion of muscular arteries in the periphery of the lung, which results in increased pulmonary vascular resistance.
D. Congenital bronchiolar cysts
   1. Unlike bronchogenic cysts, bronchiolar cysts are in communication with the more proximal parts of the bronchial tree and with distal alveolar ducts and alveoli.
   2. These cysts are usually multiple and are restricted to a single lobe.
   3. They may be filled with air, fluid, or both.
E. Congenital cystic adenomatoid malformation (CCAM)
   1. CCAM is a pulmonary maldevelopment with cystic replacement of small airways and distal lung parenchyma.
   2. There are five types of CCAM classified on the basis of the gross appearance and histologic features, but a simpler classification based on anatomic and ultrasonographic findings includes two major types: macrocystic and microcystic.
      a. In the macrocystic type, the cysts are more than 5 mm in diameter and are visible on fetal ultrasonography, and the prognosis is better.
      b. In the microcystic type, the cysts are smaller, the mass has a solid appearance, and the prognosis is worse if the mass is large and associated with mediastinal shift, polyhydramnios, pulmonary hypoplasia, or hydrops fetalis.

3. After birth, because the multiple systs are connected to the airways, the cysts fill with air, produce further compression of the adjacent lung, and result in respiratory distress.

4. Spontaneous regression of CCAM, with normal lungs at birth, can occur.

F. Alveolar capillary dysplasia (ACD)

1. In ACD, there is misalignment of the pulmonary veins.

2. ACD is characterized by inadequate vascularization of the alveolar parenchyma, resulting in reduced number of capillaries in the alveolar wall.

3. This malformation causes persistent pulmonary hypertension in the newborn and is fatal.

G. Congenital pulmonary lymphangiectasis (CPL)

1. CPL is an extremely rare condition consisting of markedly distended or dilated pulmonary lymphatics, which are found in the bronchovascular connective tissue, along the interlobular septae, and in the pleura. It may be primary, secondary, or generalized.

2. This condition has been associated with Noonan, Ulrich-Turner, and Down syndromes.

3. Primary CPL is a fatal developmental defect in which the pulmonary lymphatics fail to communicate with the systemic lymphatics. Affected infants present with respiratory distress and pleural effusions and die shortly after birth.

4. Secondary CPL is associated with cardiovascular malformations.

5. Generalized CPL is characterized by proliferation of the lymphatic spaces and occurs in the lung as part of a systemic abnormality in which multiple lymphangiomas are also found in the bones, viscera, and soft tissues.

6. Infants with CPL present with nonimmune hydrops fetalis and pleural effusions. Pleural effusions typically are chylous. Pleural effusions in the neonatal period may be serous with minimal triglycerides, particularly before enteral feeding is established.

Suggested Reading

Devine PC, Malone FD: Noncardiac thoracic anomalies. Clin Perinatol 27:865-899, 2000.

Green TP, Finder JD: Congenital disorders of the lung. In Behrman RE, Kliegman RM, Jensen HB (eds): Nelson Textbook of Pediatrics, 17th ed. Philadelphia, WB Saunders, 2004, pp 1423-1426.

Haddad GG, Pérez Fontán JJ: Development of the respiratory system. In Behrman RE, Kliegman RM, Jenson HB (eds): Nelson Textbook of Pediatrics, 17th ed. Philadelphia, WB Saunders, 2004, pp 1357-1359.

Hansen T, Corbet A, Avery ME: Malformations of the mediastinum and lung parenchyma. In Taeusch WH, Ballard RA (eds): Avery's Diseases of the Newborn, 7th ed. Philadelphia, WB Saunders, 1998, pp 668-682.

Hodson WA: Normal and abnormal structural development of the lung. In Polin RA, Fox WW (eds): Fetal and Neonatal Physiology. Philadelphia, WB Saunders, 1998, pp 1033-1046.

Wert SE: Normal and abnormal structural development of the lung. In Polin RA, Fox WW, Abman SH (eds): Fetal and Neonatal Physiology, 3rd ed. Philadelphia, WB Saunders, 2004, pp 783-794.

Principles of Mechanical Ventilation

Spontaneous Breathing

3

Emidio M. Sivieri and Vinod K. Bhutani

I. Introduction
   A. Air, like liquid, moves from a region of higher pressure to one with lower pressure.
   B. During breathing and just prior to inspiration, no gas flows because the gas pressure within the alveoli is equal to atmospheric pressure.
   C. For inspiration to occur, alveolar pressure must be less than atmospheric pressure.
   D. For expiration to occur, alveolar pressure must be higher than atmospheric pressure.
   E. Thus, for inspiration to occur, the gradient in pressures can be achieved either by lowering the alveolar pressure ("negative," "natural," spontaneous breathing) or by raising the atmospheric pressure ("positive pressure," mechanical breathing).
   F. The clinical and physiologic implications of forces that influence inspiration and expiration are discussed in this section.
II. Signals of Respiration
   A. Each respiratory cycle can be described by the measurement of three signals: driving pressure (P), volume (V), and time (Figure 3-1).
   B. The rate of change in volume over time defines flow ($\dot{V}$).
   C. The fundamental act of spontaneous breathing results from the generation of P, the inspiratory driving force needed to overcome the elastic, flow-resistive, and inertial properties of the entire respiratory system in order to initiate $\dot{V}$.
      1. This relationship has been best described by Röhrer, using an equation of motion in which the driving pressure (P) is equal to the sum of elastic (P_E), resistive (P_R), and inertial (P_I) pressure components; thus,

$$P = P_E + P_R + P_I$$

      2. In this relationship, the elastic pressure is assumed to be proportional to volume change by an elastic constant (E) representing the elastance (or elastic resistance) of the system.
      3. The resistive component of pressure is assumed to be proportional to airflow by a resistive constant (R), representing inelastic airway and tissue resistances.
      4. In addition, the inertial component of pressure is assumed to be proportional to gas and tissue acceleration ($\ddot{V}$) by an inertial constant (I). Therefore,

19

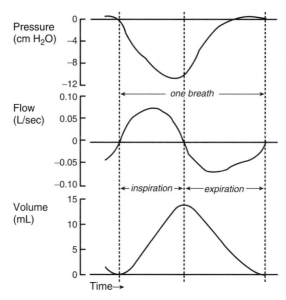

FIGURE 3-1. Graphic representation of a respiratory cycle demonstrating pressure, flow, and volume waveforms. Volume is obtained by integration (*area under the curve*) of the flow signal. (Modified from Bhutani VK, Sivieri EM, Abbasi S: Evaluation of pulmonary function in the neonate. In Polin RA, Fox WW [eds]: Fetal and Neonatal Physiology, 2nd ed. Philadelphia, WB Saunders, 1998, p 1144, with permission.)

$$P = EV + R\dot{V} + I\ddot{V}$$

5. This is a linear, first-order model in which the respiratory system is treated as a simple mechanical system (Figure 3-2), in which applied pressure P causes gas to flow through a tube (the respiratory airways) that is connected to a closed elastic chamber (alveoli) of volume V. In this ideal model, E, R, and I are assumed to be constants in a linear relationship between driving pressure and volume.

6. Under conditions of normal breathing frequencies (relatively low airflow and tissue acceleration) the inertance term is traditionally considered negligible; therefore,

$$P = EV + R\dot{V}$$

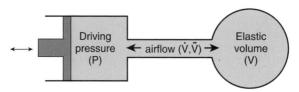

FIGURE 3-2. Linear, first-order model of the respiratory system, in which applied pressure causes gas to flow through a tube.

7. In respiratory terminology, elastance is usually replaced by compliance (C), which is a term used to represent the expandability or distensibility of a system. Because compliance is simply the reciprocal of elastance, the equation of motion can be rewritten as:

$$P = V/C + R\dot{V}$$

8. This simplified form of the Röhrer equation is the basis for most evaluations of pulmonary mechanics in which measurements of P, V, and $\dot{V}$ are used to compute the various components of respiratory system compliance, resistance, and work of breathing.

D. One can further study the nonlinear nature of the respiratory system using more advanced nonlinear models and by analyzing two-dimensional graphic plots of P-V, V-$\dot{V}$, and P-$\dot{V}$ relationships.

E. Because the inherent nature of the respiratory signals is variable (especially in premature infants), it is imperative that the signals are measured in as steady a state as feasible and over a protracted period of time (usually 2 to 3 minutes).

III. Driving Pressure

A. During spontaneous breathing, the driving pressure required to overcome elastic, airflow-resistive, and inertial properties of the respiratory system is the result of intrapleural pressure (P_{IP}) changes generated by the respiratory muscles (Figure 3-3).

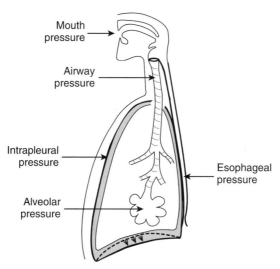

Mouth pressure
Airway pressure
Intrapleural pressure
Esophageal pressure
Alveolar pressure

FigURE 3-3. Schematic representation of components of respiratory pressures used in pulmonary function studies. Esophageal pressure approximates intrapleural pressure. (Modified from Bhutani VK, Sivieri EM, Abbasi S: Evaluation of pulmonary function in the neonate. In Polin RA, Fox WW [eds]: Fetal and Neonatal Physiology, 2nd ed. Philadelphia, WB Saunders, 1998, p 1153, with permission.)

B. During a respiratory cycle, the intrapleural and alveolar pressures both change.
   1. Just before the commencement of an inspiratory cycle, the P_{IP} is subatmospheric (−3 to −6 cm H_2O) because of the elastic recoil effect of the lung.
   2. At this time, the alveolar pressure is atmospheric (zero), because there is no airflow and thus no pressure drop along the conducting airways. At this time, the alveolar pressure is atmospheric zero, because there is no airflow and thus no pressure drop along the conducting airways.
   3. During a spontaneous inspiration, forces generated by the respiratory muscles cause the P_{IP} to further decrease, producing a concomitant fall in alveolar pressure so as to initiate a driving pressure gradient that forces airflow into the lung.
   4. During a passive expiration, the respiratory muscles are relaxed, and the P_{IP} becomes less negative.
   5. Elastic recoil forces in the now-expanded lung and thorax cause alveolar pressure to become positive and thus the net driving pressure forces air to flow out of the lungs.
   6. With forced expiration, the P_{IP} rises above atmospheric pressure.
   7. The magnitude of the change in the alveolar pressure depends on the airflow rate and the airway resistance but usually varies between 1 and 2 cm H_2O below and above atmospheric pressure during inspiration and expiration, respectively.
   8. This range of alveolar pressure change can be markedly increased with air trapping or airway obstruction.
B. Following are some physiologic observations of changes in P_{IP} during spontaneous breathing.
   1. Under some conditions respiratory airflow is zero or very close to zero:
      a. During tidal breathing, airflow is zero at end-inspiration and end-expiration, where it reverses direction (Figure 3-4).
      b. During slow static inflation, airflow can be approximated as zero.
      c. In both cases, the resistive component of driving pressure as described previously is zero or $R\dot{V} = 0$, and P_{IP} is equal to elastic pressure only:

$$P_{IP} = P_E = V/C$$

   2. The elastic component of P_{IP} can be estimated on the pressure tracing by connecting with straight lines the points of zero flow at end-expiration and end-inspiration . The vertical segment between this estimated elastic pressure line and the measured P_{IP} (solid line) represents the resistive pressure component (Figure 3-5).
   3. Resistive pressure is usually maximum at points of peak airflow, which usually occurs during mid-inspiration and mid-expiration.
   4. Transpulmonary pressure (P_{TP}) is the differential between P_{IP} and alveolar pressure. This is the portion of the total respiratory driving pressure that is attributed to inflation and deflation of the lung specifically.

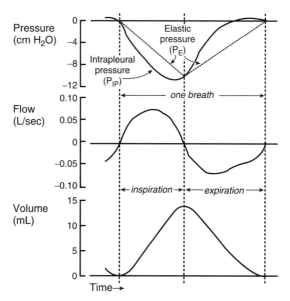

FIGURE 3-4. During tidal breathing, airflow is zero at end-inspiration and end-expiration, where it reverses direction. The pressure difference between these two points represents the net elastic pressure at end-inspiration. The elastic component of intrapleural pressure at other points can be approximated by a straight line connecting points of zero flow.

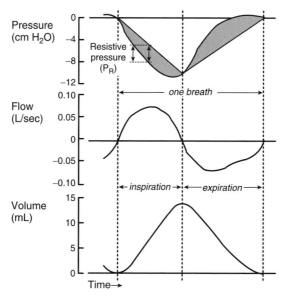

FIGURE 3-5. The elastic component of intrapleural pressure can be estimated on a pressure tracing by connecting points of zero flow at end-expiration and end-inspiration with a straight line. The vertical distance between this estimate and the measured intrapleural pressure is the resistive pressure component (*solid line*).

C. With mechanical ventilation, of course, the driving pressure is provided by the ventilator. In contrast to spontaneous breathing, in which a negative change in P_{IP} is the driving pressure for inspiration, the mechanical ventilator applies a positive pressure to an endotracheal tube. Nonetheless, in both cases there is a positive pressure gradient from the mouth to the alveoli. In both cases the P_{TP} gradient is in the same direction.

IV. Factors That Impact the Mechanics of Airflow: Factors that influence the respiratory muscles and respiratory mechanics have an effect on how air flows in and out of the lungs. These are characterized by physical, physiologic, and pathophysiologic considerations.

A. Physical factors

1. The pattern of airflow is affected by the physical properties of the gas molecules, the laminar or turbulent nature of airflow, and the dimensions of the airways, as well as the other effects described by the Poiseulle equation (see Chapter 7).

2. The elastic properties of the airway, the transmural pressure on the airway wall, and structural features of the airway wall also determine the mechanics of airflow.

3. In preterm newborns, the airways are narrower in diameter and result in a higher resistance to airflow. The increased airway compliance increases the propensity for airway collapse or distension. If a higher transmural pressure is generated during tidal breathing (as in infants with bronchopulmonary dysplasia, or during positive pressure ventilation), the intrathoracic airways are likely to be compressed during expiration (Figure 3-6).

4. During forced expiration, the more compliant airways are also likely to be compressed in presence of high intrathoracic pressure.

5. Increased distensibility of airways, as when exposed to excessive end-distending pressure, can result in increased and wasted dead space ventilation.

6. Turbulence of gas flow, generally not an issue in a healthy individual, can lead to a need for a higher driving pressure in the sick preterm infant with structural airway deformations, such as encountered in those with BPD.

B. Physiologic factors

1. The tone of the tracheobronchial smooth muscle provides a mechanism to stabilize the airways and prevent collapse.

2. An increased tone as a result of smooth muscle hyperplasia or a hyperresponsive smooth muscle should lead to a bronchospastic basis of airflow limitation.

3. The bronchomalactic airway may be destabilized in the presence of tracheal smooth muscle relaxants.

4. The effects of other physiologic factors, such as the alveolar duct sphincter tone, are not yet fully understood.

C. Pathophysiologic factors

1. Plugging of the airway lumen, mucosal edema, cohesion, and compression of the airway wall lead to alterations in tracheobronchial airflow.

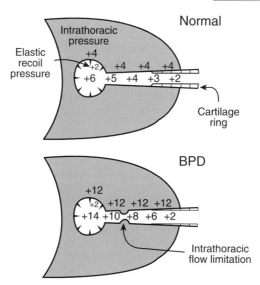

FIGURE 3-6. Schematic comparison of normal and abnormal airflow. An infant with bronchopulmonary dysplasia (BPD) has higher transmural pressure generated during tidal breathing, and thoracic airways are likely to be compressed during expiration, resulting in flow limitation. (Modified from Bhutani VK, Sivieri EM: Physiological principles for bedside assessment of pulmonary graphics. In Donn SM [ed]: Neonatal and Pediatric Pulmonary Graphics: Principles and Clinical Applications. Armonk, NY, Futura Publishing, 1998, p 63, with permission.)

    2. Weakening of the airway walls secondary to structural airway barotrauma and the consequent changes of tracheobronchomalacia also result in abnormal airflow patterns.

    3. BPD-related airflow effects have been previously described.

V. Lung Volumes: Ventilation is a cyclic process of inspiration and expiration. Total or minute ventilation (MV) is the volume of air expired each minute. The volume of air moved in or out during each cycle of ventilation is the tidal volume (V_T) and is a sum of the air in the conducting zone (V_D, or dead space volume) and the respiratory zone (V_A, or alveolar space). Thus,

$$MV = (V_A + V_D) \times \text{Frequency}$$

The process of spontaneous breathing generally occurs at about mid–total lung capacity, such that about two thirds of the total capacity is available as reserve.

A. Ventilatory volumes

    1. Tidal volume (V_T) is the volume of air inspired with each breath.

    2. Minute ventilation (MV) is the product of frequency (F, the number of tidal volumes taken per minute) and V_T.

3. Dead space volume (V_D) is the volume in which there is no gas exchange.
   a. Dead space refers to the volume within the respiratory system that does not participate in gas exchange and is often the most frequent and unrecognized cause of hypercapnia.
   b. V_D is composed of several components.
      (1) Anatomic dead space is the volume of gas contained in the conducting airway.
      (2) Alveolar dead space refers to the volume of gas in areas of "wasted ventilation"—that is, in alveoli that are ventilated poorly or are underperfused.
      (3) The total volume of gas that is not involved in gas exchange is called the physiologic dead space. It is the sum of the anatomic and alveolar dead space.
   c. In a normal person, the physiologic dead space should be equal to the anatomic dead space. For this reason, some investigators refer to physiologic dead space as pathologic dead space.
   d. Several factors can modify the dead space volume:
      (1) Anatomic dead space increases as a function of airway size and airway compliance. Because of the interdependence of the alveoli and airways, anatomic dead space increases as a function of lung volume. Similarly, dead space increases as a function of body height, bronchodilator drugs, and diseases such as BPD, tracheomegaly, and oversized artificial airways.
      (2) Anatomic dead space is decreased by reduction in the size of the airways, such as occurs with bronchoconstriction, tracheomalacia, or a tracheostomy.
4. Alveolar volume (V_A) is the volume in which gas exchange occurs:

$$V_A = V_T - V_D$$

5. Alveolar ventilation ($\dot{V}_A$) is the product of frequency and V_A.

B. Lung reserve volumes: Reserve volumes represent the maximal volume of gas that can be moved above or below a normal tidal volume (Figure 3-7). These values reflect the balance between lung and chest wall elasticity, respiratory strength, and thoracic mobility.
   1. Inspiratory reserve volume (IRV) is the maximum volume of gas that can be inspired from the peak of tidal volume.
   2. Expiratory reserve volume (ERV) is the maximum volume of gas that can be expired after a normal tidal expiration. Therefore, the reserve volumes are associated with the ability to increase or decrease tidal volume. Normal lungs do not collapse at the end of the maximum expiration.
   3. The volume of gas that remains is called the residual volume (RV).
C. Lung capacities: The capacity of the lungs can be represented in four different ways: total lung capacity, vital capacity, inspiratory capacity, and functional residual capacity (see Figure 3-7).
   1. Total lung capacity (TLC) is the amount of gas in the respiratory system after a maximal inspiration. It is the sum of all four lung

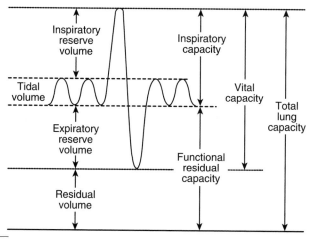

FIGURE 3-7. Graphic representation of lung volumes and capacities. (Modified from Bhutani VK, Sivieri EM: Physiological principles for bedside assessment of pulmonary graphics. In Donn SM [ed]: Neonatal and Pediatric Pulmonary Graphics: Principles and Clinical Applications. Armonk, NY, Futura Publishing, 1998, p 67, with permission.)

volumes. The normal values as well as the values of static lung volumes for term newborns are shown in Table 3-1.

2. Vital capacity (VC) is the maximal volume of gas that can be expelled from the lungs after a maximal inspiration. As such, the vital capacity is the sum of IRV + TV + ERV. Inspiratory capacity (IC) is the maximal volume of gas that can be inspired from the resting end-expiration level; therefore, it is the sum of TV + IRV.

3. Functional residual capacity (FRC) is the volume of gas in the lung when the respiratory system is at rest—that is, the volume in the lung at the end of a normal expiration that is in continuity with the airways. FRC also can also be defined as the volume of gas above which a normal tidal volume oscillates. A normal FRC makes available optimal lung mechanics and alveolar surface area for

TABLE 3-1. Normal Values for Lung Volumes in Term Newborns

Ventilatory Volumes	Static Lung Volumes
V_T: 5-8 mL/kg	RV: 10-15 mL/kg
F: 40-60 beats/min	FRC: 25-30 mL/kg
V_D: 2-2.5 mL/kg	TGV: 30-40 mL/kg
MV: 200-480 mL/min/kg	TLC: 50-90 mL/kg
V_A: 60-320 mL/min/kg	VC: 35-80 mL/kg

efficient ventilation and gas exchange. The size of the FRC is determined by the balance of two opposing forces:

a. Inward elastic recoil of the lung tending to collapse the lung
b. Outward elastic recoil of the chest wall tending to expand the lung

4. Residual volume (RV) is the volume of air remaining in the respiratory system at the end of the maximum possible expiration:

$$\text{Expiratory reserve volume (ERV)} = \text{FRC} - \text{RV}$$

D. It is important to note that thoracic gas volume (TGV) is the total amount of gas in the lung (or thorax) at end-expiration. This value differs from FRC, and the difference indicates the magnitude of air trapping.

Suggested Reading

Bancalari E: Pulmonary function testing and other diagnostic laboratory procedures in neonatal pulmonary care. In Thibeault DW Gary GA (eds): Neonatal Pulmonary Care, 2nd ed. East Norwalk, CT, Appleton-Century Crofts, 1986, pp 195-234.

Bhutani VK, Shaffer TH, Vidyasager D (eds): Neonatal Pulmonary Function Testing: Physiological, Technical and Clinical Considerations. Ithaca, NY, Perinatology Press, 1988.

Bhutani VK, Sivieri EM: Physiological principles for bedside assessment of pulmonary graphics. In Donn SM (ed): Neonatal and Pediatric Pulmonary Graphics. Principles and Clinical Applications. Armonk, NY, Futura Publishing, 1998, pp 57-79.

Bhutani VK, Sivieri EM, Abbasi S: Evaluation of pulmonary function in the neonate. In Polin RA, Fox WW (eds): Fetal and Neonatal Physiology, 2nd ed. Philadelphia, WB Saunders, 1988, pp 1143-1164.

Comroe JH. Physiology of Respiration, 2nd ed. Chicago, Year Book Medical Publishers, 1974.

Comroe JH, Forster RE, Dubois AB, et al: Clinical Physiology and Pulmonary Function Tests, 2nd ed. Chicago, Year Book Medical Publishers, 1971.

Polgar G, Promadhat V: Pulmonary Function Testing in Children. Philadelphia, WB Saunders, 1971.

Rodarte JR, Rehder K: Dynamics of respiration. In Geiger SR (ed): Handbook of Physiology, Section 3: The Respiratory System, vol III. Bethesda, MD, American Physiological Society, 1986, pp 131-144.

Stocks J, Sly PD, Tepper RS, Morgan WJ (eds): Infant Respiratory Function Testing. New York, Wiley-Liss, 1996.

West JB: Respiratory Physiology: The Essentials. Oxford, Blackwell Scientific Publications, 1974.

Pulmonary Gas Exchange

4

Vinod K. Bhutani

I. Introduction
   A. Independent pulmonary gas exchange to replace the maternal placental gas exchange mechanism needs to be established within the first few minutes of birth.
   B. In order to effect this transition, several physiologic changes occur:
      1. Adjustments in circulation
      2. Pulmonary mechanics
      3. Gas exchange
      4. Acid-base status
      5. Respiratory control
   C. Upon transition, gas exchange takes place through an air-liquid interphase of alveolar epithelium with alveolar gas in one compartment and blood in the other (vascular) compartment. An understanding of gas laws, alveolar ventilation, and pulmonary vasculature is important in facilitating optimal pulmonary gas exchange.
II. Brief Outline of Cardiopulmonary Adaptations
   A. Prior to birth, the fetus is totally dependent on the placenta (Figure 4-1) and has made cardiopulmonary adjustments for optimal delivery of

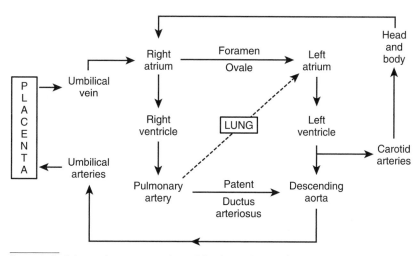

FIGURE 4-1. Schematic representation of fetal circulation. (From Bhutani VK: Extrauterine adaptations in the newborn. Semin Perinatol 1:1-12, 1997, with permission.)

29

oxygen, whereas the maternal physiology has adapted to maintain fetal normocapnia.
  B. The salient features and sequence of events that occur during fetal to neonatal transition are listed in Table 4-1.
III. Application of Gas Laws to Pulmonary Gas Exchange
  A. There are fundamental laws of physics that pertain to the behavior of gases and thereby impact on gas exchange.
  B. An understanding of these laws is specifically pertinent to the clinician in his/her ability not only to measure and interpret blood gas values but also to evaluate the impact on gas exchange during clinical conditions of hypothermia, high altitude, and the use of gas mixtures of varying viscosities and densities.
  C. A brief description of the pertinent and clinically relevant gas laws is listed in Table 4-2.
  D. One of the most fundamental relationships widely used to describe pulmonary gas exchange is summarized as:

$$P_ACO_2 = 863(\dot{V}CO_2/\dot{V}_A)$$

where, in a steady state and with negligible inspired carbon dioxide, the alveolar pressure of carbon dioxide (P_ACO_2) is proportional to the ratio of the rates of carbon dioxide elimination ($\dot{V}CO_2$) and alveolar ventilation ($\dot{V}_A$). This equation helps to summarize several of the gas laws. The applications of the laws are thus:
  1. P_ACO_2: When measured in dry gas as a percentage, Dalton law must be applied to convert the value to partial pressure. The partial pressure of carbon dioxide, rather than its percentage composition, is the significant variable because Henry law of solubility states that the gas is physically dissolved in liquid and in equilibrium with the gas phase at the same partial pressure.
  2. 863: This peculiar number is derived from the need to standardize measurements from body temperature (310° K) to standard pressure and temperature (760 mm Hg • 273° K). Based on the product 310 × (760/273), we obtain the value 863 (in mm Hg) as the constant for the relationship in the above equation.
  3. $\dot{V}CO_2/\dot{V}_A$: These values are measured at ambient temperature and pressure, saturated with water vapor (ATPS). Carbon dioxide output needs to be converted to STPD (standard temperature, pressure, dry) using Boyle and Charles laws, while alveolar ventilation has to be corrected to BTPS (body temperature, pressure and saturated with water vapor).
IV. Development of Pulmonary Vasculature
  A. The main pulmonary artery develops from the embryonic left arch.
  1. The sixth arches appear at about 32 days after conception (5-mm embryo stage) and give branches to the developing lung bud.
  2. Branches from the aorta that supply the lung bud and the right arch disappear subsequently.
  3. By 50 days (18-mm embryo stage), the adult pattern of vascularization has commenced.

TABLE 4-1. Salient Features of Extrauterine Cardiopulmonary Adaptations

Parameter	Mother (2nd trimester)	Fetus (before labor)	Newborn (before 1st breath)	Newborn (at about 6 hours)
PaO_2	80-95 mm Hg	<25 mm Hg in pulmonary artery	16-18 mm Hg	80-95 mm Hg
$PaCO_2$	~34 mm Hg	40-42 mm Hg	45-65 mm Hg	34 mm Hg
pH	~7.45	7.35-7.40	7.10-7.30	7.35-7.40
Pulmonary blood flow	Equivalent to cardiac output	13-25% cardiac output	~25% cardiac output	90-100% cardiac output
Shunts	Placental shunts	Placental shunts; foramen ovale; ductus arteriosus	Foramen ovale; ductus arteriosus; intrapulmonary shunts	Foramen ovale closed; ductus arteriosus usually closed; intrapulmonary shunts
Pulmonary mechanics	Air-filled lungs; hyperventilation	Liquid-filled lungs; FRC, 30 mL/kg	Air and fluid (16-19 mL/kg) in the lungs	Air-filled lungs; FRC, 30 mL/kg
Control of Respiration	Progesterone-mediated hyperventilation	Fetal breathing dependent more on stretch	First breath initiated by nonspecific respiratory	Rhythmic respiratory cycles based on chemoreceptors

Table 4-2. Laws that Describe Gas Behavior

Law	Description
Boyle	At constant temperature (T), a given volume (V) of gas varies inversely to the pressure (P) to which it is subjected.
Charles	Gas expands as it is warmed and shrinks as it is cooled.
Dalton	The total pressure exerted by a mixture of gases is equal to the sum of the partial pressure of each gas.
Amagat	The total volume of a mixture of gases is equal to the sum of the partial volume of each gas at the same temperature and pressure.
Henry	At constant temperature, any gas physically dissolves in a liquid in proportion to its partial pressure, although the solubility coefficient decreases with increasing temperature and differs from one gas to another.
Graham	The rate of diffusion of a gas is inversely proportional to the square root of its density.
Fick	The transfer of a solute by diffusion is directly proportional to the cross-sectional area available for diffusion and to the difference in concentration per unit of distance perpendicular to that cross-section.
Summation of Laws	
Ideal gas equation	$PV = nRT$, where R is a numerical constant.
Van der Waals equation	Refinement of the ideal gas equation based upon the attractive forces between molecules and upon the volume occupied by the molecules.
Barometric pressure and altitude	The decrease in barometric pressure is not linear; increasing altitude, weather, temperature, density of atmosphere, acceleration of gravity, etc., influence the barometric pressure.

B. Before the main pulmonary veins are developed, the vessels drain into the systemic circulation of the foregut and trachea.
   1. These connections are lost as the main pulmonary vein develops.
   2. A primitive pulmonary vein appears as a bud from the left side of the atrial chamber at about 35 days.
   3. Starting as a blind capillary, it bifurcates several times to connect with the developing lung bud.
   4. Subsequently, the first two branches are resorbed to form the left atrium at about the seventh week.
C. The branches of the pulmonary arterial system maintain a position next to the bronchial structures, as both develop during the glandular and canalicular stages of lung development.
D. By 16 weeks there is a complete set of vessels leading to the respiratory bronchioles, terminal bronchioles, and terminal sacs.

V. Onset of Pulmonary Gas Exchange
   A. The physiologic processes that facilitate the onset of postnatal
      pulmonary gas exchange are described in the series of events depicted
      in Figure 4-2.
      1. The effect of ventilation on reducing pulmonary vascular
         resistance (Fig. 4-2A)
      2. The effect of acidosis correction to enhance pulmonary blood flow
         (Fig. 4-2B)
      3. The effect of driving pressure and successful establishment of
         respiration during first breaths to achieve an optimal functional
         residual capacity (Fig. 4-2C)

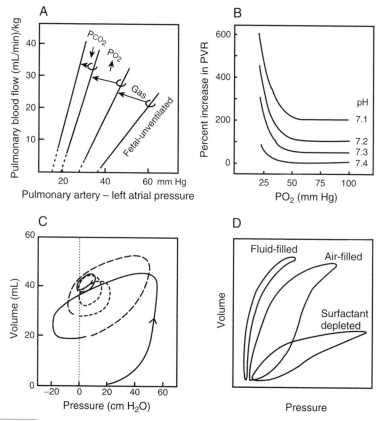

FIGURE 4-2. Physiologic processes that facilitate onset of postnatal pulmonary
gas exchange. A, Effect of ventilation on reducing pulmonary vascular resistance (PVR). B, Effects of acidosis correction on reducing PVR. C, First breaths
and establishment of optimal functional residual capacity. D, Effect of driving
pressure to maintain optimal tidal volume and work of breathing. (Modified from
Bhutani VK: Differential diagnosis of neonatal respiratory disorders. In Spitzer AR
[ed]: Intensive Care of the Fetus and Neonate. St. Louis, Mosby–Year Book, 1996,
p 500, with permission.)

      4. The effect of driving pressure to maintain optimal tidal volume and achieve the least work of breathing (Fig. 4-2D)

B. These events highlight the other series of biochemical and physiologic events that concurrently occur to successfully establish and maintain the matching of ventilation to perfusion.

C. Maladaptations delay transition to adequate pulmonary gas exchange.

D. Although it has been well established that a newborn is more likely to sustain events that lead to hypoxemia and to maintain adequate oxygenation with an inability to compensate hemodynamically, it has also been recognized that a newborn is more tolerant of hypoxemia than an adult. Reasons for occurrences of hypoxemic events include:
      1. Reduced FRC relative to the oxygen consumption
      2. Presence of intrapulmonary shunts that lead to V/Q mismatching
      3. A high alveolar-arterial oxygen gradient

E. Hypercapnia that results from an inability to maintain adequate alveolar ventilation in the face of mechanical loads also results in lower alveolar oxygen tension.

F. From a hemodynamic perspective, impaired oxygen delivery may occur because of:
      1. Low P_{50} values owing to the high oxygen affinity of fetal hemoglobin
      2. Increased blood viscosity
      3. Lower myocardial response to a volume or pressure load
      4. Inadequate regional redistribution of cardiac output

G. The relationship between arterial oxygen and carbon dioxide values and their relationship to hypoxemia and respiratory failure are shown in Figure 4-3.

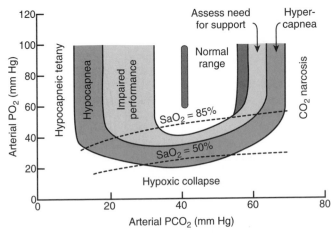

FIGURE 4-3. The relationship between alveolar oxygen and carbon dioxide values and how these relate to hypoxemia and respiratory failure. (Modified from Bhutani VK: Differential diagnosis of neonatal respiratory disorders. In Spitzer AR [ed]: Intensive Care of the Fetus and Neonate. St. Louis, Mosby–Year Book, 1996, p 501, with permission.)

  H. The effect of oxygen inhalation on the composition of alveolar and blood gas tensions is shown in Table 4-3.
VI. Optimal Pulmonary Gas Exchange
  A. Failure to establish optimal pulmonary gas exchange leads to either oxygenation or ventilation failure.
  B. Factors that impact on the adequacy of neonatal gas exchange (especially in a preterm newborn) are listed in Table 4-4.
  C. Respiratory failure can initially lead to increased respiratory effort in an attempt at compensation, followed by an inability to ventilate, or apnea.
  D. The concurrent changes in arterial oxygen and carbon dioxide gas tensions during both health and disease are shown in Figure 4-3.
VII. Physiologic Principles to Improve Pulmonary Gas Exchange
  A. The physiologic principles that may be utilized to improve oxygenation, enhance carbon dioxide elimination, and establish ventilation at optimal FRC (and thereby with the least barotrauma) are shown in Figure 4-2.
  B. Clinically relevant interventional strategies are crucial to achieve optimal gas exchange.
  C. It is also valuable to be reminded that in a healthy newborn, gas tensions are maintained in a narrow range by exquisitely sensitive feedback mechanisms of chemoreceptors and stretch receptors.

TABLE 4-3. Effect of Oxygen Inhalation (100%) on Composition of Alveolar and Blood Gas Tensions

	Inspired Dry Gas		Alveolar Gas		End Pulmonary Capillary Blood		Arterial Blood		End-Systemic Capillary Blood	
Variable	Air	O_2	Air	O_2	Air	O_2	Air	O_2	Air	O_2
PO_2 (mm Hg)	1591	760	104	673	104	673	100	640	40	53.5
PCO_2 (mm Hg)	00.3	0	40	40	40	40	40	40	46	46
PH_2O (mm Hg)	0.0	0	47	47	47	47	47	47	47	47
PN_2 (mm Hg)	600.6	0	569	0	569	0	573	0	573	0
P_{total} (mm Hg)	760	760	760	760	760	760	760	727	706	146.5*
O_2Sat (%)					98	100	98	100	75	85.5

*What happens to the total gas tension when a baby breathes 100% oxygen: the total venous gas tension is now at 146.5 mm Hg.

Table 4-4. Factors that Affect Adequacy of Neonatal Gas Exchange

Factors in Gas Exchange	Impact of Prematurity
Neural control of respiration	Immaturity
Mechanical loads: elastic and resistive	High chest wall–to–lung compliance ratio
Stability of end-expiratory lung volume	Compliant airways with pre–end-expiratory closure of airways
Ventilation-perfusion matching	Reactive pulmonary vasculature
Hemoglobin dissociation curve properties	Fetal hemoglobin characteristics
Match cardiac output to oxygen consumption	High neonatal oxygen consumption
Ability to maintain alveolar ventilation	Propensity for respiratory muscle fatigue

    D. Moreover, during fetal development, maternal physiology is significantly altered to maintain fetal normocapnia and neutral acid-base status.

    E. Thus, as clinicians assume control of the newborn's ventilation with supportive technologies, the road map for optimal pulmonary gas exchange needs to be "quality controlled" from a physiologic perspective and with the least amount of barotrauma.

Suggested Reading

Bancalari E: Pulmonary function testing and other diagnostic laboratory procedures in neonatal pulmonary care. In Thibeault DW Gary GA (eds): Neonatal Pulmonary Care, 2nd ed. East Norwalk, CT, Appleton-Century Crofts, 1986, pp 195-234.

Bhutani VK, Shaffer TH, Vidyasager D (eds): Neonatal Pulmonary Function Testing: Physiological, Technical and Clinical Considerations. Ithaca, NY, Perinatology Press, 1988.

Bhutani VK, Sivieri EM: Physiological principles for bedside assessment of pulmonary graphics. In Donn SM (ed): Neonatal and Pediatric Pulmonary Graphics. Principles and Clinical Applications. Armonk, NY, Futura Publishing, 1998, pp 57-79.

Bhutani VK, Sivieri EM, Abbasi S: Evaluation of pulmonary function in the neonate. In Polin RA, Fox WW (eds): Fetal and Neonatal Physiology, 2nd ed. Philadelphia, WB Saunders, 1988, pp 1143-1164.

Comroe JH. Physiology of Respiration, 2nd ed. Chicago, Year Book Medical Publishers, 1974.

Comroe JH, Forster RE, Dubois AB, et al: Clinical Physiology and Pulmonary Function Tests, 2nd ed. Chicago, Year Book Medical Publishers, 1971.

Polgar G, Promadhat V: Pulmonary Function Testing in Children. Philadelphia, WB Saunders, 1971.

Rodarte JR, Rehder K: Dynamics of respiration. In Geiger SR (ed): Handbook of Physiology, Section 3: The Respiratory System, vol III. Bethesda, MD, American Physiological Society, 1986, pp 131-144.

Stocks J, Sly PD, Tepper RS, Morgan WJ (eds): Infant Respiratory Function Testing. New York, Wiley-Liss, 1996.

West JB: Respiratory Physiology: The Essentials. Oxford, Blackwell Scientific Publications, 1974.

Oxygen Therapy and Toxicity 5

Win Tin

I. Introduction
  A. "The clinician must bear in mind that oxygen is a drug and must be used in accordance with well recognized pharmacologic principles; i.e., since it has certain toxic effects and is not completely harmless (as widely believed in clinical circles) it should be given only in the lowest dosage or concentration required by the particular patient." [Julius Comroe, 1945.]
  B. Oxygen is the most commonly used therapy in neonatal intensive care units, and oxygen toxicity in newborns (cicatricial retinopathy, or retrolental fibroplasia as it was formerly known) was first described more than 50 years ago.
  C. The ultimate aim of oxygen therapy is to achieve adequate tissue oxygenation, but without creating oxygen toxicity and oxidative stress.
II. Physiologic Considerations
  A. Tissue oxygenation depends on:
    1. Inspired oxygen
    2. Gas exchange mechanism within the lungs
    3. Oxygen-carrying capacity of the blood (approximately 97% of oxygen transported to the tissue is carried by hemoglobin and 3% is dissolved in plasma.)
    4. Cardiac output
    5. Local tissue edema or ischemia
  B. Fetal oxygen transport and postnatal changes
    1. Fetal hemoglobin (HbF) has higher oxygen affinity and lower P_{50} (oxygen tension at which 50% of hemoglobin is saturated at standard pH and temperature). This favors oxygen uptake from placenta to fetus, as adequate transfer of oxygen is achieved at relatively low PO_2.
    2. The high oxygen affinity of HbF, however, has a disadvantage in oxygen delivery to the fetal tissue, but this is offset by the fact that the fetal oxygen-hemoglobin saturation curve is much steeper; therefore, adequate dissociation of oxygen from hemoglobin can occur with a relatively small decrease in oxygen tension at the tissue level.
    3. The newborn infant needs more oxygen than the fetus (oxygen consumption of most animal species increases by 100% to 150% in the first few days of life); therefore, a P_{50} that is adequate for tissue oxygenation in a fetus is not enough in a newborn.

    4. Changes in both oxygen affinity and oxygen-carrying capacity occur postnatally, and in an infant born at term, P_{50} reaches adult levels by about 4 to 6 months of age.

C. Indices of oxygenation

    1. Alveolar-arterial oxygen pressure difference [P(A-a)O$_2$]: The difference in partial pressure of oxygen between alveolar and arterial levels correlates well with ventilation-perfusion (V/Q) mismatch. In a newborn who is breathing room air, this value can be as high as 40 to 50 mm Hg, and may remain high (20 to 40 mm Hg) for days. The increase in P(A-a)O$_2$ generally is caused by:

      a. Block of oxygen diffusion at the alveolar-capillary level

      b. V/Q mismatch in the lungs (from increase in physiologic dead space or from intrapulmonary shunting)

      c. Fixed right-to-left shunt (intracardiac shunting)

    2. Oxygenation index (OI): This is most frequently used clinically as well as in research studies because of its ease of calculation and is believed to be a more sensitive indicator of the severity of pulmonary illness than P(A-a)O$_2$, because mean airway pressure (Pāw) is used in its calculation ($OI = Pāw \times FiO_2/PaO_2$).

    3. Arterial-to-alveolar oxygen tension ratio (a/A ratio).

    4. There is no significant difference in the performance of these indices in predicting death and adverse respiratory outcome.

D. PaO$_2$ and O$_2$ saturation

    1. Several clinical studies have shown that fractional O$_2$ saturation >92% can be associated with PaO$_2$ values of 80 mm Hg or even higher (Fig. 5-1).

    2. Although PaO$_2$ and O$_2$ saturation are directly related, this correlation is influenced by several physiologic changes (quantity and quality of Hb, temperature, acid-base status, pCO$_2$, and concentration of 2,3 DPG).

III. Monitoring Oxygen Therapy

A. Continuous, noninvasive monitoring

    1. Pulse oxygen saturation (pulse oximetry): This is the most user-friendly method and therefore the method used most commonly for monitoring oxygen therapy, but it has limitations, mainly the failure to detect hyperoxia (see Chapter 17).

    2. Transcutaneous oxygen level (TcPO$_2$): This is the method preferred by some clinicians, particularly for monitoring in the early life of newborn infants. The accuracy depends on skin thickness and perfusion, and there is a risk of local skin burn in very premature infants.

B. Continuous, invasive monitoring (via umbilical arterial catheter)

    1. Arterial PO$_2$

    2. Blood gas analysis

C. Intermittent monitoring

    1. Arterial PO$_2$ (via umbilical arterial catheters or peripheral arterial lines)

    2. Mixed central venous PO$_2$. This value, if taken from a catheter placed in the inferior vena cava, reflects the oxygen tension of the

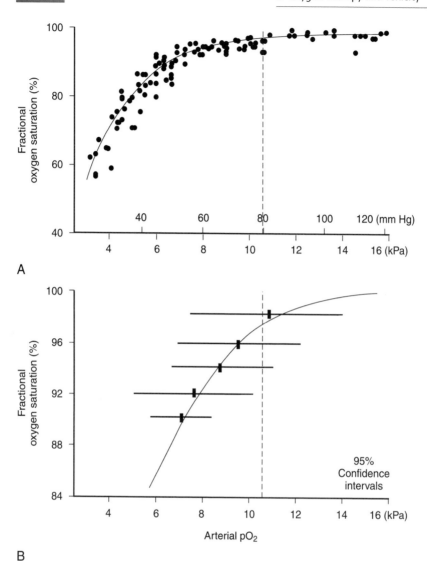

FIGURE 5-1. The relationship between fractional O_2 saturation measured with a pulse oximeter and arterial partial pressure The *dashed line* in A marks the transcutaneous oxygen level (TcPO$_2$), above which there was an increased risk of ROP in the study reported by Flynn et al in 1992. The bars in B show the range within which 95% of all measures of partial pressure varied when the oximeter read 90%, 92%, 94%, 96%, and 98% in the study reported by Brockway and Hay in 1998. (From Brockway J, Hay WW: Prediction of arterial partial pressure of oxygen with pulse oxygen saturation measurements. J Pediatr 133:63–66, 1998. Reproduced with permission from BMJ Books.)

blood that has equilibrated with the tissues and therefore can be a useful indicator of tissue oxygen delivery.

IV. Oxygen Toxicity

    A. Experimental and research work over more than a century has shown that oxygen can be toxic, and it is now clear that preterm infants are more vulnerable than other infants to the harmful effects of free oxygen radicals and oxidative stress (defined as an imbalance between pro- and antioxidant forces).

    B. Oxygen and retinopathy of prematurity (ROP): The retina is completely avascular in early fetal life. New vessels grow outward from the center around the optic nerve, controlled by vascular endothelial growth factor (VEGF) and released from normally hypoxic retinal tissue; this process is completed in utero by about 36 weeks of gestation. Treatment with supplemental oxygen in premature infants who have incompletely vascularized retinas may cause hyperoxia and vasoconstriction. This in turn leads to local hypoxia, abnormally high secretion of VEGF, and excessive proliferation of new vessels and fibrous tissue that invades the vitreous. Contraction of fibrous tissue may result in retinal detachment and visual loss. Although retinal detachment can be prevented by ablative surgery (cryo- or laser therapy), the risk of significant visual impairment remains high among infants who develop "threshold ROP" (see Chapter 69).

    C. Oxygen and bronchopulmonary dysplasia (BPD): Direct oxygen toxicity from high concentrations of inspired oxygen is an important cause of BPD. Even if inspired oxygen concentrations are not high, oxidative stress can occur and contribute to tissue injury.

    D. Oxygen and brain injury: Oxidative stress and damage to premyelinating oligodendrocytes in cerebral white matter has been proposed as a mechanism of periventricular leukomalacia, increasing the risk of cerebral palsy and cognitive deficit in preterm infants.

V. Clinical Evidence for Monitoring Oxygen Therapy

    A. There is insufficient evidence to suggest what the optimal O_2 saturation or PaO_2 values are in premature infants (who receive supplemental oxygen therapy) in order to avoid potential oxygen toxicity while providing adequate oxygen delivery to tissues.

    B. Pulse oximetry is more widely used (and is often used solely) as continuous, noninvasive monitoring for oxygen therapy, yet there remains a wide variation in O_2 saturation monitoring policies among neonatologists.

    C. Several recent observation studies have suggested that accepting lower arterial oxygen saturation (measured by pulse oximetry) is associated with lower rates of severe ROP and other neonatal complications, including BPD.

    D. The STOP-ROP trial showed that keeping saturation above 95% in very premature infants (mean gestational age, 25.4 weeks) when they were found to have developed pre-threshold ROP (mean postmenstrual age, 35 weeks) slightly reduced the risk of the progression of the disease to severe ROP requiring retinal surgery, but the benefit was seen only in those without "plus disease." However, this study also suggested that aiming to keep higher oxygen saturation was associated with significantly increased adverse pulmonary outcomes, without any benefit in growth or the eventual retinal outcome, as assessed 3 months after the expected date of delivery.

E. The BOOST trial (Askie et al, 2003) also showed that aiming to keep high oxygen saturation in chronically oxygen-dependent babies born before 30 weeks' gestation was not associated with improvement in growth and development at 1 year, and that this was associated with an increase in duration of oxygen therapy and in the use of health care resources.

VI. Summary

A. Although oxygen is the most commonly used drug in the NICU, and despite the fact that oxygen toxicity in newborns has been known for more than 50 years, clinicians remain unclear as to what is the optimal oxygenation for a preterm or ill newborn infant.

B. The current trend is toward accepting "lower" PaO_2 or O_2 saturation levels, particularly in premature infants.

C. Several other factors such as hematocrit and blood flow make major contributions to tissue oxygenation. Optimizing these factors is critical and may allow adequate oxygenation with the use of minimal supplemental oxygen.

Suggested Reading

Askie L, Henderson-Smart DJ: Restricted versus liberal oxygen exposure for preventing morbidity and mortality in preterm or low birth weight infants (Cochrane Review). In The Cochrane Library, issue 4. Chichester, UK, John Wiley & Sons, 2004.

Askie LM, Henderson-Smart DJ, Irwig L, Simpson JM: Oxygen saturation targets and outcomes in extremely preterm infants. N Engl J Med 349:959-967, 2003.

Brockway J, Hay WW: Prediction of arterial partial pressure of oxygen with pulse oxygen saturation measurements. J Pediatr 133:63-66, 1998.

Chow LC, Wright KW, Sola A: Can changes in clinical practice decrease the incidence of severe retinopathy in very low birth weight infants? Pediatrics 11:339-345, 2003.

Delivoria-Papadopoulos M , McGowan JE: Oxygen transport and delivery. In Polin RA, Fox WW, Abman SH (eds): Fetal and Neonatal Physiology. Philadelphia, WB Saunders, 2004, pp 880-889.

Flynn TJ, Bancalari E, Snyder S, et al: A cohort study of transcutaneous oxygen tension and the incidence and severity of retinopathy of prematurity. N Engl J Med 326:1050-1054, 1992.

Saugstad OD: Bronchpulmonary dysplasia—oxidative stress and antioxidants. Semin Neonatol 8:39-49, 2003.

Silverman WA: A cautionary tale about supplemental oxygen: The albatross of neonatal medicine. Pediatrics 113:394-396, 2004.

Silverman WA: Retrolental Fibroplasias: A Modern Parable. New York, Grune & Stratton, 1980.

Smith LE: Pathogenesis of retinopathy of prematurity. Semin Neonatol 8:469-473, 2003.

STOP-ROP Investigators: Supplemental therapeutic oxygen for prethreshold retinopathy of prematurity (STOP-ROP), a randomised controlled trial.1: Primary outcomes. Pediatrics 105:295-310, 2000.

Tin W, Milligan DWA, Pennefather P, Hey E: Pulse oximetry, severe retinopathy, and outcome at one year in babies of less than 28 weeks gestation. Arch Dis Child 84:F106-110, 2001.

Tin W, Wariyar U: Giving small babies oxygen: 50 years of uncertainty. Semin Neonatol 7: 361-367, 2002.

Weis CM, Cox CA, Fox WW: Oxygen therapy. In Spitzer AR (ed): Intensive Care of the Fetus and Newborn. St. Louis, Mosby, 1996, pp 538-545.

6 Respiratory Gas Conditioning and Humidification

Andreas Schulze

I. Introduction
  A. Inadequate humidification and warming of respiratory gas may lead to adverse effects within minutes to hours in infants with an artificial airway:
    1. Impaired mucociliary clearance with subsequent retention of inspissated secretions, inhaled particles, and microorganisms. Associated risks are airway clogging, atelectasis, and air leak syndromes
    2. Inflammatory and necrotic injury to the bronchial epithelium
    3. Heat loss
  B. Humidifier malfunction may also impose risks:
    1. Flushing of contaminated condensate into the airways with subsequent pneumonia
    2. Thermal injury to airways
    3. Overhydration
    4. Airway occlusion ("artificial noses," also called heat and moisture exchangers)
II. Physiology: Structure and Function of the Airway Lining
  A. Three layers cover the luminal surface of most of the upper respiratory tract and the entire tracheobronchial tree as far as the respiratory bronchioles. These layers constitute the mucociliary clearance function:
    1. A basal cellular layer of mainly ciliated epithelial cells. A variety of other cell types in this layer may each be concerned with a specific function. Serous cells, brush cells, and Clara cells produce and reabsorb aqueous fluid; goblet cells and submucosal mucus glands secrete mucus globules.
    2. An aqueous (sol) layer
    3. A viscoelastic gel (mucus) layer at the luminal surface of the airway. Neighboring cilia beat in a coordinated fashion so that waves of aligned cilia move through the airway-lining fluid, propelling mucus and entrapped particles in a cephalad direction. Dry inspired gas may dehydrate the mucus, decrease the depth of the aqueous layer, and change the viscosity gradient across the layers, all of which impair the function of the mucociliary elevator.

B. The respiratory tract functions as a countercurrent heat and moisture exchanger.

1. Inspired air gains heat and water vapor from the upper airway lining, which is partly recovered when the expired gas loses heat and water condenses on the airway surface. This recovery occurs because the upper airway temperature remains lower than core body temperature during expiration under normal physiologic circumstances. Breathing is associated with a net loss of heat and water when the expired air temperature is higher than the ambient temperature. The greater the difference in temperature between the inspired and expired gas, the greater the losses. They must be replenished by the airway epithelium, which in turn is supplied by the bronchial circulation. It is unclear under which circumstances the capacity of the airway lining to humidify cold and dry gas becomes overcharged. This capacity is likely different in health and disease.

2. The level at which the inspired air reaches core body temperature and full saturation with water vapor is called *the isothermic saturation boundary*. It is located at the level of the main bronchi during normal quiet breathing. Its position will move distally when frigid dry gas is inhaled, when minute ventilation is high, or when the upper airway is by-passed—for example, by use of a tracheostomy tube. Overall, however, under normal physiologic circumstances, only a small segment of the airway surface is exposed to a temperature below core body temperature and to less than full saturation.

3. Damage to the airway epithelial cells and their luminal coverage deprives the system of its function as a heat and moisture exchanger. Loss of this function may in turn induce structural damage in a vicious cycle that leads to penetration of the inury into the periphery of the bronchial tree.

III. Basic Physics of Humidity and Heat

A. Air can accommodate water in two different ways:

1. Nebulized water (aerosol) is a dispersion of droplets of water in air. They are visible because they scatter light (clouds) and may carry infectious agents. Deposition occurs along the tracheobroncial tree by impaction and sedimentation.The smaller the particles, the better they penetrate into more peripheral areas of the lung.

2. Vaporized water is a molecular (i.e., gaseous) distribution of water in air. It is invisible and unable to carry infectious agents. The gaseous partial pressure of water vapor is 47 mm Hg when air is fully saturated (100% relative humidity) at 37° C. This corresponds to 44 mg of water per liter of gas (absolute humidity). The term *absolute humidity* (AH) is defined as the amount of water vapor. (in milligrams) per gas volume (in liters) at a given temperature.

3. Relative humidity (RH) is the actual water vapor content of the gas volume (in milliliters) relative to the water vapor content (in milligrams) of this same gas volume at saturation at the same temperature.

4. There is a fixed relationship between AH, RH, and temperature (Fig. 6-1).

B. Air can accommodate heat in two distinct variants. The total heat content determines the capacity of inspired gas to cool or overheat the airway.

1. The air temperature represents sensible heat. Increasing the air temperature alone without adding water vapor adds very little to the total energy content of the gas. Therefore, if the respiratory gas leaves the humidifier chamber fully saturated at 37° C and is subsequently dry-heated to 40° C within the inspiratory limb of the ventilator circuit, it does not entail the risk of overheating or thermal injury of the airway.

2. The water vapor mass reflects the latent heat content. Changes in humidity represent major changes in total energy content compared to changes in air temperature alone. Therefore, vaporization consumes much energy, and thus vaporization of water from the airway lining fluid for humidification of dry inspiratory gas has a strong capacity to cool the airway even if warm gas enters the airway. Conversely, rainout (condensation of water vapor) generates energy. If it occurs inside the inspiratory limb of the ventilator circuit, the tubing may feel "nice and warm" even though the gas loses the required energy (and water vapor) content.

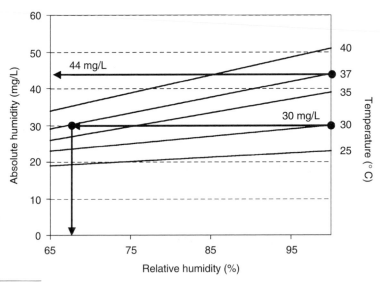

FIGURE 6-1. Relationship between absolute humidity, relative humidity, and temperature of gases. The relative humidity depends on the absolute water content and the temperature of the gas. At 37.0° C and 100% relative humidity, the respiratory gas has 44 mg/L absolute water content. If the gas is saturated (100% relative humidity) at 30.0° C, its water content will be only 30 mg/L. When the gas is then warmed to 37.0° C, its relative humidity will fall to below 70%.

IV. Inspired Gas Conditioning Devices and Procedures: Medical-grade compressed gases from cylinders or central supply systems have virtually negligible water content. It is rational to deliver the inspiratory gas at or close to core body temperature and close to full saturation with water vapor to infants with an artificial airway (nasal or pharyngeal prongs or cannula, endotracheal tube, or tracheostomy tube).

A. Heated humidifiers: The respiratory gas is warmed inside the humidification chamber to a set target temperature, and water vapor is added from the heated water reservoir. Heated-wire inspiratory circuit tubing is then used to maintain or slightly raise the gas temperature so as to prevent rainout before the gas reaches the infant. Heated humidifiers are safe and effective respiratory gas conditioning devices for short-term and long-term application in infants. However, their technology is complex, and device malfunction is not always immediately obvious. Consideration should be given to basic principles of operation common to all types of heated humidifiers:

1. The target respiratory gas condition is a temperature close to core temperature with nearly full water vapor saturation. To achieve this target, the gas must be loaded with nearly 44 mg of water/L. Knowing the circuit flow rate of the respirator, the minimum water consumption rate of the humidifier chamber to meet this target can easily be estimated and can be used to check the function of the humidifier (Fig. 6-2).

2. Rainout in the inspiratory limb of the ventilator does not prove that there is proper humidification. Major circuit condensation usually indicates a moisture loss that leads to under-humidification of the respiratory gas. This may occur if the maximum heating capacity of the heated circuit wire cannot meet requirements under specific conditions such as drafts around the tubing (air-conditioned rooms), low room temperatures, or a large outer surface area of small-diameter tubing (particularly if corrugated).

3. Rainout should also be avoided for other reasons: Condensate is easily contaminated, may be flushed down the endotracheal tube with risks of airway obstruction and nosocomial pneumonia, and may disturb the function of the respirator (particularly auto-cycling in patient-triggered ventilators). Binding the inspiratory and expiratory limbs of the tubing closely may obviate this problem.

4. The temperature probe close to the patient connection serves to monitor the respiratory gas temperature. It is commonly part of a servo-control aimed at maintaining the set gas temperature at the Wye adapter by controlling the heated-wire power output. If the temperature probe is in the presence of a heated field (incubator or radiant warmer), it may register a temperature higher than the actual respiratory gas temperature as a result of radiation or convection from the warmer environment. This may cause the servo-control to decrease the heating output of the ventilator circuit and may lead to loss of gas temperature and rainout. Insulating the temperature probe by a light reflective patch or other

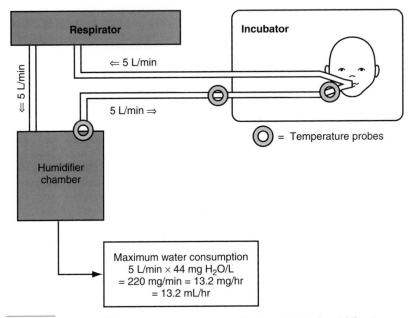

FIGURE 6-2. Position of three temperature probes of a heated-wire humidification system for infants. The user sets the target temperature to be reached at the endotracheal tube adaptor. This temperature is commonly set at or slightly above 37.0° C. The temperature inside the humidifier chamber must be high enough to vaporize an amount of water near the absolute water content of gas saturated at 37.0° C (44 mg/L absolute water content). The water consumption rate of a humidifier chamber required to reach a target respiratory gas humidity can be calculated from the circuit flow rate. Observation of this water consumption rate can be employed as a simple test of the efficiency of a humidifier.

material can improve the performance of the system. Another way to alleviate this problem is to place the temperature probe just outside the heated field and use unheated extension adapter tubing to carry the gas through the heated field to the infant. The extension tube does not need to incorporate heated wires because its temperature is maintained by the heated field. If cooler incubator temperatures are employed, as for older preterm infants, rainout will occur in the unheated segment, particularly at low circuit gas flow rates. A circuit should then be used that is equipped with a heated wire along the entire length of its inspiratory limb. Another suitable type of circuit is one with two temperature probes, one outside the heated field and another one close to the Wye adapter. These circuits can perform well over a range of incubator temperatures above and below the target respiratory gas temperature, because the heated-wire servo-control can be programmed to select the lower of the two recorded temperatures to drive the power output.

B. Artificial noses
  1. Working principle: Heat and moisture exchangers (HMEs) recover part of the heat and moisture contained in the expired air. A sponge material of low thermal conductivity inside the clear plastic housing of these devices absorbs heat and condenses water vapor during expiration for subsequent release during inspiration.
  2. Different brands may vary widely in performance characteristics. Device performance has improved recently, and further advances can be expected to facilitate neonatal applications.
     a. Some HMEs are additionally coated with bacteriostatic substances and equipped with bacterial or viral filters.
     b. Hygroscopic condenser humidifiers (HCHs) use hygroscopic compounds, such as $CaCl_2$, $MgCl_2$, and LiCl, to increase the water retention capacity.
  3. Application
     a. These devices are appropriate for short-term conventional and high-frequency mechanical ventilation in infants, such as transport or during surgical procedures.
     b. The safety and effectiveness of HMEs/HCHs for long-term mechanical ventilation is controversial in adults and has not been established in infants.
     c. HMEs/HCHs must not be used in conjunction with heated humidifiers, nebulizers, or metered dose inhalers. This may cause a hazardous increase in device resistance and/or leaching of the hygroscopic coating.
  4. Advantages of HMEs/HCHs
     a. Simplification of the ventilator circuit
     b. Passive operation without requirement of external energy and water sources
     c. No ventilator circuit condensate
     d. Low risk of circuit contamination
     e. Low expense
  5. Potential risks and drawbacks of HMEs/HCHs
     a. Depending upon the actual water load, these devices add a variable resistance and dead space to the circuit.
     b. A risk of airway occlusion from clogging with secretions or from a dislodgement of internal components has been reported for infants, even during short-term application.
     c. An expiratory air leak will impair the barrier effect of any HME/HCH against moisture loss.
  6. Measures of effectiveness of HMEs/HCHs
     a. Performance is not reliably reflected by indirect clinical measures, such as the occurrence of nosocomial pneumonia, number of endotracheal tube occlusions, or frequency of suctionings.
     b. Visual evaluation of the amount of moisture in the adapter segment between the endotracheal tube and the HME/HCH was found to closely correlate with objective measurements of the delivered humidity.

   C. Aerosol application for respiratory gas conditioning: Water or normal
       saline nebulization offers no significant benefit for inspiratory gas
       conditioning compared to the use of heated humidifiers. It may entail
       a risk of over-humidification.
       1. With appropriate use of heated humidifiers, the isothermic
           saturation boundary is close to the tip of the endotracheal tube.
           Downstream of this, aerosol particles cannot be eliminated through
           evaporation and exhalation. They will therefore become a water
           burden to the mucosa, which needs to be absorbed by the airway
           epithelium in order to maintain an appropriate periciliary fluid
           depth. An increase in depth of the airway lining fluid's aqueous layer
           may make it impossible for the cilia to reach the mucous layer and
           thus impair mucus transport. Furthermore, if the aerosol deposition
           rate exceeds absorption capacity, this may lead to increased airway
           resistance and possibly narrowing or occlusion of small airways.
           Severe systemic over-hydration subsequent to ultrasound aerosol
           therapy has been described in the term newborn and in adults.
       2. If an aerosol stream meets the airway proximal to the isothermic
           saturation boundery, the particulate water theoretically can
           contribute to the gas conditioning process by evaporation before
           and after deposition. The droplets, however, contain sensible heat
           only, and the mucosa needs to supply most of the latent heat for
           vaporization. This will cool the airway.
   D. Irrigation of the airway
       1. It is common clinical practice to instill small amounts (0.1 to 0.5 mL/kg)
           of water, normal saline solution, or diluted sodium bicarbonate
           periodically into the endotracheal tube prior to suctioning
           procedures in the belief that this provides moisture and loosens
           tenacious secretions.
       2. The safety and efficacy of this practice has not been established.
  V. Inspiratory Gas Conditioning and the Nosocomial Infection Risk
   A. There is no evidence that appropriate warming and humidifying of
       respiratory gases increases the risk of nosocomial pneumonia in
       infants with an artificial airway.
   B. The incidence of nosocomial pneumonia in adults was not increased
       when ventilator circuits were changed less frequently than every
       24 hours or even between patients only.
   C. The optimal rate of ventilator circuit changes for infants is unknown.
       Changing a ventilator circuit may disrupt ventilation in a potentially
       dangerous manner, and medical personnel may become a vector for
       cross-contamination between patients. Weekly circuit changes or no
       circuit changes at all except between patients appears to be a rational
       (although unproved) approach.

Suggested Reading

Gedeon A, Mebius C, Palmer K: Neonatal hygroscopic condenser humidifier. Crit Care Med
   15:51-54, 1987.

Kollef MH, Shapiro SD, Boyd V, et al: A randomized clinical trial comparing an extended-use hygroscopic condenser humidifier with heated-water humidification in mechanically ventilated patients. Chest 113:759-767, 1998.

Misset B, Escudier B, Rivara D, et al: Heat and moisture exchanger vs heated humidifier during long-term mechanical ventilation. A prospective randomized study. Chest 100:160-163, 1991.

Nakagawa NK, Macchione M, Petrolino HM, et al: Effects of a heat and moisture exchanger and a heated humidifier on respiratory mucus in patients undergoing mechanical ventilation. Crit Care Med 28:312-317, 2000.

Ricard JD, Le Miere E, Markowicz P, et al: Efficiency and safety of mechanical ventilation with a heat and moisture exchanger changed only once a week. Am J Respir Crit Care Med 161: 104-109, 2000.

Schiffmann H, Rathgeber J, Singer D, et al: Airway humidification in mechanically ventilated neonates and infants: A comparative study of a heat and moisture exchanger vs. a heated humidifier using a new fast-response capacitive humidity sensor. Crit Care Med 25:1755-1760, 1997.

Schulze A: Respiratory gas conditioning in infants with an artificial airway. Semin Neonatol 7:369-377, 2002.

Shelly MP, Lloyd GM, Park GR: A review of the mechanisms and methods of humidification of inspired gases. Intensive Care Med 14:1-9, 1988.

Tarnow-Mordi WO, Reid E, Griffiths P, et al: Low inspired gas temperature and respiratory complications in very low birth weight infants. J Pediatr 114:438-442, 1989.

Williams R, Rankin N, Smith T, et al: Relationship between the humidity and temperature of inspired gas and the function of the airway mucosa. Crit Care Med 24:1920-1929, 1996.

Williams RB: The effects of excessive humidity. Respir Care Clin N Am 4:215-228, 1998.

7 Pulmonary Mechanics

Emidio M. Sivieri and Vinod K. Bhutani

I. Introduction
   A. The structural and physiologic characteristics of the neonatal respiratory system are unique and may act as impediments to normal respiration.
   B. These mechanical characteristics are the elastic and resistive properties of the respiratory system and the forces that cause airflow.
   C. The energy for ventilating the lungs is supplied by the active contraction of the respiratory muscles, and these are required to overcome the elastic recoil of the lungs and the frictional resistance to airflow in the conducting airways.

II. Elastic Properties
   A. The elastic properties of the lung parenchyma are dependent on the elasticity of pulmonary tissues, gas exchange spaces, smooth muscle, connective tissue, and the vascular tissue. Equally important as tissue elasticity is the recoil effect from surface tension forces at the alveolar liquid–air interface. The elastic properties of the airways depend on the smooth muscle, tissue properties, and fibrocartilaginous structure, whereas the elastic properties of the thorax depend on the rib cage, intercostal muscle, diaphragm, and tissues of the chest wall. These forces are interdependent, maintain a complex balance, and are influenced by the respiratory cycle and position of the body.
   B. Elasticity is the property of matter such that if a system is disturbed by stretching or expanding it, the system will tend to return to its original position when all external forces are removed. Like a spring, the tissues of the lungs and thorax stretch during inspiration, and when the force of contraction (respiratory muscular effort) is removed, the tissues return to their resting position. The resting position or lung volume is established by a balance of elastic forces. At rest, the elastic recoil forces of the lung tissues exactly equal those of the chest wall and diaphragm. This occurs at the end of every normal expiration when the respiratory muscles are relaxed, and the volume remaining in the lungs is the functional residual capacity.
   C. The visceral pleura of the lung is separated from the parietal pleura of the chest wall by a thin film of fluid, creating a potential space between the two structures. In a normal newborn, at the end of expiration the mean pressure in this space (i.e., the intrapleural pressure) is 3 to 6 cm H_2O less than atmospheric pressure. This pressure results from the equal and opposite retractile forces of the

lungs and chest wall and varies during the respiratory cycle, becoming more negative during active inspiration and more positive during expiration. During normal breathing, the pressure within the lungs is dependent on the airway and tissue frictional resistive properties in response to airflow. Because there is no net movement of air at end-expiration and at end-inspiration, pressure throughout the lung at these times is in equilibrium with atmospheric air.

D. Lung compliance
1. If pressure is sequentially decreased (made more subatmospheric) around the outside of an excised lung, the lung volume increases.
2. When the pressure is removed from around the lung, it returns to its resting volume.
3. This elastic behavior of the lungs is characterized by the pressure-volume curve (Fig. 7-1A). Note that the pressure-volume curve during inspiration is different from that during expiration.
4. This difference is typical of non-ideal elastic systems and is called the hysteresis of the system.
5. The ratio of change in lung volume to change in distending pressure defines the compliance of the lungs:

$$\text{Lung compliance} = \text{change in lung volume} / \text{change in transpulmonary pressure}$$

where transpulmonary pressure (P_{TP}) is the net driving pressure to expand the lungs only and is defined as the difference between alveolar pressure and intrapleural pressure. Intrapleural pressure cannot easily be measured directly, but it can be approximated by measuring the intraesophageal pressure.
6. By definition, lung compliance is a static characteristic obtained while the respiratory system is in a passive state and there is no airflow.
   a. This can be achieved in infants by numerous, well-proven, static techniques.
   b. Using special dynamic techniques, lung compliance can also be measured during uninterrupted spontaneous breathing or mechanical ventilation.
   c. Compliance obtained in this manner is termed dynamic compliance.
7. Although the pressure-volume relationship of the lung is not linear over the entire lung volume range, the compliance (of slope $\Delta V/\Delta P$) may be close to linear over the normal range of tidal volumes beginning at functional residual capacity (Fig. 7-1F). Thus, for a given change in pressure, volume will increase in proportion to lung compliance, or $\Delta V = C/\Delta P$.
   a. When lung compliance is decreased, the lungs are stiffer and more difficult to expand.
   b. When lung compliance is increased, the lung becomes easier to distend and thus is more compliant.

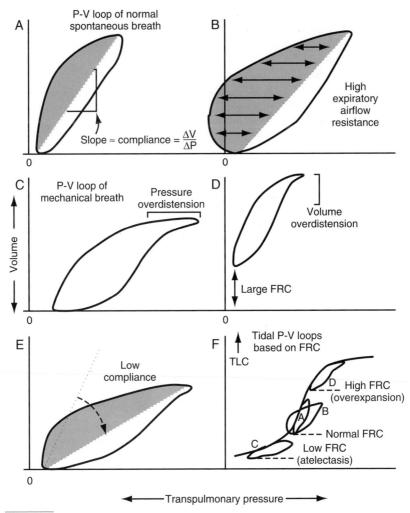

FIGURE 7-1. Pressure-volume (P-V) curves demonstrating elastic behavior of the lungs. A, Normal spontaneous breath. B, High expiratory airflow resistance. C, Mechanical breath with pressure overdistention. D, Mechanical breath with volume overdistention and large functional residual capacity (FRC). E, Low compliance with clockwise shift of axis. F, Tidal pressure-volume loops based on the functional residual capacity. TLC, total lung capacity. (Modified from Bhutani VK, Sivieri EM: Physiological principles for bedside assessment of pulmonary graphics. In Donn SM [ed]: Neonatal and Pediatric Pulmonary Graphics: Principles and Clinical Applications. Armonk, NY, Futura Publishing, 1998, p 70, with permission.)

8. Lung compliance and pressure-volume relationships are determined by the interdependence of elastic tissue elements and alveolar surface tension. Tissue elasticity is dependent on elastin and collagen content of the lung.
9. A typical value for lung compliance in a young healthy newborn is 1.5 to 2.0 mL/cm H_2O/kg.
   a. This value is dependent on the size of the lung (mass of elastic tissue).
   b. As may be expected, the compliance of the lung increases with development as the tissue mass of the lung increases.
   c. When comparing values in different subjects, lung compliance should be normalized for lung volume by dividing by the functional residual capacity. This ratio is called the specific lung compliance.
10. The surface-active substance (surfactant) lining the alveoli of the lung has a significant physiologic function.
   a. Surfactant lowers surface tension inside the alveoli, thereby contributing to lung stability by reducing the pressure necessary to expand the alveoli.
   b. Alveolar type II cells contain osmophilic lamellar bodies that are associated with the transformation of surfactant.
   c. Impaired surface activity, such as occurs in premature infants with RDS, typically results in lungs that are stiff (low compliance) and prone to collapse (atelectasis).
11. In bronchopulmonary dysplasia, the areas of fibrosis and scarring lead to a reduction in lung compliance. In these conditions, the baby has to generate a higher driving pressure to achieve a similar tidal volume or hypoventilation will occur.

E. Total respiratory system compliance
   1. If the driving pressure is measured across the entire respiratory system (transthoracic pressure), then for a given volume change we obtain the compliance of the combined lung and chest wall together:

   $$\text{Total compliance} = \text{change in lung volume}/\text{change in transthoracic pressure}$$

   where, in a passive respiratory system, transthoracic pressure is the differential between alveolar and atmospheric pressure.
   2. In a newborn connected to a mechanical ventilator, the transthoracic pressure can be measured simply as the airway pressure applied at the mouth or endotracheal tube.

F. Chest wall compliance
   1. Like the lung, the chest wall is elastic.
   2. If air is introduced into the pleural cavity, the lungs will collapse inward and the chest wall will expand outward:

   $$\text{Chest wall compliance} = \text{volume change}/\text{change in intrathoracic pressure}$$

where the intrathoracic pressure is the pressure differential across the chest wall to atmosphere. Because it is difficult to measure chest wall pressure directly, chest wall compliance may be measured indirectly where

Elastance of the respiratory system = elastance of lungs
+ elastance of chest wall

Thus,

1/Total lung compliance = 1/lung compliance
+ 1/chest wall compliance

3. As previously discussed, there is a balance of elastic recoil forces at rest (end of expiration) such that the lungs maintain a stable functional residual capacity (Fig. 7-2).
   a. In the newborn, the chest wall compliance is higher than that of the adult.
   b. The chest wall is more compliant at earlier stages of gestation.
   c. Even if the lungs have a normal elastic recoil and compliance, the FRC will be lower, because the chest wall will be unable to balance the elastic forces.
   d. The preterm newborn is therefore destined to have a lower FRC, and this state is aggravated if the FRC is decreased further because of disease states.

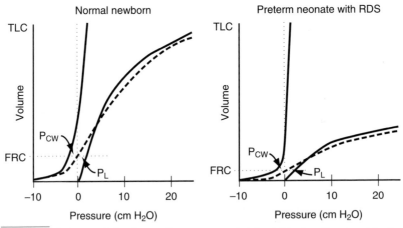

FIGURE 7-2. Balance of elastic recoil at rest to maintain stable functional residual capacity (FRC). *Left*, Normal newborn; chest wall compliance is higher than that of the adult. *Right*, Preterm newborn with RDS. Chest wall is even more compliant and aggravated by the disease state, and FRC is lower. P_{CW}, pressure (chest wall); P_L, pressure (lung); TLC, total lung capacity. (Modified from Bhutani VK, Sivieri EM: Physiological principles for bedside assessment of pulmonary graphics. In Donn SM [ed]: Neonatal and Pediatric Pulmonary Graphics: Principles and Clinical Applications. Armonk, NY, Futura Publishing, 1998, p 72, with permission.)

III. Resistive Properties
  A. Non-elastic properties of the respiratory system characterize its resistance to motion.
  B. Because motion between two surfaces in contact usually involves friction or loss of energy, resistance to breathing occurs in any moving part of the respiratory system.
  C. These resistances include frictional resistance to airflow, tissue resistance, and inertial forces.
    1. Lung resistance results predominantly (80%) from airway frictional resistance to airflow.
    2. Tissue resistance (19%) and inertia (1%) also influence lung resistance.
  D. Airflow through the airways requires a driving pressure generated by changes in alveolar pressure.
  E. When alveolar pressure is less than atmospheric pressure (during spontaneous inspiration), air flows into the lung; when alveolar pressure is greater than atmospheric pressure, air flows out of the lung.
  F. By definition, resistance to airflow is equal to the resistive component of driving pressure (P_R) divided by the resulting airflow ($\dot{V}$); thus,

$$\text{Resistance} = P_R/\dot{V}$$

  G. When determining pulmonary resistance (tissue and airway), the resistive component of the measured transpulmonary pressure is used as the driving pressure (Fig. 7-3).
  H. To obtain airway resistance alone, the differential between alveolar pressure and atmospheric pressure is used as the driving pressure.
  I. Under normal tidal breathing conditions, there is a linear relationship between airflow and driving pressure.
    1. The slope of the flow vs. pressure curve changes as the airways narrow, indicating that the patient with airway obstruction has a greater resistance to airflow.
    2. The resistance to airflow is greatly dependent on the size of the airway lumen.
    3. According to the Poiseuille law, the pressure (ΔP) required to achieve a given flow ($\dot{V}$) for a gas having viscosity η and flowing through a rigid and smooth cylindrical tube of length L and radius r is given as:

$$\Delta P = (\dot{V}\,8\eta L)/(\pi r^4)$$

    Therefore, resistance to airflow is defined as:

$$\Delta P/\dot{V} = (8\eta L)/(\pi r^4)$$

    4. Thus, the resistance to airflow increases by a power of four with any decrease in airway diameter.

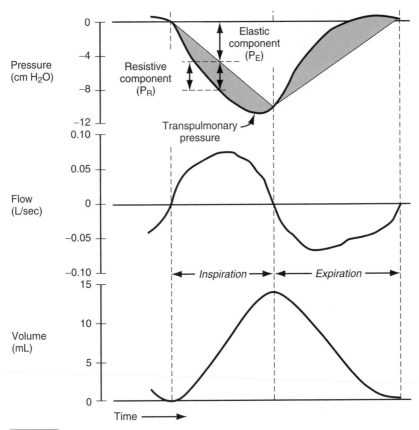

Figure 7-3. The relative elastic and resistive components of transpulmonary pressure recorded from a typical single spontaneous breath. Pulmonary resistance is determined by simultaneous measurements of the resistive component of pressure and the flow signal.

    5. Because the newborn airway lumen is approximately half that of the adult, the neonatal airway resistance is about 16-fold that of the adult. Normal airway resistance in a term newborn is approximately 20 to 40 cm $H_2O/L/s$, which is about 16-fold the value observed in adults (1 to 2 cm $H_2O/L/s$).

J. Nearly 80% of the total resistance to airflow occurs in large airways up to about the fourth to fifth generation of bronchial branching.

    1. The patient usually has large airway disease when resistance to airflow is increased.

    2. Because obstruction can occur without being readily detected in the smaller airways, which contribute only a small proportion of total airway resistance, they have been designated the "silent zone" of the lung.

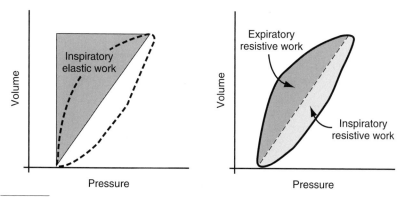

FIGURE 7-4. Work of breathing is calculated as the area under the pressure-volume curve (*shaded areas*).

IV. Inertial Properties: Inertial forces generally are considered negligible in normal tidal breathing and when considering a linear model of respiration. However, with use of high-airflow mechanical ventilation and high-frequency ventilation, and in severe airway disease, inertial forces must be considered.

V. Work of Breathing

A. The true work of breathing may be expressed as the energy required by the respiratory muscles when moving a given tidal volume of air into and out of the lungs. For obvious reasons, this type of work is difficult to determine accurately, whereas the actual mechanical work done by or in the lungs is much easier to measure. The mechanical work expended in compressing or expanding a given volume is obtained from the integral product of the applied pressure and the resulting volume change, or:

$$\text{Work} = \int P \, dV$$

TABLE 7-1. Calculated Respiratory Parameters

Parameter	Units	Adult	Newborn	Newborn with RDS	Newborn with BPD
Pulmonary compliance	mL/cm H_2O/kg	2.5-3	2-2.5	<0.6	<1.0
Chest wall compliance	mL/cm H_2O	<1	>4	–	–
Pulmonary resistance	cm H_2O/L/sec	1-2	20-40	>40	>150
Resistive work	g-cm/kg	<10	20-30	30-40	>40

TABLE 7-2. Mean Normal Values of Neonatal Pulmonary Function during the First Month

Author	Study Year	GA (wks)	Age (days)	V_T (mL/kg)	FRC (mL/kg)	C_{DYN} (mL/ cm H_2O)	R (cm H_2O/ L/sec)
Berglund/ Karlberg	1956	Term	7		27		
Cook et al	1957	Term	1-6	5.3		5.2	29
Swyer et al	1960	Term	1-11	6.7		4.9	26
Polgar	1961	Term	1-17		52.6	5.7	18.8*
Strang/ McGrath	1962	Term	1-6		49.5		
Nelson et al	1963	Preterm Term	1-16 2-4		38.7 27		
Feather/Russell	1974	Term	1-3			3.7	42
Ronchetti et al	1975	34	4-28		29.5		
Taeusch et al	1976	Term	4-6	7.2		3.7	
Adler/Wohl	1978	Term	2-5			3.5	
Mortola et al	1984	Term	1-4	6.2		3.8	
Taussig et al	1982	Term	1-9		31.4		
Migdal et al	1987	34 Term	1-28 1-29			2.4 3.2	
Anday et al	1987	28-30	2-3 5-7	5.9 6.6		2.0 2.3	50 exp 70 exp
Gerhardt et al	1987	31-36 Term	3-30 6-16		16.7 17.1	2.2 3.6	87 exp 58 exp
Abbasi/ Bhutani	1990	28-34	2-3	6.3		2.4	54
Sivieri et al	1995	27-40 26-37 23-32	2-30 2-30 1-22		23.4 21.5 RDS 18.9 BPD		

GA, gestational age; V_T, tidal volume; FRC, functional residual capacity; C_{DYN}, dynamic lung compliance; R, pulmonary resistance; exp, expiratory; RDS, infants with respiratory distress syndrome; BPD, infants who developed bronchopulmonary dysplasia.

B. This value is simply the area under the applied pressure vs. volume curve for any gas. Therefore, by integrating the transpulmonary pressure curve over volume, the pulmonary work of breathing is easily calculated (Fig. 7-4). This mechanical work can be partitioned into elastic and resistive components:

1. Elastic work is that portion needed to overcome elastic resistance to inflate the lungs. Under normal conditions, this work is stored as potential energy and is used in restoring the system to its resting volume.

2. Resistive work is that portion needed to overcome airway and tissue frictional resistances. The hysteresis of the pressure-volume relationship represents the resistive work of breathing and can be further partitioned into inspiratory and expiratory components.

C. Normally, the elastic energy stored during inspiration is sufficient to provide the work needed to overcome expiratory frictional resistance.

1. In babies with obstructive airway disease, the expiratory component of resistive work of breathing is increased (see Fig. 7-1B).

2. The units of work of breathing correspond to the units of pressure times volume (cm $H_2O \cdot L$), or equivalently, force times distance (kg $\cdot$ m), and is usually expressed as the work per breath or respiratory cycle.

VI. Some Reference Values

A. Calculated values of both elastic and resistive properties determined in adult and term newborns are listed in Table 7-1. These are compared to values obtained in infants with respiratory distress syndrome and bronchopulmonary dysplasia.

B. Table 7-2 lists values of neonatal pulmonary function parameters during the first month collected by several investigators over several decades of work in this area.

Suggested Reading

Bancalari E: Pulmonary function testing and other diagnostic laboratory procedures in neonatal pulmonary care. In Thibeault DW, Gary GA (eds): Neonatal Pulmonary Care, 2nd ed. East Norwalk, CT, Appleton-Century Crofts, 1986, pp 195-234.

Bhutani VK, Shaffer TH, Vidyasager D (eds): Neonatal Pulmonary Function Testing: Physiological, Technical and Clinical Considerations. Ithaca, NY, Perinatology Press, 1988.

Bhutani VK, Sivieri EM: Physiological principles for bedside assessment of pulmonary graphics. In Donn SM (ed): Neonatal and Pediatric Pulmonary Graphics. Principles and Clinical Applications. Armonk, NY, Futura Publishing, 1998, pp 57-79.

Bhutani VK, Sivieri EM, Abbasi S: Evaluation of pulmonary function in the neonate. In Polin RA, Fox WW (eds): Fetal and Neonatal Physiology, 2nd ed. Philadelphia, WB Saunders, 1988, pp 1143-1164.

Comroe JH: Physiology of Respiration, 2nd ed. Chicago, Year Book Medical Publishers, 1974.

Comroe JH, Forster RE, Dubois AB, et al: Clinical Physiology and Pulmonary Function Tests, 2nd ed. Chicago, Year Book Medical Publishers, 1971.

Polgar G, Promadhat V: Pulmonary Function Testing in Children. Philadelphia, WB Saunders, 1971.

Rodarte JR, Rehder K: Dynamics of respiration. In Geiger SR (ed): Handbook of Physiology, Section 3: The Respiratory System, vol III. Bethesda, MD, American Physiological Society, 1986, pp 131-144.

Stocks J, Sly PD, Tepper RS, Morgan WJ (eds): Infant Respiratory Function Testing. New York, Wiley-Liss, 1996.

West JB: Respiratory Physiology: The Essentials. Oxford, Blackwell Scientific Publications, 1974.

Basic Principles of Mechanical Ventilation

8

Waldemar A. Carlo,
Namasivayam Ambalavanan, and
Robert L. Chatburn

I. Introduction: The ventilatory needs of a patient depend largely on the mechanical properties of the respiratory system and the type of abnormality in gas exchange.

II. Pulmonary Mechanics
   A. The mechanical properties of the lungs are a determinant of the interaction between the ventilator and the infant.
   B. A pressure gradient between the airway opening and alveoli drives the flow of gases.
   C. The pressure gradient necessary for adequate ventilation is largely determined by compliance and resistance.

III. Compliance
   A. Compliance describes the elasticity or distensibility of the lungs or respiratory system (lungs plus chest wall).
   B. It is calculated as follows:

$$\text{Compliance} = \frac{\Delta \text{ volume}}{\Delta \text{ pressure}}$$

   C. Compliance in infants with normal lungs ranges from 3 to 5 mL/cm H_2O/kg.
   D. Compliance in infants with RDS is lower and often ranges from 0.1 to 1 mL/cm H_2O/kg.

IV. Resistance
   A. Resistance describes the ability of the gas-conducting parts of the lungs or respiratory system (lungs plus chest wall) to resist airflow.
   B. It is calculated as follows:

$$\text{Resistance} = \frac{\Delta \text{ pressure}}{\Delta \text{ flow}}$$

   C. Resistance in infants with normal lungs ranges from 25 to 50 cm H_2O/L/sec. Resistance is not markedly altered in infants with RDS or other acute pulmonary disorders but can be increased to 100 cm H_2O/L/sec or more by small endotracheal tubes.

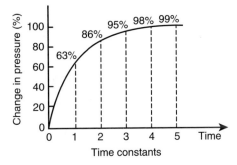

FIGURE 8-1. Percentage change in pressure in relation to the time (in time constants) allowed for equilibration. As a longer time is allowed for equilibration, a higher percentage change in pressure will occur. The same rules govern the equilibrium for step changes in volume. Changes in pressure during inspiration and expiration are illustrated. (Modified from Carlo WA, Chatburn RL: Assisted ventilation of the newborn. In Carlo WA, Chatburn RL [eds]: Neonatal Respiratory Care, 2nd ed. Chicago, Year Book Medical Publishers, 1988, p 323, with permission.)

V. Time Constant
   A. The time constant is the time (expressed in seconds) necessary for the alveolar pressure (or volume) to reach 63% of a change in airway pressure (or volume) (Fig. 8-1).
   B. It is calculated as follows:

$$\text{Time constant} = \text{compliance} \times \text{resistance}$$

For example, if an infant has a lung compliance of 2 mL/cm H_2O (0.002 L/cm H_2O) and a resistance of 40 cm H_2O/L/sec, the time constant is calculated as follows:

$$\text{Time constant} = 0.002 \text{ L/cm } H_2O \times 40 \text{ cm } H_2O/\text{L/sec}$$

$$= 0.080 \text{ sec}$$

Note that in the calculation of the time constant, compliance is not corrected for unit of weight.
   C. A duration of inspiration or expiration equivalent to 3 to 5 time constants is required for a relatively complete inspiration or expiration. Thus, in the infant described above, inspiratory and expiratory duration should be around 240 to 400 msec each (or 0.24 to 0.4 seconds).
   D. The time constant will be shorter if compliance is decreased (e.g., in patients with RDS) or if resistance is decreased. The time constant will be longer if compliance is high (e.g., large infants with normal lungs) or if resistance is high (e.g., infants with chronic lung disease).
   E. Patients with a short time constant ventilate well with short inspiratory and expiratory times and high ventilatory frequency, whereas patients with a long time constant require longer inspiratory and expiratory times and lower rates.

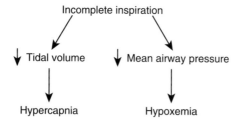

FIGURE **8-2.** Effect of incomplete inspiration on gas exchange. (From Carlo WA, Greenough A, Chatburn RL: Advances in mechanical ventilation. In Boynton BR, Carlo WA, Jobe AH [eds]: New Therapies for Neonatal Respiratory Failure: A Physiologic Approach. Cambridge, UK, Cambridge University Press, 1994, p 137, with permission.)

F. If inspiratory time is too short (i.e., a duration shorter than approximately 3 to 5 time constants), there will be a decrease in tidal volume delivery and mean airway pressure (Fig. 8-2).

G. If expiratory time is too short (i.e., a duration shorter than approximately 3 to 5 time constants), the result will be gas trapping and inadvertent positive end-expiratory pressure (PEEP) (Fig. 8-3).

H. Although the respiratory system is often modeled as being composed of a single compliance and a single resistance, it is known that the mechanical properties vary with changes in lung volume, even within a breath. Furthermore, the mechanical characteristics of the respiratory system change somewhat between inspiration and expiration. In addition, lung disease can be heterogeneous, and thus mechanical characteristics can vary in different areas of the lungs.

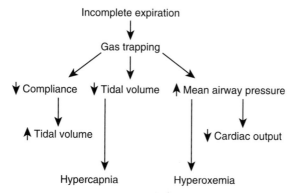

FIGURE **8-3.** Effect of incomplete expiration on gas exchange. (From Carlo WA, Greenough A, Chatburn RL: Advances in mechanical ventilation. In Boynton BR, Carlo WA, Jobe AH [eds]: New Therapies for Neonatal Respiratory Failure: A Physiologic Approach. Cambridge,UK, Cambridge University Press, 1994, p 137, with permission.)

VI. Equation of Motion
  A. The pressure necessary to drive the respiratory system is the sum of the elastic, resistive, and inertial components and can be calculated as follows:

$$P = 1/C\ V + R\dot{V} + I\ddot{V}$$

where P is pressure, C is compliance, V is volume, R is resistance, $\dot{V}$ is flow, $\ddot{V}$ is the rate of change in flow, and I is inertance.
  B. Because the inertial component is small at physiologic flows, the last component ($I\ddot{V}$) can be neglected
  C. The equation of motion can be used to derive estimates of compliance and resistance. For example, between points of $\dot{V} = 0$ (points of no flow), the pressure gradient results from compliance.

VII. Gas Exchange
  A. Hypercapnia and hypoxemia occur during respiratory failure.
  B. Although impairment in CO_2 elimination and O_2 uptake and delivery may coexist, some conditions may affect gas exchange differentially.

VIII. Gas Exchange during Transition to Extrauterine Life
  A. Hemodynamic changes during transition to extrauterine life
    1. Systemic vascular resistance increases
    2. Pulmonary vascular resistance decreases
    3. Pulmonary blood flow increases
  B. Blood gas values in the perinatal period

	At birth	At age 10 min
PaO_2 (mm Hg)	15-20	46-57
$PaCO_2$ (mm Hg)	49-76	40-47

IX. Determinants of Pulmonary Gas Exchange
  A. Composition and volume of alveolar gas
  B. Composition and volume of mixed venous blood
  C. Mechanisms of gas exchange
X. Composition of Inspired and Alveolar Gases
  A. Partial pressure of oxygen in dry air (PO_2):

$$PO_2 = \text{fractional content} \times \text{total gas pressure}$$

If barometric pressure = 760 mm Hg, then

$$PO_2 = 0.21 \times 760 \text{ mm Hg}$$
$$= 160 \text{ mm Hg}$$

  B. Partial pressure of oxygen in humidified air (PiO_2)

$$PiO_2 = \text{fractional content} \times (\text{total gas pressure} - \text{water vapor pressure})$$
$$= 0.21 \times (760 - 47 \text{ mm Hg})$$
$$= 149 \text{ mm Hg}$$

C. Partial pressure of oxygen in humidified alveolar gas

Partial pressure of alveolar $O_2 = PiO_2 - P_ACO_2$ $(FiO_2 + [1 - FiO_2]/R)$

where P_ACO_2 is alveolar PCO_2 and R is the respiratory quotient. Because CO_2 diffuses very well through the alveoli, $P_ACO_2 \approx PaCO_2$. If barometric pressure = 760 mm Hg and water vapor pressure = 47 mm Hg, and if $FiO_2 = 100$, then

$$PiO_2 = 713$$

If FiO_2 is 1.00, then

$$(FiO_2 + [1 - FiO_2]/R) = 1.0$$

and

$$P_AO_2 = 713 - 40 = 673 \text{ mm Hg}$$

If FiO_2 is 0.21, then

$$P_AO_2 = 149 - 40 \ (0.21 + [1-0.21]/0.8) = 100 \text{ mm Hg}$$

XI. Composition of Mixed Venous Blood
   A. Mixed venous PO_2 (P_VO_2) depends on arterial O_2 content, cardiac output, and metabolic rate.
   B. Oxygen content of blood per 100 mL:

Dissolved $O_2 = 0.003$ mL O_2 per mm Hg PaO_2
Hb-bound $O_2 = O_2$Sat $\times$ 1.34/g Hb $\times$ Hb concentration

For example, in 1 kg of infant blood (volume $\approx$ 100 mL), with PaO_2 = 100 mm Hg (O_2Sat = 100%, or 1.0), and Hb = 17 mg/dL:

$$
\begin{aligned}
O_2 \text{ content} &= \text{Hb-bound } O_2 + \text{dissolved } O_2 \\
&= 1.00 \times (1.34 \times 17) + (0.003 \times 100) \\
&= 22.78 + 0.3 \text{ mL } O_2 \\
&= 23.08 \text{ mL } O_2
\end{aligned}
$$

C. CO_2 content of blood: CO_2 is carried in three forms:
   1. Dissolved in plasma and red cells
   2. As bicarbonate
   3. Bound to hemoglobin
XII. Hypoxemia: The pathophysiologic mechanisms responsible for hypoxemia are in the following order of relative importance in newborns: ventilation-perfusion mismatch, shunt, hypoventilation, and diffusion limitation (Figs. 8-4, 8-5, and 8-6).

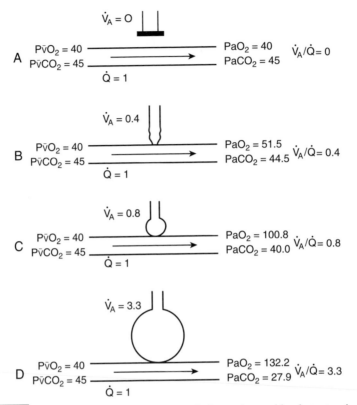

FIGURE 8-4. Effects of various ventilation-perfusion ratios on blood gas tensions.
A, Direct venoarterial shunting ($\dot{V}_A/\dot{Q} = 0$). B, Alveolus with a low $\dot{V}_A/\dot{Q}$ ratio.
C, Normal alveolus. D, Underperfused alveolus with high $\dot{V}_A/\dot{Q}$ ratio. (From
Krauss AN: Ventilation-perfusion relationships in neonates. In Thibeault DW,
Gregory GA [eds]: Neonatal Pulmonary Care, 2nd ed. Norwalk, CT,
Appleton-Century-Crofts, 1986, p 127, with permission.)

A. Ventilation-perfusion (V/Q) mismatch: V/Q mismatch is an
   important cause of hypoxemia in newborns. Supplemental oxygen
   can largely overcome the hypoxemia resulting from V/Q mismatch.
B. Shunt: Shunt is a common cause of hypoxemia in newborns.
   A shunt may be physiologic, intracardiac (e.g., PPHN and congenital
   cyanotic heart disease), or pulmonary (e.g., atelectasis). It can be
   thought of as a V/Q = 0, and supplemental O_2 cannot reverse the
   hypoxemia.
C. Hypoventilation: Hypoventilation results from a decrease in tidal
   volume or respiratory rate. During hypoventilation, the rate of
   oxygen uptake from the alveoli exceeds its replenishment.

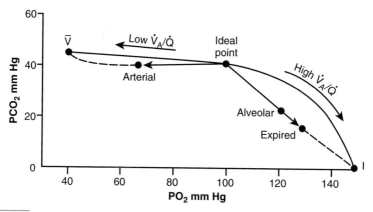

FIGURE 8-5. O_2-CO_2 diagram showing the arterial, ideal, alveolar, and expired points. The curved line indicates the PO_2 and the PCO_2 of all lung units having different ventilation-perfusion ratios. (From West JB: Gas exchange. In West JB [ed]: Pulmonary Pathophysiology: The Essentials. Baltimore, Williams & Wilkins, 1977, p 27, with permission.)

Thus, alveolar PO_2 falls and PaO_2 decreases. It can be thought of as low V/Q, and supplemental O_2 can overcome the hypoxemia easily. Causes of hypoventilation include depression of respiratory drive, weakness of the respiratory muscles, restrictive lung disease, and airway obstruction.

D. Diffusion limitation: Diffusion limitation is an uncommon cause of hypoxemia, even in the presence of lung disease. Diffusion limitation occurs when mixed venous blood does not equilibrate with alveolar gas. Supplemental O_2 can overcome hypoxemia secondary to diffusion limitation.

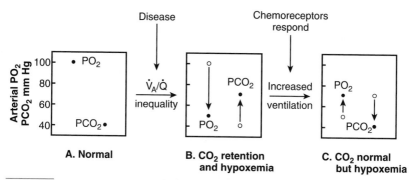

FIGURE 8-6. PO_2 and PCO_2 in different stages of ventilation-perfusion inequality. Initially, there must be both a fall in oxygen and a rise in carbon dioxide tensions. However, when the ventilation to the alveoli is increased, the PCO_2 exchange increases. In West JB [ed]: Pulmonary Pathopysiology: The Essentials. Baltimore, Williams & Wilkins, 1977, p 30, with permission.)

XIII. Oxygenation during Assisted Ventilation
   A. Oxygenation may be largely dependent on lung volume, which in turn depends on mean airway pressure (Fig. 8-7).
   B. On a pressure ventilator, any of the following will increase mean airway pressure: increasing inspiratory flow, increasing peak inspiratory pressure (PIP), and increasing the inspiratory-to-expiratory (I:E) ratio or PEEP.
   C. Mean airway pressure may be calculated as follows:

$$\text{Mean airway pressure} = K(\text{PIP} - \text{PEEP})\,[T_I/(T_I + T_E)] + \text{PEEP}$$

   where K is a constant that depends on the shape of the early inspiratory part of the airway pressure curve (K ranges from approximately 0.8 to 0.9 during pressure-limited ventilation); T_I is inspiratory time; and T_E is expiratory time. For the same change in mean airway pressure, increases in PIP and PEEP increase oxygenation more. A very high mean airway pressure transmitted to the intrathoracic structures may impair cardiac output and thus decrease oxygen transport despite an adequate PaO_2.

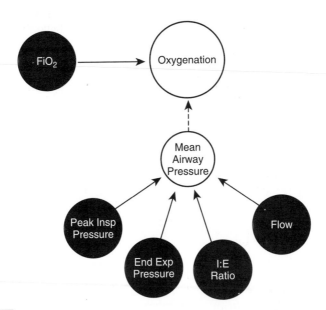

FIGURE 8-7. Determinants of oxygenation during pressure-limited, time-cycled ventilation. *Shaded circles* represent ventilator-controlled variables. *Solid lines* represent the simple mathematical relationships that determine mean airway pressure and oxygenation, whereas the *dashed lines* represent relationships that cannot be quantified. (From Carlo WA, Greenough A, Chatburn RL: Advances in mechanical ventilation. In Boynton BR, Carlo WA, Jobe AH [eds]: New Therapies for Neonatal Respiratory Failure: A Physiologic Approach. Cambridge, UK, Cambridge University Press, 1994, p 134, with permission.)

XIV. Hypercapnia: The pathophysiologic mechanisms responsible for hypercapnia are V/Q mismatch, shunt, hypoventilation, and increased physiologic dead space. The physiologic dead space results in part from areas of inefficient gas exchange because of low perfusion (wasted ventilation). Physiologic dead space includes ventilation to conducting airways and alveolar spaces not perfused (i.e., anatomic dead space).

XV. CO_2 Elimination during Assisted Ventilation

A. CO_2 diffuses easily into the alveoli and its elimination depends largely on the total amount of gas that comes in contact with the alveoli (alveolar ventilation). Minute alveolar ventilation is calculated from the product of the frequency (per minute) and the alveolar tidal volume (tidal volume minus dead space).

$$\text{Minute alveolar ventilation} = \text{frequency} \times (\text{tidal volume} - \text{dead space})$$

B. On a volume-cycled (volume-targeted) ventilator the tidal volume is preset. On a pressure-controlled ventilator, the tidal volume depends on the pressure gradient between the airway opening and the alveoli; this is peak inspiratory pressure (PIP) minus the positive end-expiratory pressure (PEEP), or amplitude (ΔP).

C. Depending on the time constant of the respiratory system (and the ventilator), a very short inspiratory time (T_I) may reduce the tidal volume and a very short expiratory time (T_E) may cause gas trapping and inadvertent PEEP and consequently may also reduce tidal volume (see above).

D. Fig. 8-8 illustrates the relationships of ventilator controls, pulmonary mechanics, and minute ventilation.

XVI. Blood Gas Analysis: A careful interpretation is essential for appropriate respiratory care (Table 8-1, Figs. 8-9 and 8-10; also see Chapter 18).

A. Respiratory acidosis (low pH, high $PaCO_2$, normal HCO_3^-) can result from:

1. V/Q mismatch, shunt, and/or hypoventilation
2. Secondary renal compensation
   a. Reduced bicarbonate excretion
   b. Increased hydrogen ion excretion

B. Respiratory alkalosis (high pH, low $PaCO_2$, normal HCO_3^-) can result from:

1. Hyperventilation
2. Secondary renal compensation
   a. Increased bicarbonate excretion
   b. Retention of chloride
   c. Reduced excretion of acid salts and ammonia

C. Metabolic acidosis (low pH, normal $PaCO_2$, low HCO_3^-) can result from:

1. Increased acid production
2. Impaired acid elimination
3. Secondary pulmonary compensation—hyperventilation with decreased $PaCO_2$

D. Metabolic alkalosis (high pH, normal $PaCO_2$, high HCO_3^-) can result from:
   1. Excessive $NaHCO_3$ administration, diuretic therapy, and loss of gastric secretions
   2. Secondary pulmonary compensation—hypoventilation

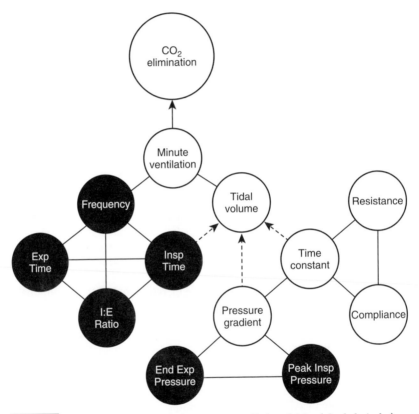

Figure 8-8. Relationships among ventilator-controlled variables (*shaded circles*) and pulmonary mechanics (*unshaded circles*) that determine minute ventilation during time-cycled, pressure-limited ventilation. Relationships between circles joined by *solid lines* are mathematically derived. The *dashed lines* represent relationships that cannot be precisely calculated without considering other variables such as pulmonary mechanics. Alveolar ventilation can be calculated from the product of tidal volume and frequency when dead space is subtracted from the former. (From Carlo WA, Greenough A, Chatburn RL: Advances in mechanical ventilation. In Boynton BR, Carlo WA, Jobe AH [eds]: New Therapies for Neonatal Respiratory Failure: A Physiologic Approach. Cambridge, UK, Cambridge University Press, 1994, p 133, with permission.)

TABLE 8-1 Blood Gas Classifications

Classification	pH	PaCO$_2$	HCO$_3^-$	BE
Respiratory Disorder				
Uncompensated acidosis	↓	↑	N	N
Partly compensated acidosis	↓	↑	↑	↑
Compensated acidosis	N	↑	↑	↑
Uncompensated alkalosis	↑	↓	N	N
Partly compensated alkalosis	↑	↓	↓	↓
Compensated alkalosis	N	↓	↓	↓
Metabolic Disorder				
Uncompensated acidosis	↓	N	↓	↓
Partly compensated acidosis	↓	↓	↓	↓
Uncompensated alkalosis	↑	N	↑	↑
Partly compensated alkalosis	↑	↑	↑	↑
Compensated alkalosis	N	↑	↑	↑

BE, base excess; ↑, elevated values; ↓, depressed values; N, normal.
From Carlo WA, Chatburn RL: Assessment of neonatal gas exchange. In Carlo WA, Chatburn RL (eds): Neonatal Respiratory Care, 2nd ed. Chicago, Year Book Medical Publishers, 1988, p 51, with permission.

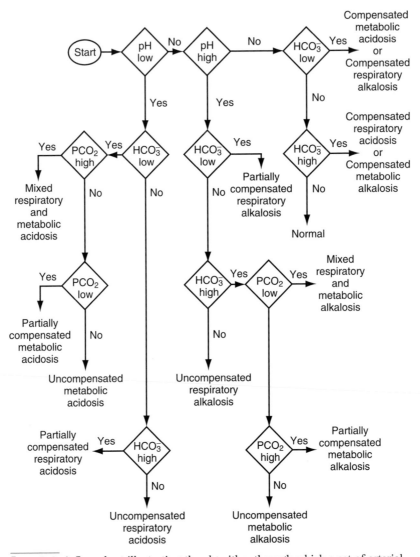

FIGURE 8-9. A flow chart illustrating the algorithm through which a set of arterial blood gas values may be interpreted. (From Chatburn RL, Carlo WA: Assessment of neonatal gas exchange. In Carlo WA, Chatburn RL [eds]: Neonatal Respiratory Care, 2nd ed. Chicago, Year Book Medical Publishers, 1988, p 56, with permission.)

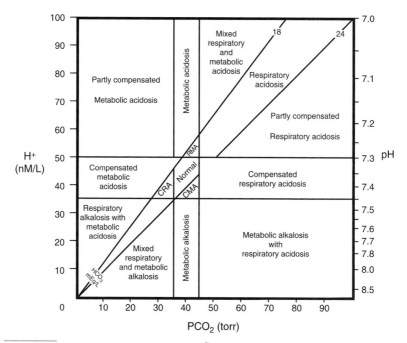

FIGURE 8-10. A neonatal acid-base map. CRA, compensated respiratory acidosis; CMA, compensated metabolic acidosis; RMA, mixed respiratory and metabolic acidosis. (From Chatburn RL, Carlo WA: Assessment of neonatal gas exchange. In Carlo WA, Chatburn RL [eds]: Neonatal Respiratory Care, 2nd ed. Chicago, Year Book Medical Publishers, 1988, p 58, with permission.)

Suggested Reading

Carlo WA, Chatburn RL: Assisted ventilation of the newborn. In Carlo WA and Chatburn RL (eds): Neonatal Respiratory Care, 2nd ed. Chicago, Year Book Medical Publishers, 1988 pp 320-346.

Carlo WA, Greenough A, Chatburn RL: Advances in conventional mechanical ventilation. In Boynton BR, Carlo WA, Jobe AH (eds): New Therapies for Neonatal Respiratory Failure: A Physiologic Approach. Cambridge, UK, Cambridge University Press, 1994, pp 131-151.

Donn SM (ed): Neonatal and Pediatric Pulmonary Graphics: Principles and Clinical Applications. Armonk, NY, Futura Publishing, 1997.

Greenough A, Milner AD (eds): Neonatal Respiratory Disorders. London, Arnold Publishers, 2003.

Krauss AN: Ventilation-perfusion relationship in neonates. In Thibeault DW, Gregory GA (eds): Neonatal Pulmonary Care, 2nd ed. Norwalk, CT, Appleton-Century-Crofts, 1986, p 127.

Mariani GL, Carlo WA: Ventilatory management in neonates. Controversies in Neonatal Pulmonary Care 25:33-48, 1998.

Spitzer AR, Fox WW: Positive-pressure ventilation: Pressure-limited and time-cycled ventilators. In Goldsmith JP, Karotkin EH (eds): Assisted Ventilation of the Neonate, 4th ed. Philadelphia, WB Saunders, 2004, pp 167-186.

West JB: Gas exchange. In West JB (ed): Pulmonary Pathophysiology—The Essentials. Baltimore, Williams & Wilkins, 1977, p 32.

9

Classification of Mechanical Ventilation Devices

Waldemar A. Carlo
Namasivayam Ambalavanan, and
Robert L. Chatburn

I. Introduction: Ventilators can be classified by the variables that are controlled (e.g., pressure or volume), as well as those that start (or trigger), sustain (or limit), and end (cycle) inspiration and those that maintain the expiratory support (or baseline pressure).

II. Control Variables: A ventilator can be classified as a pressure, volume, or flow controller (Fig. 9-1). Ventilators control more than one variable at different times.

    A. Pressure controller: This type of ventilator controls either: (1) airway pressure, making it rise above the body surface pressure (i.e., positive pressure ventilator); or (2) body surface pressure, making it fall below the airway pressure (i.e., negative pressure ventilator).

    B. Volume controller: This type of ventilator controls and measures the tidal volume generated by the ventilator despite changes in loads. In the past, the usefulness of this type of ventilator has been limited in newborns because the control variable was regulated near the ventilator and not near the patient, resulting in a tidal volume lower than the preset value. Microprocessor and sensor technology has corrected this.

    C. Flow controller: This type of ventilator controls the tidal volume but does not measure it directly. A ventilator is a flow controller if the gas delivery is limited by flow.

    D. Time controller: This type of ventilator controls the timing of the ventilatory cycle but not the pressure or volume. Most high-frequency ventilators are time controllers.

III. Phase Variables: The ventilatory cycle has four phases: (1) the change from expiration to inspiration (trigger); (2) inspiratory limit; (3) the change from inspiration to expiration (cycle); and (4) expiration (baseline pressure) (Fig. 9-2).

    A. Trigger

        1. One or more variables in the equation of motion (i.e., pressure, volume, flow, and time) is measured by the ventilator and is used to trigger (or start) inspiration.

        2. Inspiration begins when one of these variables reaches a preset value.

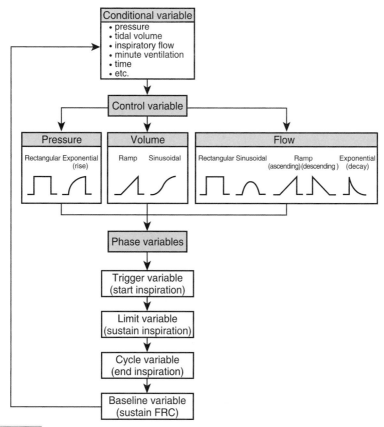

FIGURE 9-1. Application of the equation of motion to the respiratory system. A common waveform for each control variable is shown. Pressure, volume, flow, and time are also used as phase variables that determine the characteristics of each ventilatory cycle (e.g., trigger sensitivity, inspiratory time, baseline pressure). This emphasizes that each breath may have a different set of control and phase variables, depending on the mode of ventilation desired. (From Chatburn RL: Classification of mechanical ventilators. In Branson RD, Huess DR, Chatburn RL [eds]: Respiratory Care Equipment. Philadelphia, JB Lippincott, 1995, p 280, with permission.)

3. The most common trigger variables are time (i.e., after a pre-defined time, the ventilator is triggered to start inspiration as in intermittent mandatory ventilation) and pressure (i.e., when an inspiratory effort is detected as a change in the end-expiratory pressure, the ventilator is triggered to start inspiration, as in patient-triggered ventilation). Flow-triggering involves less effort by the patient and is more commonly used in infant ventilators.

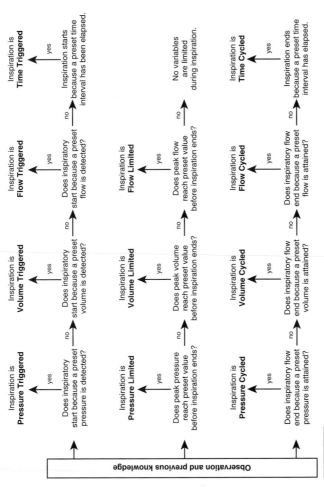

FIGURE 9-2. Criteria for determining the phase variables during a ventilator-supported breath. (From Chatburn RL: Classification of mechanical ventilators. In Branson RD, Huess DR, Chatburn RL [eds]: Respiratory Care Equipment. Philadelphia, JB Lippincott, 1995, p 280, with permission.)

B. Limit
1. Pressure, volume, and flow increase during inspiration.
2. A limit variable restricts the inspiratory increase to a preset value but does not limit the duration.
3. Many neonatal ventilators are pressure limited.
C. Cycle
1. The cycle variable is used to end inspiration.
2. Many neonatal ventilators, including high-frequency ventilators, are time-cycled.
3. Changes in airway flow may also be used to terminate the inspiratory phase and cycle into expiration.
D. Baseline: The baseline variable maintains expiratory pressure and expiratory lung volume (e.g., positive end-expiratory pressure).
IV. Ventilatory Modes: This classification of mechanical ventilation devices can be applied to the various ventilatory modes (Table 9-1).

TABLE 9-1. Ventilatory Modes

Mode	Mandatory				Spontaneous			
	Control	Trigger[a]	Limit	Cycle	Control	Trigger	Limit	Cycle
Control	Flow[b]	Time	Volume Flow	Volume Time	NA[c]	NA	NA	NA
A/C or CMV[d]	Flow	Pressure Volume Time	Volume Flow	Volume Time	NA	NA	NA	NA
IMV (continuous flow)	Pressure Flow	Time	Volume Flow	Volume Time	–[e]	–	–	–
SIMV (continuous flow)	Pressure Flow	Pressure Volume Flow Time	Pressure Volume Flow Time	Volume Time	–	–	–	–
SIMV (demand flow)	Pressure Flow	Pressure Volume Flow Time	Pressure Volume Flow Time	Volume Time	Pressure Flow	Pressure	Pressure	Pressure

TABLE 9-1. Ventilatory Modes—cont'd

	Mandatory—cont'd			Spontaneous—cont'd		
PS	—	—	—	Pressure	Pressure	Flow
PS + SIMV	Pressure Flow	Pressure Volume Flow Time	Time	Pressure Flow	Pressure	Flow
CAP or CPAP (continuous flow)	—	—	—	—	Pressure	—
CAP or CPAP (demand flow)	—	—	—	Pressure Flow	Pressure	—
PC	Pressure	Pressure	Time	NA	NA	—

[a]Whether or not a breath is patient-triggered depends on the sensitivity setting and the magnitude of the patient's inspiratory effort.

[b]For the purposes of this table, flow control is equivalent to volume control. Baseline PEEP is assumed to be available for all modes.

[c]NA, not applicable.

[d]A/C, assist/control; CMV, conventional mandatory ventilation; IMV, intermittent mandatory ventilation; PS, pressure support; SIMV, synchronized mandatory ventilation; CAP, constant airway pressure; CPAP, continuous positive airway pressure; PC, pressure control.

[e]Ventilator does not respond.

From Carlo WA, Greenough A, Chatburn RL: Advances in Conventional Mechanical Ventilation. New Therapies for Neonatal Respiratory Failure: A Physiologic Approach. Cambridge, UK, Cambridge University Press, 1994, p 144, with permission.

Suggested Reading

Carlo WA, Greenough A, Chatburn RL: Advances in conventional mechanical ventilation. In Boynton BR, Carlo WA, Jobe AH (eds): New Therapies for Neonatal Respiratory Failure: A Physiologic Approach, Cambridge, UK, Cambridge University Press, 1994, pp 131-151.

Chatburn RL: Classification of mechanical vventilators. In Branson RD, Hess DR, Chatburn RL (eds): Respiratory Care Equipment. Philadelphia, JB Lippincott, 1995, pp 264-293.

Ventilator Parameters

10

Waldemar A. Carlo,
Namasivayam Ambalavanan, and
Robert L. Chatburn

I. Peak Inspiratory Pressure (PIP)
   A. Physiologic effects
      1. PIP in part determines the pressure gradient between the onset and end of inspiration and thus affects the tidal volume and minute ventilation.
      2. During volume ventilation, an increase in tidal volume corresponds to an increase in PIP during pressure ventilation. If tidal volume is not measured, initial PIP can be selected based on observation of chest wall movement and magnitude of breath sounds.
   B. Gas exchange effects
      1. An increase in PIP will increase tidal volume, increase CO_2 elimination, and decrease $PaCO_2$.
      2. An increase in PIP will increase mean airway pressure and thus improve oxygenation.
   C. Side effects
      1. An elevated PIP may increase the risk of barotrauma, volutrauma, and bronchopulmonary dysplasia/chronic lung disease.
      2. There is increasing evidence that lung injury is primarily caused by large tidal volume delivery and lung overdistention.
      3. It is important to adjust PIP based on lung compliance and to ventilate with relatively small tidal volumes (e.g., 3 to 5 mL/kg).
II. Positive End-Expiratory Pressure (PEEP)
   A. Physiologic effects
      1. PEEP in part determines lung volume during the expiratory phase, improves ventilation-perfusion mismatch, and prevents alveolar collapse.
      2. PEEP contributes to the pressure gradient between the onset and end of inspiration, and thus affects the tidal volume and minute ventilation.
      3. A minimum "physiologic" PEEP of 2 to 3 cm H_2O should be used in most newborns.
   B. Gas exchange effects
      1. An increase in PEEP increases expiratory lung volume (FRC capacity) during the expiratory phase and thus improves ventilation-perfusion matching and oxygenation in patients whose disease state reduces expiratory lung volume.

2. An increase in PEEP will increase mean airway pressure and thus improve oxygenation in patients with this type of disease.

3. An increase in PEEP will also reduce the pressure gradient during inspiration and thus reduce tidal volume, reduce CO_2 elimination, and increase $PaCO_2$.

C. Side effects

1. An elevated PEEP may overdistend the lungs and lead to decreased lung compliance, decreased tidal volume, less CO_2 elimination, and an increase in $PaCO_2$.

2. Although use of low to moderate PEEP may improve lung volume, a very high PEEP may cause overdistention and impaired CO_2 elimination secondary to decreased compliance and gas trapping.

3. A very high PEEP may decrease cardiac output and oxygen transport.

III. Frequency (or Rate)

A. Physiologic effects: The ventilator frequency (or rate) in part determines minute ventilation, and thus, CO_2 elimination. Ventilation at high rates (≥ 60/min) frequently facilitates synchronization of the ventilator with spontaneous breaths. Spontaneous breathing rates are inversely related to gestational age and the time constant of the respiratory system. Thus, infants with smaller and less compliant lungs tend to breathe faster.

B. Gas exchange effects: When very high frequencies are used, the problem of insufficient inspiratory time or insufficient expiratory time may occur (see below).

C. Side effects: Use of very high ventilator frequencies may lead to insufficient inspiratory time and decreased tidal volume or insufficient expiratory time and gas trapping.

IV. Inspiratory Time (T_I), Expiratory Time (T_E), and Inspiratory-to-Expiratory Ratio (I:E Ratio)

A. Physiologic effects

1. The effects of T_I and T_E are strongly influenced by their relationship to the inspiratory and expiratory time constants.

TABLE 10-1. Desired Blood Gas Goal and Corresponding Ventilator Parameter Changes

Desired Goal	Ventilator Parameter Change				
	PIP	PEEP	Frequency	I:E Ratio	Flow
Decrease $PaCO_2$	↑	↓	↑	–	±↑
Increase $PaCO_2$	↓	↑	↓	–	±↑
Decrease PaO_2	↓	↓	–	↓	±↑
Increase PaO_2	↑	↑	–	↑	±↑

–, Not applicable; ±, may or may not.

2. A T_I as long as 3 to 5 time constants allows relatively complete inspiration.
3. A T_I of 0.2 to 0.5 sec is usually adequate for newborns with RDS.
4. Use of a longer T_I generally does not improve ventilation or gas exchange.
5. A very prolonged T_I may lead to ventilator asynchrony.
6. A very short T_I will lead to decreased tidal volume.
7. Infants with a long time constant (e.g., with chronic lung disease) may benefit from a longer T_I (approximately 0.6 to 0.8 sec).

B. Gas exchange effects
   1. Changes in T_I, T_E, and I:E ratio generally have modest effects on gas exchange.
   2. A sufficient T_I is necessary for adequate tidal volume delivery and CO_2 elimination.
   3. Use of relatively a long T_I or high I:E ratio improves oxygenation slightly.

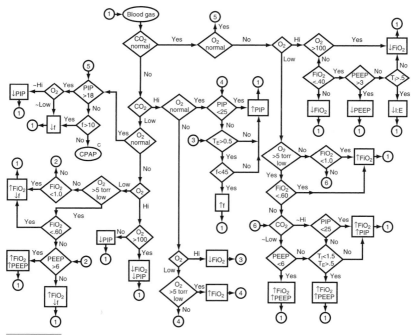

FIGURE 10-1. Algorithm showing simplified flow chart used to optimize pressure-limited mechanical ventilation of infants with RDS. *Diamonds* call for decisions; *squares* indicate types and directions of ventilator setting changes. Flow chart is followed until a square is reached. If a number other than 1 is reached, re-enter the algorithm as appropriate. See Table 10-2 for explanation of abbreviations. (From Chatburn RL, Carlo WA, Lough MD: Clinical algorithm for pressure-limited ventilation of neonates with respiratory distress syndrome. Respir Care 28:1579, 1983, with permission.)

    C. Side effects: A very short T_I or T_E can lead to insufficient times and decrease tidal volume and increase gas trapping, respectively.

V. Inspired Oxygen Concentration (FiO_2)

    A. Physiologic effects

       1. Changes in FiO_2 alter alveolar oxygen pressure, and thus, oxygenation.

       2. Because both FiO_2 and mean airway pressure determine oxygenation, the most effective and less adverse approach should be used to optimize oxygenation.

       3. When FiO_2 is above 0.6 to 0.7, increases in mean airway pressure are generally warranted.

       4. When FiO_2 is below 0.3 to 0.4, decreases in mean airway pressure are generally preferred.

    B. Gas exchange effects: FiO_2 directly determines alveolar PO_2 and thus PaO_2.

    C. Side effects: A very high FiO_2 can damage the lung tissue, but the absolute level of FiO_2 at which it is toxic has not been determined.

VI. Flow

    A. Changes in flow rate have not been well studied in infants, but they probably impact arterialblood gases minimally as long as a sufficient flow is used (which is generally the case with most ventilators).

    B. Inadequate flow may contribute to air hunger, asynchrony, and increased work of breathing.

    C. Excessive flow may contribute to turbulence, inefficient gas exchange, and inadvertent PEEP.

VII. Summary

    A. Depending on the desired change in blood gases, the following ventilator parameter changes shown in Table 10-1 can be performed.

    B. A suggested management algorithm for RDS is shown in Figure 10-1 (also see Table 10-2).

TABLE 10-2. Abbreviations and Symbols Used in the Flow Chart in Figure 10-1

CO_2	Arterial carbon dioxide tension (mm Hg)
O_2	Arterial oxygen tension (mm Hg)
FiO_2	Fraction of inspired oxygen
PIP	Peak inspiratory pressure (cm H_2O)
P̄aw	Mean airway pressure (cm H_2O)
PEEP	Positive end-expiratory pressure (cm H_2O)
CPAP	Continuous positive airway pressure without mechanical ventilation (cm H_2O)
I:E	Ratio of inspiratory to expiratory time
f	Ventilator frequency (breaths/min). Unless otherwise specified, a change in frequency should be accompanied by a change in I:E to maintain the same T_I, so that tidal volume remains constant
T_I	Inspiratory time (sec)
T_E	Expiratory time (sec)
Hi	The variable in the decision symbol is above normal range
Low	The variable in the decision symbol is below normal range
~Hi	The variable in the decision symbol is at the high end of normal
~Low	The variable in the decision symbol is at the low end of normal
↑	Increase
↓	Decrease
>	Greater than
<	Less than
Torr	Unit of pressure; 1 torr = 1 mm Hg

From Carlo WA, Chatburn RL: Assisted Ventilation of the newborn. In Carlo WA, Chatburn RL (eds): Neonatal Respiratory Care, 2nd ed. Chicago, Year Book Medical Publishers, 1988 p 339, with permission.

Suggested Reading

Donn SM (ed): Neonatal and Pediatric Pulmonary Graphics: Principles and Clinical Applications. Armonk, NY, Futura Publishing, 1997.

Greenough A: Respiratory support. In Greenough A, Roberton NRC, Milner AD (eds): Neonatal Respiratory Disorders. New York, Oxford University Press, 1996, pp 115-151.

Mariani GL, Carlo WA: Ventilatory management in neonates. Controversies in Neonatal Pulmonary Care 25:33-48, 1998.

Spitzer AR, Fox WW: Positive-pressure ventilation: Pressure-limited and time-cycled ventilators. In Goldsmith JP, Karotkin EH (eds): Assisted Ventilation of the Neonate, 3rd ed. Philadelphia, WB Saunders, 1996, pp 167-186.

Procedures and Techniques

Clinical Examination

11

Avroy A. Fanaroff and Jonathan M. Fanaroff

I. Normal Physical Findings
   A. Respiratory rate 40 to 60 breaths/min
      1. Irregular with pauses of ≤5 seconds in REM sleep
      2. Regular in non-REM sleep; rate is 5 to 10 breaths/min slower than in REM sleep or when awake
      3. No dyspnea
      4. No intercostal retractions
      5. No subcostal retractions
      6. No grunting (an expiratory noise produced by sudden relaxation of the laryngeal adductors at the end of expiration)
   B. Pulse rate 120 to160 bpm
      1. Sinus arrhythmia is rare in the newborn.
      2. Pulses are easy to feel; some reduction in leg pulses is common if neonate is ≤48 hours old. Femoral pulses may be impalpable, reduced, or delayed, with coarctation of the aorta. In any infant with suspected heart disease, blood pressure should be measured in all four limbs. A difference of >15 mm Hg between the upper (higher) and lower extremities is significant. Bounding pulses are characteristic of patent ductus arteriosus.
      3. Interpreting the heart rate is best done in conjunction with measurement of the respiratory rate and SaO_2.
         a. Episodes of desaturation are mostly transient or a movement artifact, but if more severe and prolonged may be accompanied by bradycardia.
         b. An increase in heart rate may be observed with movement/ crying, respiratory distress, anemia, hypovolemia, fever, infection, pain, fluid overload, and arrhythmia.
         c. Slowing of the heart may be seen with hypoxia, hypothermia, seizures, heart block, and, rarely, raised intracranial pressure.
         d. Monitor artifacts may also produce bradycardia. The clinical diagnosis of neonatal sepsis is preceded by abnormal heart rate characteristics of transient decelerations and reduced variability.
   C. First and second heart sounds are often single; S_2 splits are seen by 48 hours in 75% of infants.
   D. Murmurs are common in the first few days.
   E. Blood pressure (Fig. 11-1)

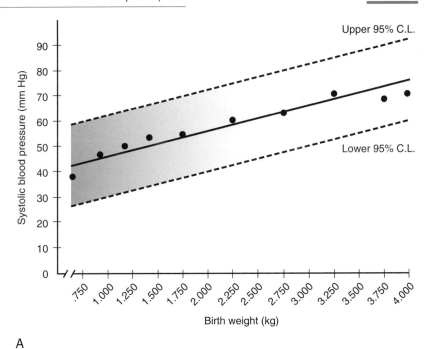

A

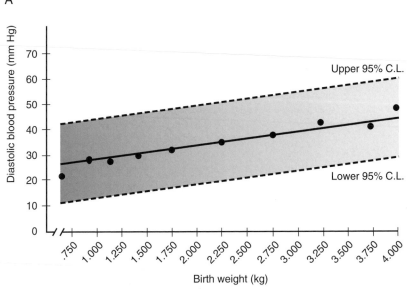

B

FIGURE 11-1. Linear regression of mean systolic (A) and diastolic (B) blood pressure on birth weight in 329 infants admitted to the NICU on day 1 of life is plotted. C.L., Confidence limits. (From Zubrow AB, Hulman S, Kushner H, et al: Determinants of blood pressure in infants admitted to neonatal intensive care units: A prospective multicenter study. J Perinatol 15:470-479, 1995. Copyright, the Nature Publishing Group, reprinted with permission.)

II. Clinical Examination of the Cardiorespiratory System
   A. The four classic components should be followed:
      1. Observation
      2. Palpation
      3. Percussion
      4. Auscultation: Murmurs are common in healthy newborns.
         Their source may be pulmonary branch stenosis, patent ductus
         arteriosus, tricuspid regurgitation, and other congenital cardiac
         lesions.
   B. Careful visual as well as auditory observation of the newborn is
      important.
   C. Cardinal signs of respiratory distress:
      1. Intercostal, subcostal, and substernal retractions
      2. Nasal flaring
      3. Expiratory grunting
      4. Tachypnea >60/min
      5. Cyanosis
         a. Peripheral cyanosis (extremities) is common in normal
            infants.
         b. Central cyanosis (lips and tongue) signifies >5 g/dL
            of desaturated hemoglobin and is significant (pulse
            oximeter <90%).
         c. The most common causes of cyanosis are heart disease,
            pulmonary disease, and methemoglobinemia. The
            underlying cause of cyanosis must be determined. If cyanosis
            is relieved by oxygen administration, the most likely cause is
            pulmonary disease.
III. Respiraton Rate
   A. Rates >60 breaths/min are abnormal.
   B. Very fast rates may have a better prognosis because they occur in
      more mature babies with a good respiratory pump able to sustain
      the tachypnea.
   C. Slow irregular rates <30 breaths/min with or without gasping are
      ominous, as are apneic periods in term infants.
   D. Remember that tachypnea is a very nonspecific finding and
      can be caused by:
      1. Pulmonary disease
      2. Cardiac disease
      3. Sepsis
      4. Anemia
      5. Metabolic academia of any cause
      6. Fever
      7. CNS pathology
      8. Stress (e.g., after feeding or crying)
IV. Dyspnea
   A. Distortion of the chest by the powerful attempts of the muscles
      of respiration to expand noncompliant lungs is one of the most
      significant findings in parenchymal lung disease.

B. With anemia, acidemia, cyanotic heart disease, or fever, there is often tachycardia without dyspnea.

C. Preterm babies (<1.5 kg) in non-REM sleep when muscle tone is low show mild intercostal and subcostal retractions.

D. Other features of dyspnea include:

   1. Flaring of the alae nasi. By enlarging the nostrils there is a reduction in nasal resistance, enhancing air flow.

   2. "See-saw" respiration—abdominal expansion (from diaphragmatic contraction) at the same time as sternal retractions.

   3. Intercostal and subcostal retractions.

   4. Retractions (suprasternal, intercostal, and subcostal) result from the compliant rib cage being drawn in on inspiration by the diaphragm as the infant attempts to generate high intrathoracic pressures in order to ventilate poorly compliant lungs.

V. Interaction with Positive Pressure Ventilation

A. In the early stages of severe lung disease, especially RDS, the baby may breathe out of phase with the ventilator. This compromises oxygenation and increases the risk of air leaks. Synchronization of the ventilator to the baby's own respiratory effort has been shown to decrease time on the ventilator and assists weaning.

B. In ventilated babies, a sign of recovery is that they breathe faster than the ventilator; this becomes part of the weaning process as the ventilator rate is reduced, with or without one of the support modes of ventilation.

C. In both situations (sick or convalescing babies) it is important to count the ventilator rate as well as the baby's spontaneous ventilation rate.

D. If the baby's condition has deteriorated rapidly, is the chest moving at all with the ventilator? It if is not, this may suggest a blocked or dislodged endotracheal tube. Always consider pneumothorax in an infant whose condition has deteriorated rapidly.

VI. Apnea and Gasping: When counting the respiratory rate, note if there are any pauses lasting more than 5 seconds, or if there are any gasping respirations (both very abnormal), as opposed to normal sighs (deep inspirations against the normal background respiratory pattern).

VII. General Appearance

A. Does the baby look ill or well? Multiple factors to assess are:

   1. Color—pallor, cyanosis, plethora

   2. Level of activity

   3. Cry

   4. Eye opening

   5. Posture

   6. Edema

   7. Perfusion

   8. Dysmorphic features

B. Edema: Leaky capillaries in ill babies lead to subcutaneous edema as well as pulmonary edema.

C. Perfusion

   1. Pallor (capillary refill time >3 seconds)

   2. Nonspecific illness
   3. Anemia
   4. Hypotension
   5. Shock (septic or other)
   6. Visible veins in skin (especially in preterm infants)
      a. Hypercapnia
      b. Nonspecific severe illness with shock (e.g., extensive hemorrhage)
   D. Cyanosis
      1. Assessed from lips, mucous membranes (acrocyanosis is peripheral cyanosis of hands and feet; common and rarely significant); May be difficult to see in nonwhite races (even in mucosa).
      2. Cyanosis results from >5.0 g/dL desaturated hemoglobin.
         a. Seen in normally oxygenated polycythemic babies
         b. Difficult to detect in very anemic babies
      3. In an oxygen-enriched environment, oxygen may be absorbed through the skin, making the baby look pink although central cyanosis may be present.
   E. Saturation
      1. Because clinical signs of hypoxemia are unreliable, if in doubt initially check oxygen saturation (SpO_2) by pulse oximetry (quick and easy) and if necessary confirm hypoxemia by arterial blood gas analysis.
      2. An arterial oxygen tension of 60 to 90 mm Hg results in a saturation of 94% to 98%; changes of 1% to 2% usually reflect a PaO_2 change of 6 to 12 mm Hg. Below 40 mm Hg, the saturation falls to less than 90%.
      3. Saturations >95% are normal in term babies.
      4. Note that SpO_2 does not correct for abnormal hemoglobin as in methemoglobinemia—the baby is blue but saturation is high.
VIII. Clubbing: Rarely seen in babies
  IX. Venous Pressure
   A. Observe venous pulsation in the neck for evidence of congestive heart failure.
   B. Prominent pulsation in the neck may be observed with vein of Galen arteriovenous malformation.
   C. Auscultation of the head will reveal a bruit.
   X. Other Systems
   A. Abdomen
      1. Distention
         a. Large amount of gas in the stomach after positive pressure ventilation, especially with mask and bag
         b. Enlarged liver from heart failure, hepatitis, or metabolic disorder
         c. Liver pushed down by hyperinflated chest or tension pneumothorax
         d. Enlarged spleen, kidneys, or other abdominal mass
         e. Retention of urine secondary to drugs, CNS disease
      2. Scaphoid strongly suggests congenital diaphragmatic hernia

      B. Central Nervous System
        1. Seizures
        2. Tense fontanel when the newborn is not crying (suggests increased intracranial pressure)
        3. Abnormal tone
        4. Abnormal level of consciousness (e.g., irritability, lethargy, coma)

XI. Auditory Observations
    A. Listen to the baby. If the baby is crying vigorously, he or she is unlikely to be seriously ill.
    B. Three important auditory clues:
        1. Grunting—a pathognomonic feature of neonatal lung disease—is expiration against a partially closed glottis that traps alveolar air and maintains FRC.
        2. Stridor, usually inspiratory
            a. Upper airway problems (laryngomalacia is the commonest)
            b. Glottic and subglottic injury or postintubation edema
            c. Local trauma following overvigorous laryngeal instrumentation
            d. Congenital subglottic stenosis
            e. Vascular rings, hemangiomas, hamartomas (rare)
        3. "Rattle"—the bubbling of gas through secretions in the oropharynx. Often an ominous sign in a baby with severe CNS injury as well as lung disease.
        4. Excessive drooling suggests esophageal atresia with fistula.

XII. Palpation
    A. Not usually of much help. The following may be noted:
        1. Mediastinal shift (trachea, apical beat) with air leak, diaphragmatic hernia, collapse (consolidation)
        2. Tense abdomen (tension pneumothorax or pneumoperitoneum)
        3. Subcutaneous emphysema following air leaks
        4. Pulses
            a. Pulses should be checked in all four limbs if there is any suspicion of cardiac disease and should be documented by blood pressure measurements.
            b. Bounding pulses are a feature of an increased cardiac output, often with a left-to-right shunt. In the preterm infant, this may be the first sign of a PDA.
        5. Cardiac precordial activity
        6. Thrills (very rare in the neonatal period; if present, always significant)

XIII. Percussion
    A. Increased resonance may be seen with a pneumothorax and occasionally with severe PIE.
    B. Decreased resonance accompanies pleural effusions.
    C. Decreased resonance with marked collapse/consolidation
        1. Pneumonia
        2. ETT in one bronchus
    D. Decreased resonance with congenital diaphragmatic hernia

XIV. Auscultation
  A. Always use the small neonatal stethoscope. It can be difficult to apply to the chest of a preterm newborn in a way that excludes extraneous noise, and trial and error will identify whether the bell or diaphragm is best in a given situation. Use whichever gives the best acoustic seal.
  B. Another problem is that babies, particularly preterm infants, wiggle when the stethoscope is placed on the chest, making cardiac examination difficult. The trick is to hold the prewarmed stethoscope in the same place; after 10 to 15 seconds, the baby habituates to the stimulus and lies still.
  C. Breath sounds are conducted through the upper torso of the newborn, and the smaller the baby, the greater the conduction. Even with the neonatal stethoscope head it is difficult to be certain about where air is going. Two common (and very serious) auscultation mistakes:
    1. Failing to realize during mechanical ventilation that air is going in and out of the stomach rather than the lungs.
    2. Failing to realize that only one lung is being ventilated (particularly if there is some mediastinal shift).
XV. Air Entry
  A. The breath sounds in newborns with normal lungs can be heard in both inspiration and expiration, being slightly louder and longer in inspiration. In other words, part of the expiratory phase, which is physiologically longer, is silent.
  B. A general reduction in air entry is heard with:
    1. Any severe lung disease (e.g., RDS)
    2. An occluded ETT
  C. Unilateral decrease in air entry—any unilateral lung disease, which will usually require a chest radiograph for further evaluation.
    1. Pneumonia
    2. Air leak
    3. Pleural effusion
    4. Misplaced ETT/spontaneous extubation
XVI. Other Sounds
  A. There should be no rales or crepitations (discontinuous sounds) and no rhonchi (continuous sounds). The other common sound heard on auscultating the chest of a preterm baby is water bubbling in the ventilator tubing in which it has condensed. Clearly, it is impossible to do a successful clinical examination under these circumstances. The tubing should be transiently disconnected from the ventilator circuit and emptied.
  B. Crepitations occur in:
    1. Pneumonia
    2. Aspiration
    3. Heart failure (PDA and other)
    4. Massive pulmonary hemorrhage
    5. Chronic lung disease
    6. Meconium aspiration (stickier and louder)

C. Rhonchi occur with:
1. Retained secretions during mechanical ventilation
2. Meconium aspiration
3. Chronic lung disease
D. None of these findings is specific. They indicate a lung disease that requires further evaluation, initially by radiography.
E. Bowel sounds in the chest are a specific finding of congenital diaphragmatic hernia.

XVII. Cardiac Auscultation
A. Heart sounds: The ready availability of echocardiography has blunted the need for sophisticated auscultatory diagnostic skills for the newborn. The following, however, should always be noted:
1. S_1 and S_2 are usually single in the first 24 to 48 hours, with splitting of S_2 being present in 75% of babies by 48 hours.
2. A gallop rhythm (S_3 and S_4) is always abnormal, usually indicating heart failure.
B. Innocent murmurs are very common in the first 24 to 48 hours. Characteristics include:
1. Grade 1-2/6 mid-systolic at the left sternal edge
2. No ejection clicks
3. May occur in babies with normal pulses (especially femoral— document by blood pressure measurements).
4. May occur in babies with an otherwise normal clinical examination.
C. Significant murmurs are more likely to be heard in babies >48 hours of age. Characteristics include:
1. Pansystolic ± diastolic ± thrills
2. Grade 3/6 or more and harsh
3. Best heard at upper left sternal edge (e.g., PDA)
4. Abnormal S_2 (not splitting) ± gallop rhythm
5. Early or mid-systolic click
6. Decreased femoral pulses with murmur heard at back
7. Other signs of illness (heart failure, shock, and cyanosis)
D. Any baby with these features needs urgent evaluation (radiography, ECG, and echocardiogram). The absence of murmurs or auscultatory abnormality in the first 48 to 72 hours does not exclude serious or even fatal heart disease.

XVIII. Transillumination (see Chapter 21)
A. A bright light source applied to the chest wall can be a useful and effective way of detecting a collection of intrapleural air, typically a pneumothorax, but large cysts, severe PIE, and marked lobar emphysema may also transilluminate. To be effective, the light source has to be very bright (ideally a fiberoptic source), the area around the baby needs to be very dark, and some experience is required to differentiate the normal halo of light (0.5 to 0.1 cm) around the probe from increased transillumination caused by a small collection of air. In cases in which the whole hemithorax lights up, the diagnosis is easy.

    B. The technique is more useful in smaller babies in whom the light is transmitted into the pleural cavity much more easily than in term babies with a thick layer of subcutaneous fat.

XIX. Blood Pressure

    A. The readily available automatic blood pressure recording devices now make this a routine part of the assessment of all newborns.

    B. Attention to the following details is important:

       1. Baby is quiet and not recently crying.

       2. Cuff covers 75% of the distance between the axilla and the elbow.

       3. Bladder virtually encircles the arm.

       4. A similar cuff size is appropriate for the upper arm and the calf.

    C. In ill preterm babies the oscillometric device may overestimate the true blood pressure; if there is any doubt about systolic pressure accuracy, direct measurement from an indwelling arterial catheter may be indicated.

    D. Summary: In the newborn, the circulation is assessed by:

       1. Blood pressure measurement: Normative values are available for term infants, but there is less reliable data for very-low-birth-weight infants (see Fig. 11-1). Blood pressure may correlate poorly with systemic blood flow and circulating volume. Cerebral blood flow is critical.

       2. Heart rate: Tachycardia from hypovolemia is common, and bradycardia is a late sign of shock.

       3. Temperature gap (between abdomen and toes) >2° C may suggest shock, but also may be caused by a cold environment and infection without shock.

       4. Capillary refill time >3 seconds is abnormal.

       5. Acid-base status (increased lactate with circulating insufficiency).

       6. Echocardiographic evaluation of cardiac function.

Suggested Reading

Arlettaz R, Archer N, Wilkinson AR: Natural history of innocent heart murmurs in newborn babies: controlled echocardiographic study. Arch Dis Child Fetal Neonatal Ed 78:F166-F170, 1998.

Farrer KF, Rennie JM: Neonatal murmurs: Are senior house officers good enough? Arch Dis Child Fetal Neonatal Ed 88:F147-F151, 2003.

Frommelt MA: Differential diagnosis and approach to a heart murmur in term infants. Pediatr Clin North Am 51:1023-1032, 2004.

Greenough A, Greenall F: Observation of spontaneous respiratory interaction with artificial ventilation. Arch Dis Child 63:168-171, 1988.

Yi MS, Kimball TR, Tsevat J, et al: Evaluation of heart murmurs in children: Cost-effectiveness and practical implications. J Pediatr 141:504-511, 2002.

12 Neonatal Resuscitation

Janet M. Rennie

I. Anticipating Resuscitation: "*Time* is of the utmost importance. *Delay* is damaging to the infant. *Act* promptly, accurately and gently." [Virginia Apgar] Some form of resuscitation is required in about 5% to 10% of all deliveries; about 2 per 100 newborn infants require intubation. A person trained in the basic skills of resuscitation with sole responsibility for the baby should be present at all deliveries, but an individual with advanced resuscitation skills should be present at the following types of deliveries (the list is not exhaustive):
   A. Preterm delivery
   B. Multiple deliveries
   C. Breech delivery
   D. Instrumental or operative delivery (unless elective cesarean section)
   E. Meconium staining
   F. Fetal distress (whether cesarean section or vaginal delivery)
II. Normal Postnatal Transition: Most babies establish independent breathing and circulation quickly after birth, crying lustily and becoming pink within a few minutes. During this period of time the baby normally:
   A. Clears lung liquid from the trachea and alveoli.
   B. Establishes a functional residual volume with the aid of surfactant.
   C. Reduces pulmonary vascular resistance (oxygenation, nitric oxide, prostaglandins).
   D. Increases pulmonary blood flow, and reverses intra- and extracardiac shunts (foramen ovale and ductus arteriosus).
III. Equipment Needed for Resuscitation
   A. A warm, well-lit area in which resuscitation can take place
   B. A heater
   C. Towels, gloves; hat for baby
   D. Immediate access to a telephone or intercom
   E. An assured oxygen supply with a suitable pressure valve to limit pressure
   F. A supply of medical gases
   G. A suction device with a range of catheter sizes
   H. Laryngoscopes with back-up bulbs and batteries; assorted blades
   I. Endotracheal tubes ranging from 2.5 to 4.5 mm with stylets
   J. A mask resuscitation system with masks of various sizes
   K. All systems capable of providing respiratory support should have protective "blow-off devices." However, in case high pressures are

needed on an individual basis, the resuscitator should be able to override such a device.

  L. Equipment for placing a peripheral and/or umbilical venous catheter

  M. Scissors

  N. Stethoscope

  O. Timing device

  P. Fluids and drugs (sodium bicarbonate, naloxone, epinephrine, dextrose, saline)

IV. Assessing the Infant after Birth

  A. Start the clock.

  B. Receive the baby, remove any wet wraps, and dry the baby with a warm towel.

  C. Place the infant on the resuscitation surface, cover with a warm towel, and assess breathing, heart rate, and color.

  D. Babies fall into one of three categories at this point:

   1. Pink, breathing spontaneously and regularly, heart rate >100; active tone

   2. Cyanotic, breathing irregularly, heart rate >100; some tone

   3. White, floppy, not breathing, heart rate <100

V. The Apgar Score (Table 12-1): The Apgar score can be helpful in categorizing infants at this stage. A score of >3 means that advanced resuscitation is required immediately and is an indication to call for help.

VI. Initiating Resuscitation

  A. Babies who are pink, breathing regularly, and with a good heart rate should be returned to their mothers as soon as possible, without any further intervention.

  B. If the baby falls into one of the other categories previously described, and respiration is not established, resuscitation should be started.

  C. Babies who are blue but with a good heart rate usually respond to simple resuscitation.

  D. Babies who are white, floppy, and not breathing will most likely need full resuscitation with intubation and chest compression following the "A, B, C, D" approach outlined in Section VII.

  E. Optimally, two people should be dedicated to the resuscitation of a baby in this situation. Call for help immediately if you are single-handed in this situation.

TABLE 12-1. The Apgar Score

	Score	0	1	2
A	Appearance	Pale or blue	Body pink but extremities blue	Pink
P	Pulse rate	Absent	<100	>100
G	Grimace	Nil	Some	Cry
A	Activity (muscle tone)	Limp	Some flexion	Well flexed
R	Respiratory Effort	Absent	Hypoventilation	Good

VII. The "A, B, C, D" of Resuscitation
  A. Airway
    1. Make sure the airway is clear.
    2. Position the baby supine with the jaw drawn forward.
    3. Gently suction the mouth, and then the nose if secretions are present. Many babies will resuscitate themselves once the airway is clear.
    4. Do not insert the suction catheter too far into the oropharynx or it will induce a vagal response including bradycardia and apnea.
    5. Do not suction for more than 5 seconds at a time.
    6. Suction is particularly important for depressed babies born through meconium-stained fluid, but is not required for those who remain vigorous.
  B. Breathing
    1. If resuscitation does not commence rapidly, try gentle stimulation, such as rubbing the soles of the feet and drying the body with a towel.
    2. If respirations do not commence within 20 seconds or remain irregular, the baby will require artificial lung inflation.
    3. Choose a face mask that fits over the baby's mouth and nose but does not overhang the chin or cover the eyes. Masks with cushioned rims are preferable because it is easier to make a tight seal.
    4. Hold the mask over the face, making a tight seal.
    5. Begin to inflate the lungs with the Y piece (easier and better; can provide sustained inflation) or self-inflating bag.
    6. Never, ever, connect a baby directly to the "wall" oxygen supply, which is at a dangerously high pressure. Hospital gas supplies must be passed through a pressure-reducing system before being delivered to babies via a T piece or bag and mask. Babies have died from an air leak caused by high-pressure gas delivered this way.
    7. Ventilate at 30 to 40 breaths per minute, giving the first few breaths a long (2-second) inflation time ("rescue breaths").
      a. The first few breaths need to overcome surface tension.
      b. The pressure given should be enough to move the chest wall (about 20 cm water, although the first few breaths may need to be 30 to 40 cm water pressure).
      c. Watch to see that the chest moves and listen to the heart rate, which should rise rapidly.
      d. If the heart rate remains low or falls in spite of adequate ventilation, the baby will need intubation and external chest compression.
      e. In an emergency, oral intubation is generally preferred. Take care to use the correct tube size and to insert it to the appropriate depth (see Chapter 13).
  C. Circulation
    1. Chest compressions should be administered if the heart rate is <60 bpm for more than 30 seconds despite adequate assisted ventilation.
    2. A baby who needs chest compressions should be intubated.

3. The recommended method for external chest compression in babies is to encircle the chest with both hands at the level of the lower third of the sternum and compress the sternum with the thumbs.
4. Aim to compress the chest by about a third of the anteroposterior diameter, at a rate of about 120 compressions per minute.
5. Chest compressions should be sufficiently deep to generate a palpable pulse.
6. Coordinate chest compression with ventilation; inflate the lungs after every third compression (ratio of 3:1).

D. Drugs: Drugs are used rarely, when there is no response after intubation and ventilation and chest compression. If the baby remains white, is not breathing, and has a heart rate of 60 bpm or less, drugs can sometimes achieve a "jump start" of the system. The ideal route is via the umbilicus.
1. Epinephrine, 0.1 to 0.3 mL/kg 1:10,000 by IV or ETT.
2. Sodium bicarbonate, 2 mL/kg IV (4.2%); baby must be ventilating effectively.
3. Dextrose, 2 mL/kg, 10% solution.
4. Naloxone may be used if the mother was given opiate analgesia >6 hours before delivery. Use 100 µg/kg. The dose may need to be repeated. Do *not* give if there is a history or suspicion of maternal drug abuse, as it may initiate immediate neonatal withdrawal syndrome.
5. Calcium: There is no evidence that calcium is useful in resuscitation.

VIII. Monitoring the Response to Resuscitation
A. Resuscitation does not end with the baby achieving a good heart rate and spontaneous breathing.
B. Observations should continue and a decision made as to whether it is safe for the baby to remain with the mother or whether the baby should be admitted to the nursery for observation.
C. Any baby who has required resuscitation should have early glucose screening until stable.

IX. Reasons for Failure to Respond to Resuscitation
A. There is a leak in the system delivering oxygen or air to the baby.
B. The endotracheal tube is in the esophagus.
C. Hemorrhagic shock—consider blood transfusion.
D. Sepsis, including pneumonia
E. Pneumothorax
F. Pleural effusion
G. Pulmonary hypoplasia—may respond to high ventilatory pressures
H. Laryngeal abnormality, choanal atresia, Pierre Robin sequence
I. Congenital diaphragmatic hernia
J. Congenital heart disease
K. Spinal cord injury

X. Ceasing Resuscitation
A. This decision should be made only by a senior physician.

B. If there has been no spontaneous cardiac output after 15 minutes of resuscitation, further attempts should be stopped.

C. If the baby has a heart beat but is not making respiratory effort, artificial ventilation should continue while further information is obtained.

XI. Documentation: Good records are vital

    A. Condition at birth, color/tone/respiration

    B. Time to first gasp; time to regular respiration, cry

    C. Heart rate at the start and at intervals: time when heart rate rose >100 bpm

    D. Apgar scores at 5-minute intervals to supplement the preceding observations (but not to replace them)

    E. Time commencing bag and mask ventilation; duration

    F. Time at tracheal intubation, duration of intubation, length of ETT at the lips or nares

    G. Umbilical cord pH; specify whether arterial or venous (include other blood gas parameters, if available)

    H. Drugs given; dose, route, and time

    I. Names and designations of personnel; times of their arrival

    J. Reasons for any delay

    K. Information given to the parents

XII. Controversies in Resuscitation

    A. Concern has been expressed regarding the possibility that resuscitation with 100% oxygen may cause damage from release of free radicals and from cerebral vasoconstriction. Trials have been conducted comparing resuscitation with room air and 100% oxygen. A meta-analysis of these trials concluded that at present there is insufficient evidence to recommend switching to air as the routine resuscitation gas. Hospitals who choose to use room air should continue to provide 100% oxygen as a back-up, because a one fourth of the babies who were initially resuscitated with air eventually required oxygen.

    B. Resuscitation of extremely preterm babies can be contentious. This is a job for an experienced neonatologist, who should meet the parents *beforehand* if at all possible. Occasionally it is considered appropriate to offer comfort care only to a baby of very early gestation who is not vigorous at birth. The reported success rate of full CPR in the delivery room when applied to this group varies, with some units claiming good results and others reporting a gloomy prognosis (see Chapter 74).

    C. Cooling: Therapeutic hypothermia is under investigation as a potential treatment in babies following severe intrapartum asphyxia. At the present time, there is no indication to commence cooling at birth, and the aim should be to maintain normothermia during resuscitation. Hyperthermia should be avoided.

    D. Babies who are born through meconium-stained fluid but who are vigorous do not require aggressive suctioning of the oropharynx or tracheal intubation. Babies who are depressed at birth should have the airways cleared of meconium before commencing active resuscitation (see Chapter 50).

Suggested Reading

Halliday HL, Sweet D: Endotracheal intubation at birth for preventing morbidity and mortality in vigorous, meconium-stained infants born at term. Cochrane Review Library, issue 3, 2002. www.Cochranelibrary.net.

Kattwinkel J (ed): Neonatal Resuscitation Textbook. Dallas, American Heart Association/American Academy of Pediatrics, 2000.

Kattwinkel J, Niermeyer S, Nadkarni V, et al: ILCOR advisory statement. Eur J Pediatr 158:345-358, 1999.

Royal College of Paediatrics and Child Health, Royal College of Obstetricians and Gynaecologists: Resuscitation of Babies at Birth. London, BMJ Publishing Group, 1997.

Tan A, Schulze A, O'Donnell CPF, Davis PG: Air versus oxygen for resuscitation of infants at birth. Cochrane Review Library, issue 3, 2004. www.Cochranelibrary.net.

13 Laryngoscopy and Endotracheal Intubation

Sam W. J. Richmond

I. Endotracheal Tube Diameter
  A. Birth weight vs size of tube (internal diameter, mm)

Up to 1000 g	2.5
1001-2000 g	3.0
2001-3000 g	3.5
>3000 g	3.5-4.0

  B. Birth weight vs tube length measured in cm at lip for orotracheal intubation

Up to 1000 g	7
1001-2000 g	8
2001-3000 g	9
>3000 g	10

  C. Birth weight vs tube length in cm for nasal intubation

750 g	7
1000 g	7.5
1500 g	8.5
2000 g	9.5
3000 g	10.5
4000 g	12

II. Administration of Anesthesia or Analgesia: Anesthesia or analgesia should be provided except in emergency situations. Give medication for pain relief (e.g., morphine) and sedation (e.g., midazolam), and prepare a suitable paralyzing agent (e.g., succinyl choline or atracurium).

III. Laryngoscopy and Oral Intubation
  A. Position all the equipment you need close by and prepare a means of securing the ETT once it is in place.
  B. Position the baby on a firm flat surface. Place a small roll or blanket under the baby's shoulders so as to lift them (not the head) about 1.5 inches (3 cm) off the surface. Extend the baby's neck slightly beyond the neutral position.
  C. Open the baby's mouth with the index finger of your right hand. Holding the laryngoscope in your left hand, insert the blade carefully into the right side of the baby's mouth while looking along the blade.
  D. Move the laryngoscope into the center by pushing the tongue over to the left side of the mouth.

E. Position yourself so that you can see comfortably along the laryngoscope blade. If the blade is pushed in too far, all you will see is the esophagus; you must then withdraw the blade slightly to allow the larynx to drop into view from above. Alternatively, if the blade is not in far enough, you may see little except the tongue and the roof of the mouth: you must advance the blade gently until you can see the epiglottis.

F. Once you have found the epiglottis, place the tip of the blade at the base where it meets the tongue (the vallecula). Lift the laryngoscope gently upward. This will open the mouth further and gently compress the tongue and will bring the larynx into view from behind the epiglottis. Slight external downward pressure on the cricoid should bring the larynx into the center of the field of view. Do not lever the end of the laryngoscope blade forward by pressing backward on the baby's upper jaw, as this may damage the alveolus and developing teeth.

G. Bring the ETT in from the right-hand corner of the mouth and keep the curve of the tube horizontal so as not to obscure the view of the larynx. Visualize the vocal cords through the groove in the laryngoscope blade. If necessary, wait for the cords to relax. Insert the tube 1 to 2 cm through the cords.

H. Tape or otherwise fix the ETT in place immediately while it is still optimally positioned. Most ETTs are marked in centimeters from the tip; make a note of the length at the upper lip.

I. Inflate the lung using a controlled inflation device. Watch the chest to check that it is moving appropriately and listen at the mouth to check that there is no significant leak around the ETT.

IV. Oral Intubation without a Laryngoscope: Oral intubation using a finger rather than a laryngoscope is possible. Skilled practitioners can place a tube in a baby with normal anatomy in 3 to 5 seconds.

A. Insert the index finger of the left hand into the baby's mouth, with the palmar surface sliding along the tongue. Use the little finger if the baby is small.

B. Slide the finger along the tongue until it meets the epiglottis. This feels like a small band running across the root of the tongue.

C. Slide the finger a little further until its tip lies behind and superior to the larynx and the nail touches the posterior pharyngeal wall.

D. Slide the tube into the mouth between your finger and the tongue until the tip lies in the midline at the root of the distal phalanx of your finger.

E. At this point, place your left thumb on the baby's neck just below the cricoid cartilage in order to grasp the larynx between the thumb on the outside and the fingertip on the inside.

F. While the thumb and finger steady the larynx, use the right hand to advance the tube a short distance, about 1 to 2 cm.

G. A slight "give" can sometimes be felt as the tube passes into the larynx *but no force is needed for insertion.*

H. When the tube is in the trachea, the laryngeal cartilages can be felt to encircle it. If it has passed into the esophagus, it can be felt between the finger and the larynx.

V. Nasal Intubation: Nasal intubation is not normally used for emergency intubation, but many units prefer to place tracheal tubes nasally for ventilation. Nasal intubation is therefore most commonly carried out as an elective procedure in an orally intubated baby.

  A. Ensure that the baby is well oxygenated in preparation for the procedure.

  B. Give medication for pain relief (e.g., morphine) and sedation (e.g., midazolam) and prepare a suitable paralyzing agent (e.g., atracurium).

  C. Position the baby supine with the shoulders supported on a small roll of toweling (see preceding section) with the neck slightly extended beyond the neutral position.

  D. Give the paralyzing agent (optional).

  E. Take a small feeding tube, narrow enough to fit inside the intended ETT, remove the flared end, and lubricate the other end. Lift up the tip of the nose and pass the tube down one nostril, directing it toward the back of the mouth until it has passed through the nose into the nasopharynx. Remember that the nasal passages follow the line of the palate, not the line of the nasal bone.

  F. Choose an appropriately sized tube, cut it to the proper length (see chart in Section I), and attach the appropriate connector.

  G. Lubricate the end of the ETT, thread it over the feeding tube, and insert it through the nostril and into the nasopharynx.

  H. Remove the feeding tube.

  I. Loosen the attachments of the oral tube and have an assistant prepare to remove it when requested.

  J. Visualize the larynx with the oral tube in place, using a laryngoscope. Identify the nasal tube within the nasopharynx.

  K. Ask an assistant to remove the oral tube. Pick up the nasal tube with a small pair of Magill or crocodile forceps and position the end of the tube in the laryngeal opening.

  L. It may not be possible to advance the tip of the nasal tube directly into the larynx because the tube, approaching from the nasopharynx rather than from the oropharynx, is likely to be at an angle to the line of the trachea. Gently flexing the neck while pushing the tube into the nose may suffice to correct this. Alternatively, if you take hold of the tube connector at the nose and gently twist it clockwise through about 120 degrees while maintaining some forward pressure, the tube will slip gently through the cords.

  M. Fix the tube in place and continue ventilation.

VI. Confirm Tube Position

  A. Clinical

    1. Equality of breath sounds

    2. No large leak

    3. Good chest excursions, symmetrical

    4. Appropriate physiologic responses (HR, RR, SaO$_2$)

  B. Radiologic

    1. Radiograph should always be obtained for initial intubation.

    2. Obtain with head and neck in *neutral* position.

    3. Optimal position is midway between the glottis and carina.

    C. Capnography may also be helpful.

    D. Disposable end-tidal CO_2 detectors are now available to confirm that the tube is in the trachea.

VII. Replacing the ETT

    A. Despite meticulous post-extubation care, use of methylxanthines, and a trial of CPAP, about 20% to 25% of babies require re-intubation. The immediate goal is to re-intubate and provide assisted ventilation in order to stabilize the infant's cardiopulmonary status.

    B. The following factors, singularly or in combination, should alert the caregiver that a trial of extubation is failing:

        1. Clinical manifestation of respiratory muscle fatigue, such as progressive hypercapnia or apnea

        2. Major cardiovascular collapse

        3. Increasing base deficit and developing respiratory or metabolic acidosis

        4. Increasing FiO_2 requirement (>0.6) to achieve PaO_2 or oxygen saturation in the normal range

    C. Suggested protocol for reintubation

        1. Stabilization with pre-oxygenation and bag and mask ventilation.

        2. Select optimal size (and length) of the ETT.

        3. Before fixation, determine correct placement by assessing air entry, chest wall movement, and improvement in SaO_2 and HR. If in doubt, obtain a chest radiograph.

        4. Use of premedication (see Chapter 61).

           a. Sedation

           b. Muscle relaxants should only be used with an experienced neonatologist present. Do not paralyze the baby unless you are confident the airway can be maintained and hand ventilation provided.

           c. When practical, premedication prior to intubation in the newborn offers the following potential advantages:

               (1) Increased hemodynamic stability

               (2) Faster intubation

               (3) Less hypoxemia

               (4) Less rise in intracranial pressure

        5. Adjunctive or reversal agents

           a. Atropine: Given prior to anesthesia to reduce secretions and prevent bradycardia and hypotension. Intravenous bolus will produce an effect in 30 seconds that will last for up to 12 hours.

           b. Neostigmine: Reverses the effects of nondepolarizing muscle relaxants.

    D. Changing an indwelling tube

        1. Prepare new ETT and adjunctive equipment (e.g., tape, stylet, adhesives).

        2. Remove tape and adhesive from existing ETT but stabilize tube position manually while doing so.

        3. Visualize the glottis by direct laryngoscopy.

        4. Hold new tube in the right hand.

5. Ask assistant to remove old ETT and quickly insert new ETT to desired depth.
6. Secure new ETT when successful placement is confirmed clinically.
7. A radiograph is necessary only if there is a question about suitable placement.

Suggested Reading

Donn SM, Blane CE: Endotracheal tube movement in the preterm infant: Oral versus nasal intubation. Ann Otol Rhinol Laryngol 1985;94:18-20.

Donn SM, Faix RG: Special procedures used in resuscitation. In Donn SM (ed): The Michigan Manual—A Guide to Neonatal Intensive Care, 2nd ed. Armonk, NY, Futura Publishing, 1997, pp 10-11.

Donn SM, Kuhns LR: Mechanism of endotracheal tube movement with change of head position in the neonate. Pediatr Radiol 9:37-40, 1980.

Woody NC, Woody HB: Direct digital intubation for neonatal resuscitation. J Pediatr 1968;73:47-58.

Vascular Access

14

Steven M. Donn and Barbara S. Steffes

I. Umbilical Artery Catheterization
  A. Indications
   1. Monitoring arterial blood gases
      a. $F_iO_2 \geq 0.4$
      b. Unreliable capillary samples
      c. Continuous monitoring
   2. Need for invasive blood pressure monitoring
  B. Procedure
   1. This is an elective procedure.
   2. Use sterile technique.
   3. Catheterize vessel after cutdown technique, using 3.5 F (<1500 g) or 5 F catheter.
   4. Preferred position of tip:
      a. High (T_7-T_{10})
      b. Low (L_3-L_4)
   5. Confirm position radiographically.
   6. Secure with tape bridge and (optional) sutures.
  C. Complications
   1. Blood loss
   2. Infection
   3. Thromboembolic events
      a. Digit necrosis
      b. NEC
      c. Renal artery thrombosis
      d. Spinal cord injury (rare)
   4. Vasospasm
   5. Vessel perforation
   6. Air embolus
   7. Hypertension
  D. Removal
   1. When F_iO_2 is <0.4 and decreasing
   2. When noninvasive blood pressure monitoring is adequate
   3. At first signs of complication
  E. Comments
   1. Confirm position. A malpositioned UAC can have life-threatening consequences.
   2. Remember that samples obtained from the UAC are postductal.
   3. Never infuse pressor agents through a UAC.

    4. When removing, withdraw last 5 cm *very* slowly. Watch for pulsations to stop.

    5. Controversy exists regarding infusion of TPN and certain medications through a UAC.

    6. Inadequate line clearing prior to sampling may result in spurious laboratory results.

II. Umbilical Vein Catheterization

  A. Indications

    1. Emergent need for vascular access (i.e., resuscitation)

    2. Need for central venous line

      a. Pressure monitoring

      b. TPN or hypertonic glucose administration

      c. Frequent blood sampling in unstable patient without other access

    3. Exchange transfusion

  B. Procedure

    1. Use Sterile technique.

    2. Direct cutdown approach is required.

    3. Use umbilical catheter (5.0 F (preterm); 8.0 F (term) for exchange transfusion in term infant); do not use feeding tube except as last resort.

    4. Preferred positions

      a. Low—Insert 4 to 6 cm to achieve blood return if using for resuscitation or exchange transfusion.

      b. High—Tip should be above diaphragm and below right atrium in the vena cava for indwelling use.

    5. Confirm position radiographically.

    6. Secure with tape and (optional) sutures.

  C. Complications

    1. Blood loss

    2. Infection

    3. Vessel perforation

    4. Thromboembolic events

    5. Air embolus

    6. Liver necrosis (see below)

    7. NEC (may be related to procedures such as exchange transfusion rather than to the catheter itself)

  D. Removal

    1. When no longer needed or when other central venous access is achieved

    2. At first signs of complications

    3. When procedure is completed

    4. May be pulled directly

  E. Comments

    1. Avoid infusion or injection of hypertonic solutions (e.g., sodium bicarbonate) unles catheter tip is above diaphragm. This may cause hepatic necrosis.

    2. CVP monitoring may provide useful trend data regarding intravascular fluid status and hemodynamics.

3. There is a recent trend in increased longer-term use in ELBW infants.
4. Inadequate line clearing prior to sampling may result in spurious laboratory results.

III. Peripheral Artery Catheterization
  A. Indications generally are the same as for UAC when umbilical access is unavailable or cannot be achieved.
  B. Procedure
    1. Preferred sites
      a. Radial artery
      b. Posterior tibial artery
    2. Assess for adequate collateral circulation.
    3. Prepare site thoroughly using antiseptic solution.
    4. Cannulate vessel percutaneously.
    5. Secure catheter with tape.
    6. Check for blood return, pulse waveform, and adequacy of distal circulation.
  C. Complications
    1. Infection
    2. Blood loss
    3. Thromboembolic events
    4. Ischemic injury
  D. Removal
    1. At first sign of complications
    2. When no longer indicated
  E. Comments
    1. Transillumination may be helpful in locating vessel.
    2. Keep patency by infusing continuously but slowly. Use low tonicity fluid (i.e., 0.45% sodium chloride). Many centers prefer use of low-dose heparin (0.5 to 1.0 units/mL) to decrease risk of clotting.
    3. Tne brachial artery should not be cannulated (inadequate collateral circulation), and the femoral artery should be used only as a last resort.
    4. Cerebral infarction has been reported following superficial temporal artery cannulation, and thus this vessel should not be used.

IV. Peripheral Intravenous Catheters
  A. Indications
    1. To provide partial or total fluids and/or nutrition when gastrointestinal nutrition is not possible.
    2. Used when central access is unnecessary or unattainable.
  B. Procedure
    1. Visualize, palpate, and/or use transillumination to select vessel for cannulation. Suggested order of preference for vessels to cannulate:
      a. Dorsal venous plexus of back of hand
      b. Median antebrachial, accessory, or cephalic veins of forearm
      c. Dorsal venous plexus of foot
      d. Basilic or cubital veins of antecubital fossa
      e. Small saphenous or great saphenous veins of ankle
      f. Supratrochlear, superficial temporal, or posterior auricular veins of scalp

    2. Apply tourniquet if placing in extremity.

    3. Clean area with antiseptic.

    4. Attach syringe to cannula and test patency by passing small amount of saline through syringe, then detach syringe.

    5. Hold needle parallel to vessel, in direction of blood flow.

    6. Introduce needle into skin a few millimeters distal to the point of entry into the vessel. Introduce needle into the vessel until blood flashback appears in the cannula.

    7. Remove stylet and advance needle into vessel.

    8. Remove tourniquet.

    9. Infuse a small amount of saline to assure patency then attach IV tubing.

C. Special considerations

    1. Placement should not be near area of skin loss or infection or across joints, if possible, because of problems with joint immobilization.

    2. Care should be taken to ensure that vessel is a vein and not an artery.

      a. Note color of blood obtained from vessel.

      b. Look for blanching of skin over vessel when fluid is infused, suggesting arterial spasm.

      c. When attempting scalp vein cannulation, shave area of head where IV needle is to be placed. Avoid sites beyond hairline.

D. Complications

    1. Phlebitis

    2. Infection

    3. Hematoma

    4. Embolization of formed clot with vigorous flushing

    5. Air embolus

    6. Infiltration of subcutaneous tissue by IV fluid. Infiltration may cause:

      a. Superficial blistering

      b. Sloughing of deep layers of skin that may require skin grafting

      c. Subcutaneous tissue calcification due to infiltration of calcium-containing IV solutions

Suggested Reading

Donn SM: Vascular catheters. In Donn SM (ed): The Michigan Manual of Neonatal Intensive Care, 3rd ed. Philadelphia, Hanley & Belfus, 2003, pp 46-49.

Feick HJ, Donn SM: Vascular access and blood sampling. In Donn SM, Faix RG (eds): Neonatal Emergencies. Mt. Kisco, NY, Futura Publishing, 1991, pp 31-50.

Workman EL, Donn SM: Intravascular catheters. In Donn SM, Fisher CW (eds): Risk Management Techniques in Perinatal and Neonatal Practice. Armonk, NY, Futura Publishing, 1996, pp 531-549.

Tracheostomy

15

Steven M. Donn

I. Description: Creation of an artificial airway through the trachea for the purposes of establishing either airway patency below an obstruction or an airway for prolonged ventilatory support.

II. Indications
   A. Emergent
      1. Upper airway malformations
      2. Upper airway obstructions
   B. Elective
      1. Prolonged ventilatory support
         a. Chronic lung disease
         b. Neurologic or neuromuscular dysfunction
      2. Subglottic stenosis following endotracheal intubation

III. Preparation
   A. Rarely needed for emergent tracheostomy because of obstructive lesion that precludes use of endotracheal intubation.
   B. Baby should be intubated.
   C. Generally should be performed in operating room because of availability of:
      1. General anesthesia
      2. Optimal lighting
      3. Facilities for suction
      4. Proper exposure
      5. All necessary equipment

IV. Technique
   A. Position baby supine, with head and neck maximally extended. Use towel roll or sandbag.
   B. Identify cricoid cartilage by palpation of tracheal rings.
   C. Make short (1.0 cm) transverse skin incision over second tracheal ring.
   D. Dilate incision with hemostat.
   E. Deepen incision using needle point cautery.
   F. Maintain meticulous hemostasis.
   G. Separate strap muscles using fine hemostat.
   H. Expose trachea by dividing isthmus of thyroid gland using cautery, if necessary.
   I. Make longitudinal incision in trachea (by cautery) through second and third tracheal rings. Do not excise tracheal cartilage, which would lead to loss of tracheal support and stricture formation.

J. Place silk ties on each side to facilitate placement of tracheostomy tube and postoperative replacement.

K. Withdraw ETT until it is visualized just proximal to incision.

L. Insert tracheostomy tube. Choose a size that requires minimal pressure to insert; avoid metal tubes. Remove ETT.

M. Assess proper fit by manual ventilation through tracheostomy tube. If leak is large, replace with bigger tube.

N. Secure tube with tapes around neck. These should be padded and can be tightened during neck flexion.

O. Trachea may be irrigated with 2.0 mL saline and suctioned.

P. Auscultate chest; obtain radiograph.

V. Postoperative Care

A. Minimize movement of head and neck for 3 to 5 days to establish stoma. Sedation and analgesia are strongly recommended.

B. Frequent suctioning and humidification are required until stoma is established.

C. Caretakers must know how to replace tube if it becomes dislodged or occluded.

D. Removal should be accomplished in intensive care unit setting.

VI. Ex Utero Intrapartum Treatment (EXIT) Procedure

A. Performed in selected centers to manage various forms of fetal airway obstruction such as:
1. Neck masses
2. Congenital high airway obstruction syndrome (CHAOS)
3. Intrathoracic masses
4. Unilateral pulmonary agenesis and diaphragmatic hernia

B. The Procedure
1. Requires multidiscipline team
   a. Obstetrics
   b. Neonatology
   c. Pediatric anesthesiology
   d. Radiology
   e. Nursing
2. Tocolytic (indomethacin) given to mother
3. Maternal rapid sequence intubation after anesthesia
4. Maintain uterine relaxation and maternal blood pressure with:
   a. Inhalational agents
   b. Terbutaline or intravenous nitroglycerine
5. Fetal anesthesia with pancuronium and fentanyl
6. Maternal laparotomy
7. Ultrasound to map placental borders
8. Hysterotomy
9. Exposure of fetal head
10. Attempt intubation
11. Clamp and cut cord, deliver infant
12. EXIT to ECMO has also been successfully reported

Suggested Reading

Coran AG: Tracheostomy. In Donn SM, Faix RG (eds): Neonatal Emergencies, Mount Kisco, NY, Futura Publishing, 1991, pp 247-251.

Coran AG, Behrendt DM, Weintraub WH, et al: Surgery of the Neonate. Boston, Little, Brown, 1978, pp 31-35.

Hirose S, Harrison MR: The ex utero intrapartum treatment (EXIT) procedure. Semin Neonatol 8:207-214, 2003.

Monitoring the Ventilated Patient

Continuous Monitoring Techniques

16

Christian F. Poets

I. Transcutaneous Partial Pressure of Oxygen (TcPO$_2$) Monitoring
   A. Principles of operation
      1. Electrodes consist of a platinum cathode and a silver reference anode encased in an electrolyte solution and separated from the skin by an O$_2$-permeable membrane.
      2. Electrodes are heated to improve oxygen diffusion and to arterialize the capillary blood.
      3. Oxygen is reduced at the cathode, generating an electric current proportional to the O$_2$ concentration in the capillary bed underneath the sensor.
      4. Sensors require a warm-up period of 10 to 15 minutes after application and have to be calibrated every 4 to 8 hours.
   B. Factors influencing measurements
      1. Sensor temperature
         a. Good agreement with PaO$_2$ only at 44° C, but at this temperature site changes are necessary every 2 to 4 hours.
         b. At lower sensor temperatures, as PaO$_2$ increases, the difference between PaO$_2$ and TcPO$_2$ increases.
      2. Probe placement
         a. The TcPO$_2$ monitor will underread PaO$_2$ if the sensor is placed on a bony surface, if pressure is applied on the sensor, or if too much contact gel is used.
         b. With patent ductus arteriosus and right-to-left shunt, TcPO$_2$ will be higher on the upper than on the lower half of the thorax.
      3. Peripheral perfusion
         a. TcPO$_2$ depends on skin perfusion. If the latter is reduced—e.g. from hypotension, anemia, acidosis (pH <7.05), hypothermia, or marked skin edema—TcPO$_2$ will be falsely low.
         b. If underreading of PaO$_2$ occurs, check patient for the the aforementioned conditions.
      4. Skin thickness
         a. There is close agreement with PaO$_2$ only in newborns.
         b. Beyond 8 weeks of age, TcPO$_2$ will be only 80% of PaO$_2$.
      5. Response times: In vivo response time to a sudden fall in PaO$_2$ is 16 to 20 seconds.
   C. Detection of hypoxemia and hyperoxemia: Sensitivity to these conditions (at 44° C sensor temperature) is approximately 85%.

II. Pulse Oximetry (SpO$_2$)
   A. Principles of operation
      1. The ratio of the absorbance of red and infrared light sent through a tissue correlates with the proportion of oxygenated to deoxygenated hemoglobin in the tissue.
      2. Conventional oximeters determine the arterial component within this absorbance by identifying the peaks and troughs in the absorbance over time, thereby obtaining a "pulse-added" absorbance that is independent of the absorbance characteristics of the nonpulsating parts of the tissue.
      3. Next-generation instruments use additional techniques.
         a. One recently developed technology scans through all red-to-infrared ratios found in the tissue, determines the intensity of these, and chooses the right-most peak of these intensities, which will correspond to the absorbance by the arterial blood in the tissue.
         b. This tecnology also uses frequency analysis, time domain analysis, and adaptive filtering to establish a noise reference in the detected physiologic signal, thereby improving the ability to separate signal and noise.
      4. All instruments have built-in algorithms to associate their measured light absorbance with empirically determined SaO$_2$ values.
   B. Factors influencing measurements
      1. Probe placement
         a. The light-receiving diode must be placed exactly opposite the emitting diode.
         b. Both must be shielded against ambient light and must not be applied with too much pressure.
         c. Light by-passing the tissue can cause both falsely high and falsely low values.
         d. The sensor site must be checked every 6 to 8 hours.
         e. Highly flexible sensors (usually disposable) provide better skin contact and thus better signal-to-noise ratio.
      2. Peripheral perfusion
         a. Most oximeters require a pulse pressure >20 mm Hg or a systolic blood pressure >30 mm Hg to operate reliably.
         b. Performance at low perfusion is substantially better with next-generation instruments.
      3. Response times
         a. Response times depend upon the averaging time used.
         b. Longer averaging times may reduce alarm rates but will increase response time and will hide the true severity of short-lived hypoxemic episodes.
      4. Movement artifacts
         a. Most frequent cause of false alarms.
         b. Their occurrence has been reduced with next-generation instruments, but potentially at the cost of unreliable detection of true alarms.

      c. May be identified from analysis of the pulse waveform signal or via a signal quality indicator displayed by some instruments.

   5. Other hemoglobins and pigments

      a. Methemoglobin (MetHb) will cause SpO_2 readings to tend toward 85%, independent of SaO_2.

      b. Carboxyhemoglobin (COHb) will cause overestimation of SaO_2 by 1% for each percentage of COHb in the blood.

      c. Fetal hemoglobin (HbF) and bilirubin do not affect pulse oximeters, but may lead to an underestimation of SaO_2 by co-oximeters.

      d. In patients with dark skin, SpO_2 values may be falsely high, particularly during hypoxemia.

   6. Algorithms

      a. These may vary among brands and even among different software versions from the same manufacturer.

      b. Some instruments subtract a priori the typical levels of COHb, MetHb, etc., in healthy nonsmoking adults from their measurements and will thus display SpO_2 values that are 2% to 3% lower than those displayed by other instruments.

C. Detection of hypoxemia and hyperoxemia

   1. In the absence of movement, pulse oximeters have a high sensitivity for the detection of hypoxemia.

   2. Because of the shape of the O_2 dissociation curve, they are less well suited for detecting hyperoxemia.

   3. The upper alarm limits at which hyperoxemia can be reliably avoided with different instruments range from 88% to 95%, although the upper limit of most next-generation instruments is at the high end of this range.

III. Transcutaneous Partial Pressure of Carbon Dioxide ($TcPCO_2$) Monitoring

A. Principles of operation

   1. A $TcPCO_2$ sensor consists of a pH-sensing glass electrode and a silver-silver chloride reference electrode, covered by a hydrophobic CO_2-permeable membrane from which they are separated by a sodium bicarbonate–electrolyte solution.

   2. As CO_2 diffuses across the membrane, there is a pH change in the electrolyte solution ($CO_2 + H_2O/HCO_3^- + H^+$), which is sensed by the glass electrode.

   3. All instruments have built-in correction factors, because their uncorrected measurements will be 50% higher than $PaCO_2$.

   4. Instruments must be calibrated at regular intervals and require a run-in time of 10 to 15 minutes following site changes.

B. Factors influencing measurements

   1. Sensor temperature

      a. Optimal sensor temperature is 42° C.

      b. If sensors are used in combination with a $TcPO_2$ sensor, a sensor temperature of 44° C can be used without jeopardizing the precision of the $TcPCO_2$ measurement.

    2. Sensor placement and skin thickness.
      a. $TcPCO_2$ measurements are relatively independent of sensor site and skin thickness.
      b. $TcPCO_2$ may be falsely high if pressure is applied on the sensor.
    3. Peripheral perfusion.
      a. $TcPCO_2$ may be falsely high in severe shock.
      b. Precision may be affected if $PaCO_2$ is >45 mm Hg and/or arterial pH is <7.30, but there is no systematic over- or underestimation of $PaCO_2$ under these conditions.
    4. A 90% response time to a sudden change in $PaCO_2$ is between 30 and 50 seconds.
  C. Detection of hypocarbia and hypercarbia: Sensitivity to both hypocarbia and hypercarbia is 80% to 90%.
IV. End-Tidal Carbon Dioxide ($ETCO_2$) Monitoring (Capnometry)
  A. Principles of operation
    1. An infrared beam is directed through a gas sample, and the amount of light absorbed by the CO_2 molecules in the sample is measured.
    2. This is proportional to the CO_2 concentration in the sample.
  B. Factors influencing measurements
    1. Gas sampling technique
      a. Mainstream capnometers
        (1) The CO_2 analyzer is built into an adapter that is placed in the breathing circuit.
        (2) Advantage: Fast response time (10 msec), therefore reliable even at high respiratory rates.
        (3) Disadvantage: 1 to 10 mL extra dead space; risk of tube kinking.
      b. Sidestream capnometers aspirate the expired air via a sample flow.
        (1) Advantages: No extra dead space; can be used in nonintubated patients.
        (2) Disadvantages: Risk of dilution of expired gas by entrainment of ambient air at the sampling tube–patient interface; longer response time; falsely low values at high respiratory rates (>60 breaths/min).
    2. Influence of V/Q mismatch
      a. $ETCO_2$ will only approximate $PaCO_2$ if
        (1) CO_2 equilibrium is achieved between end-capillary blood and alveolar gas.
        (2) $ETCO_2$ approximates the average alveolar CO_2 during a respiratory cycle.
        (3) Ventilation-perfusion relationships are uniform within the lung.
      b. These conditions are rarely achieved in patients with respiratory disorders.
      c. The reliability of an $ETCO_2$ measurement can be assessed from the expiratory signal: this must have a steep rise, a clear end-expiratory plateau, and no detectable CO_2 during inspiration.

V. Chest Wall Movements
   A. Impedance plethysmography
      1. Changes in the ratio of air to fluid in the thorax, occurring during the respiratory cycle, create changes in transthoracic impedance.
      2. Cannot be used to quantify respiration.
      3. May be heavily influenced by cardiac and movement artifacts.
   B. Inductance plethysmography
      1. Changes in the volume of the thoracic and abdominal compartment create changes in inductance, which is registered via abdominal and thoracic bands.
      2. The sum of these changes is proportional to tidal volume.
      3. Several methods have been developed to calibrate the systems so that tidal volume can be quantified. (This however, only works if the patient does not shift position.)
   C. Strain gauges (usually mercury in silicon rubber) sense respiratory efforts by measuring changes in electrical resistance in response to stretching. These measurements, however, are not reproducible enough to quantify tidal volume.
   D. Pressure capsules detect movements of an infant's diaphragm by means of an air-filled capsule that is taped to the abdomen and connected to a pressure transducer via a narrow air-filled tube.
      1. The outward movement of the abdomen during inspiration compresses the capsule to produce a positive pressure pulse that is interpreted as a breath.
      2. Thistechnique is predominantly used in apnea monitors and trigger devices for infant ventilators and is not suitable for quantifying tidal volume.
VI. Electrocardiography (ECG)
   A. The ECG records electrical depolarization of the myocardium.
   B. During continuous monitoring, only the heart rate can be determined with sufficient precision; any analysis of P and T waves, axis, rhythm or QT times requires a printout and/or a 12-lead ECG.

Suggested Reading

Bernet-Buettiker V, Ugarte MJ, Frey B, et al: Evaluation of a new combined transcutaneous measurement of PCO_2/pulse oximetry oxygen saturation ear sensor in newborn patients. Pediatrics 115:e64-e68, 2005 [Epub 2004 Dec 15].

Bohnhorst B, Peter CS, Poets CF: Detection of hyperoxaemia in neonates: Data from three new pulse oximeters. Arch Dis Child Fetal Neonatal Ed 87:F217-F219, 2002.

Di Fiore JM: Neonatal cardiorespiratory monitoring techniques. Semin Neonatol 9:195-203, 2004.

Meyers PA, Worwa C, Trusty R, Mammel MC: Clinical validation of a continuous intravascular neonatal blood gas sensor introduced through an umbilical artery catheter. Respir Care 7:682-687, 2002.

Poets CF, Martin R: Noninvasive determination of blood gases. In Stocks J, Sly PD, Tepper RS, Morgan WJ (eds): Infant Respiratory Function Testing. New York, John Wiley & Sons, 1996, pp 411-444.

17 Clinical Issues Regarding Pulse Oximetry

Win Tin and Samir Gupta

I. Introduction
   A. Noninvasive monitoring of oxygenation has become a standard procedure in neonatology.
   B. Pulse oximetry (SpO_2) is based on using the pulsatile variations in optical density of tissues in the red and infrared wavelengths to compute SaO_2 without need for calibration.
   C. The method was invented in 1972 by Takuo Aoyagi, and its clinical use was first reported in 1975 by Susumu Nakajima, a surgeon, and his associates.

II. Advantages
   A. Saturation is a basic physiologic determinant of tissue oxygen delivery.
   B. No warm-up or equilibration time.
   C. Immediate and continuous readout.
   D. Pulse-by-pulse detection of rapid or transient changes in saturation.
   E. Substantially lower maintenance.
   F. Skin burns from probe are very rare, compared to transcutaneous monitoring.
   G. Minimal effect of motion, light, perfusion and temperature with the advent of "signal extraction technology" in pulse oximetry.

III. Disadvantages
   A. Fails to detect hyperoxia at functional saturation of more than 94%, and thus slow weaning of oxygen as high PaO_2 is not recognized.
   B. Not reliable in cases of severe hypotension or marked edema.
   C. Older pulse oximeters may provoke unnecessary evaluation of transient, clinically insignificant desaturations.

IV. Terminology in Pulse Oximetry
   A. Functional and fractional saturation
      1. Functional saturation: Any forms of hemoglobin in the sample that do not bind oxygen in a reversible way are not included in calculating functional hemoglobin saturation. The pulse oximeter can measure functional saturation from only two forms of hemoglobin, oxyhemoglobin (HbO_2) and deoxyhemoglobin (Hb), which is calculated by:

$$\text{Functional saturation} = \frac{HbO_2}{HbO_2 + Hb} \times 100$$

2. Fractional saturation: Fractional saturation is defined as the ratio of the amount of hemoglobin saturated with oxygen to all other forms of hemoglobin, including dyshemoglobin (COHb and MetHb). The co-oximeters found in blood gas laboratories measure fractional saturation because they use many wavelengths of light and are thus able to measure all types of hemoglobin present in a patient's blood:

$$\text{Fractional saturation} = \frac{HbO_2}{HbO_2 + Hb + COHb + MetHb} \times 100$$

3. Pulse oximeters can measure only functional saturation. Some instruments display fractional saturation measurements that are derived by subtracting 2% from the functional saturation. It is important to be aware of what the instrument is reading.

B. Bias and precision: The normal level of dyshemoglobin is <2%. The mean of the difference (error) between oxygen saturation and oxyhemoglobin (SaO_2 and HbO_2) measured by co-oximetry is called *bias,* and the standard deviation of this is called *precision.*

V. Practical Considerations

A. Oxyhemoglobin dissociation curve and pulse oximetry: See Chapter 5 (oxygen therapy).

B. Presence of abnormal hemoglobins (dyshemoglobin)

1. Carboxyhemoglobin: SpO_2 is overestimated in the presence of COHb (e.g., neonatal jaundice).

2. Methemoglobin: SpO_2 decreases in proportion to the percentage of MetHb present.

C. Reduced perfusion states

1. Hypothermia does not cause a problem if the temperature is >30° C.

2. Hypovolemia may cause loss of signal (but presence of signal does not indicate adequate perfusion).

D. Anemia does not cause a problem as long as Hb is >5g /dL.

E. Effect of dyes

1. Bilirubin has no influence unless there is acute hemolysis (COHb).

2. Meconium staining of skin can cause falsely low SpO_2 readings.

F. Venous pulsations (e.g., tricuspid regurgitation) may cause falsely low SpO_2 readings.

G. An abnormal absorption spectrum of hemoglobin (e.g., Hb Köln) may affect the reliability of pulse oximetry, but this is extremely rare.

VI. Technical Considerations

A. Calibration and accuracy

1. Quality of signal: Before interpreting an SpO_2 reading, the quality of signal received by probe should be confirmed by a good plethysmographic waveform and/or heart rate similar to that seen on an ECG monitor.

2. Differing software among brands: There are small differences between the measurements obtained with different brands of pulse oximeters.

   3. Inaccuracy increases when saturation is less than 75% to 80%:
      The bias and precision between SpO_2 and HbO_2 measured by
      co-oximetry is:
      • 0.5% and 2.5%, respectively, when SpO_2 is >90%
      • 1.9% and 2.7%, respectively, when SpO_2 is 80% to 90%
      • 5.8% and 4.8%, respectively, when SpO_2 is <80%
   B. Delay of response
      1. Response time is faster if the probe is centrally placed; detection is
         50% to 60% earlier by sensors placed centrally (ear, cheek, tongue)
         than by sensors placed peripherally (finger, toe).
      2. Delay depends on averaging time. The shortest averaging time
         should be selected, although this usually increases sensitivity to
         motion.
   C. Motion artifact: The performance of pulse oximeters is affected by
      motion. To overcome this, several brands of pulse oximeters are now
      equipped with new algorithms that cancel a noise signal that is
      common to both wavelengths.
   D. Interference from other light sources
      1. Fluctuating light sources: Shielding the probe with cloth or
         opaque material can overcome the problem of light interference.
      2. Incorrectly placed probe (optical shunt or penumbra effect): Part
         of the light is transmitted without any tissue absorption. This can
         occur if too large a probe is used.
   E. Electrical or magnetic interface
      1. When using pulse oximetry in the MRI suite, care should be taken
         to use specially designed equipment in order to avoid interference
         with SpO_2 or even burns (ferrous metals).
      2. Electrocautery can cause failure of pulse oximetry.
VII. Rules for the Optimal Use of Pulse Oximetry
   A. Verify probe integrity before use.
   B. Avoid mixing probes and monitors of different brands.
   C. Check the quality of signal received by the probe (good waveform or
      true heart rate).
   D. Maintain probe positioning under direct visual control.
   E. Consider the physiologic limitations of SpO_2 and interpret
      accordingly.
   F. In case of doubt, check patient's condition.
   G. Check arterial blood gas if saturation is persistently below 80%.
   H. Remember that a high SaO_2 reading may indicate significant
      hyperoxemia.

Suggested Reading

Hay WW Jr, Rodden DJ, Collins SM, et al: Reliability of conventional and new pulse oximetry
   in neonatal patients. J Perinatol 22:360-366, 2002.
Morgan C, Newell SJ, Ducker DA, et al: Continuous neonatal blood gas monitoring using
   a multiparameter intra-arterial sensor. Arch Dis Child 80:F93-F98, 1999.
Moyle JTB, Hahn CEW, Adams AP (eds): Principles and Practice Series: Pulse Oximetry. London,
   BMJ Books, 1998.

Poets CF, Southhall DP: Noninvasive monitoring of oxygenation in infants and children: Practical considerations and areas of concern. Pediatrics 3:737-746, 1994.

Richardson DK, Eichenwald EC: Blood gas monitoring and pulmonary function tests. In Cloherty JP, Stark AR (eds): Manual of Neonatal Care. New York, Lippincott-Raven, 1998, pp 354-355.

Veyckemans F: Equipment, monitoring and environmental conditions. In Bissonnette B, Dalens BJ (eds): Pediatric Anesthesia—Principles and Practice. New York, Mc Graw-Hill, 2002, pp 442-445.

18 Interpretation of Blood Gases

David J. Durand

I. Physiology of Gas Exchange
  A. Oxygenation: The movement of O_2 from the alveoli into the blood is dependent on ventilation-perfusion matching. Ventilation-perfusion matching is abnormal if:
    1. Pulmonary blood flows past unventilated alveoli, causing an intrapulmonary right-to-left shunt. In newborns, this is typically caused by atelectasis. The treatment for atelectasis is positive pressure, which opens previously unventilated alveoli and decreases intrapulmonary shunting.
    2. Blood flows right to left through the foramen ovale or patent ductus arteriosus, causing an extrapulmonary right-to-left shunt. This sort of extrapulmonary shunt typically is caused by elevated pulmonary vascular resistance (pulmonary hypertension) and can be treated by decreasing pulmonary vascular resistance (e.g., with inhaled nitric oxide).
  B. Ventilation: The movement of CO_2 from the blood into the alveoli is dependent on alveolar ventilation. Alveolar ventilation is the product of alveolar volume and respiratory rate. Thus, any change in ventilatory strategy that results in an increase in alveolar volume and/or respiratory rate will improve ventilation and decrease $PaCO_2$.
  C. Acid-base status (see Table 8-1)
    1. The pH of arterial blood is determined primarily by:
      a. $PaCO_2$
      b. Lactic acid, produced by anaerobic metabolism
      c. Buffering capacity, particularly the amount of bicarbonate in the blood
    2. Respiratory acidosis occurs when an increase in $PaCO_2$ causes a decrease in pH. Respiratory alkalosis occurs when a decreases in $PaCO_2$ causes an increase in pH.
    3. Metabolic acidosis occurs when there is either an excess of lactic acid, or a deficiency in the buffering capacity of the blood, causing a decrease in pH. It is reflected in an increased base deficit, also termed a decreased base excess.
    4. If $PaCO_2$ remains persistently elevated, the pH will gradually return to normal as a result of a gradual increase in bicarbonate in the blood, termed *compensatory metabolic alkalosis*.

Conversely, a patient with a persistently low $PaCO_2$ will gradually develop *compensatory metabolic acidosis.*

5. In patients with an intact respiratory drive, persistent metabolic acidosis will result in hyperventilation, termed *compensatory respiratory alkalosis.*

6. Most ELBW infants have immature renal tubular function in the first week of life and spill bicarbonate in the urine, leading to a metabolic acidosis. Administration of extra base in the intravenous fluids will correct this but is a controversial practice.

7. If an infant has severe hypoxemia and/or decreased tissue perfusion, anaerobic metabolism will cause the accumulation of lactic acid, and result in metabolic acidosis. This should be treated by improving the underlying problem rather than by administering additional base. Direct measurement of lactic acid is now readily available and is a useful tool for monitoring infants with significant tissue hypoperfusion (e.g., septic or cardiogenic shock).

II. Oxygen Content of Blood

A. Oxygen is carried in the blood in two ways:

1. Dissolved in plasma: In the normal infant (or adult), the amount of oxygen dissolved in plasma is trivial compared to the amount of oxygen that is bound to Hb. Approximately 0.3 mL O_2 is dissolved in 100 mL plasma per 100 mm Hg or 100 torr PO_2.

2. Bound toHb: The amount of O_2 that is carried in the blood bound to Hb is dependent on both the Hb concentration and the Hb saturation (SaO_2). In the normal infant with an Hb level of 15 g/100 mL and and an SaO_2 of 100%, approximately 20 mL O_2 is bound to the Hb in 100 mL of blood.

B. Significantly increasing PaO_2 beyond that which is needed to fully saturate Hb will slightly increase the amount of O_2 dissolved in plasma but will not increase the amount of O_2 bound to Hb.

C. The PaO_2 that is required to fully saturate Hb is dependent on the oxygen-Hb dissociation curve (Fig. 18-1). This curve is dependent on many factors, including the relative amount of fetal Hb in the blood (fetal Hb is fully saturated at a lower PaO_2 than is adult Hb). For this reason, SaO_2 is a better indicator of the amount of oxygen in the blood than is PaO_2.

III. Oxygen Delivery and Mixed Venous Oxygen Saturation

A. The amount of oxygen delivered to the tissues depends on the amount of oxygen in the blood (CaO_2) and cardiac output (CO).

1. Assume that an average infant has a CaO_2 of 20 mL O_2/100 mL blood and a CO of 120 mL/kg/min.

2. Therefore, the amount of oxygen available for delivery to the body can be calculated as the product of CaO_2 and CO. Thus,

$$(20 \text{ mL O}_2/100 \text{ mL blood}) \times (120 \text{ mL/kg/min})$$
$$= 24 \text{ mL O}_2/\text{kg/min available for delivery to tissues}$$

B. Under stable conditions, oxygen consumption for the average infant is approximately 6 mL/kg/min.

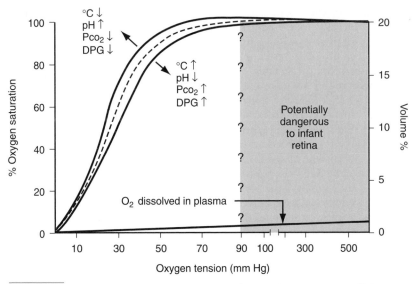

FIGURE 18-1. The oxygen-Hb dissociation curve. (From Klaus MH, Fanaroff AA: Care of the High Risk Neonate. Philadelphia, WB Saunders, 1986, p 173. Used by permission.)

C. If an infant is delivering oxygen to the systemic circulation at a rate of 24 mL/kg/min and is utilizing oxygen at a rate of 6 mL/kg/min, then 25% of the oxygen in the blood is utilized by the tissues; 75% of the oxygen (18 mL/kg/min) is not utilized by the tissues; therefore, the blood returning to the right atrium from the systemic circulation is 75% saturated. This is the normal mixed venous oxygen saturation (SvO_2) in a healthy infant.

   1. SvO_2 is the saturation of blood as it enters the pulmonary artery. This can be measured directly with a pulmonary artery catheter in older patients, and can be approximated by a sample of blood from the right atrium in infants without the use of a pulmonary artery catheter. SvO_2 is referred to as "mixed" venous blood, because it represents the average of the blood returning to the right atrium from the superior vena cava and the inferior vena cava.

   2. SvO_2 is an important measurement in patients with questionable CO. A low SvO_2 (<75%) means that an unusually large fraction of the available oxygen has been extracted by the tissues. This usually occurs when the amount of oxygen delivered to the tissues is less than normal.

   3. Causes of low SvO_2 include inadequate oxygenation of the blood, anemia, and low CO. The presence of low SvO_2 in a patient with normal SaO_2 and normal Hb is diagnostic of CO which is inadequate to meet tissue oxygen demands.

4. SvO_2 typically is used to monitor the adequacy of tissue perfusion in patients receiving ECMO and can be useful in any patient when adequacy of CO is uncertain.

IV. Errors in Blood Gas Measurements
  A. An air bubble in a blood gas sample will cause the blood to equilibrate with room air.
    1. $PaCO_2$ will be artificially lowered.
    2. PaO_2 will move closer to the partial pressure of O_2 in room air (approximately 140 mm Hg or 18.7 kPa, depending on altitude and humidity).
  B. Dilution of a blood gas sample with IV fluid of any sort will cause both CO_2 and O_2 to diffuse from the blood into the diluting fluid.
    1. PaO_2 will be artificially lowered.
    2. $PaCO_2$ will be artificially lowered.
    3. Because of the buffering capability of the blood, pH will not change as much as will $PaCO_2$. The combination of relatively normal pH and decreased $PaCO_2$ will appear to be respiratory alkalosis with metabolic acidosis.
  C. If a blood gas sample is kept for a long period at room temperature, the blood cells will continue to metabolize oxygen and produce CO_2.
  D. Most blood gas machines calculate SaO_2 from PaO_2, assuming that all of the Hb is adult Hb. In an infant with a significant amount of fetal Hb, this calculated value will be much lower than the actual measured SaO_2.
  E. Capillary blood gas values are frequently assumed to approximate arterial blood gas values. However, there is marked variation in the correlation of capillary and arterial values. Capillary blood gases should be interpreted with caution.
  F. Blood gases obtained by arterial puncture or capillary stick are painful and disturb the infant, frequently causing agitation, desaturation, or hyperventilation. These readings should be interpreted with caution.

V. Clinical Interpretation of Blood Gases: Blood gas values, by themselves, convey relatively little information; they must be interpreted in a clinical context. When interpreting blood gas results, a number of factors must be assessed simultaneously.
  A. How hard is the infant working to breathe?
    1. A normal blood gas result in an infant who is clearly struggling to breathe is not necessarily reassuring.
    2. An elevated $PaCO_2$ in an infant with chronic lung disease who is comfortable is not necessarily concerning.
  B. Does a recent change in blood gas values represent a change in the patient, or is it an artifact?
  C. If a blood gas result is used to make decisions about ventilator strategy, how much of the total respiratory work is being done by the patient, and how much is being done by the ventilator?
  D. Where is the patient in the course of the disease? A $PaCO_2$ of 65 mm Hg (8.7 kPa) may be of great concern in an infant in the first few hours of life but perfectly acceptable in an infant with chronic lung disease.

E. When deciding whether to obtain a blood gas sample, ask yourself whether you will learn anything from it that you cannot learn from a clinical examination of the patient.

VI. Target Ranges for Blood Gases: A wide range of blood gas values is seen in newborn infants, depending upon gestational age, postnatal age, and disease state. In most infants with respiratory disease, the goal is not to make blood gases entirely normal, but to keep them within an acceptable "target range." There are few controlled data to guide the choice of these "target ranges"; instead, they have gradually evolved and are continuing to evolve.

A. pH: In most newborns, the goal is to keep the arterial pH between 7.25 and 7.40. However, in some infants it is appropriate to allow an arterial pH as low as 7.20. An alkalotic pH (>7.40) should almost always be avoided.

B. $PaCO_2$: In the healthy newborn, a normal $PaCO_2$ is approximately 35 to 40 mm Hg. However, infants with any significant lung disease will hypoventilate and develop an elevated $PaCO_2$ and respiratory acidosis. In recent years, there has been a gradual shift toward tolerating higher $PaCO_2$ levels, an approach that is termed "permissive hypercarbia." Partly because the data suggest a link between hypocarbia and decreased cerebral blood flow and resultant possible brain injury, $PaCO_2$ levels much below 40 should be avoided. With time, respiratory acidosis will be matched by compensatory metabolic alkalosis, and the arterial pH will move toward the normal range. Because of the complex interaction of disease severity, ventilatory support, and duration of hypercapnea, many clinicians find it easier to define a "target pH" rather than a "target $PaCO_2$."

C. PaO_2:PaO_2 is not nearly as important a physiologic parameter as oxygen saturation and, because of the variable amount of fetal Hb in an infant's blood, is widely variable. Many neonatologists now think of oxygenation only in terms of SaO_2, not in terms of PaO_2.

D. SaO_2: In the healthy term infant SaO_2 is close to 100%. However, the oxygen content of blood is adequate for tissue oxygen delivery at much lower levels of SaO_2. In patients with cyanotic heart disease, a persistent SaO_2 of 70% to 75% is often sufficient to ensure adequate tissue oxygenation. Although there are limited data supporting this practice, there has been a gradual trend toward acceptance of lower SaO_2 values in infants with lung disease.

E. Base deficit: In the healthy term infant, the base deficit is usually around 3 to 5 mEq/L. However, base deficit is a calculated value and can vary significantly. In most patients with a base deficit between 5 and 10 mEq/L, assuming good tissue perfusion on clinical examination, no acute intervention is needed. A base deficit in this range in a very preterm infant may suggest renal bicarbonate wasting and may prompt an increase in the amount of base administered in the maintenance fluids. A base deficit >10 mEq/L should prompt a careful examination of the infant for signs of underperfusion. In an infant with a significant base deficit and clinical underperfusion, correcting the cause of the underperfusion should be the primary goal. In most cases, correcting the underlying cause of metabolic acidosis is far more effective than is administering extra base.

Suggested Reading

Ambalavanan N, Carlo W: Hypocapnia and hypercapnia in respiratory management of newborn infants. Clin Perinatol 28:517-531, 2001.

Clark JS, Votteri B, Ariagno RL, et al: Noninvasive assessment of blood gases. Am Rev Respir Dis 145:220-232, 1992.

Courtney SE, Weber KR, Breakie LA, et al: Capillary blood gases in the neonate: A reassessment and review of the literature. Am J Dis Child 144:168-172, 1990.

Dennis RC, Ng R, Yeston NS, Statland B: Effect of sample dilutions on arterial blood gas determinations. Crit Care Med 13:1067-1068, 1985.

Dudell G, Cornish JD, Bartlett RH: What constitutes adequate oxygenation? Pediatrics 85:39-41, 1990.

Kim EH, Cohen RS, Ramachandran P: Effect of vascular puncture on blood gases in the newborn. Pediatr Pulmonol 10:287-290, 1991.

Tin W: Optimal oxygen saturation for preterm babies. Do we really know? Biol Neonate 85:319-325, 2004.

19 Neonatal Graphic Monitoring

Joanne J. Nicks

I. Indications
   A. Optimizing mechanical ventilation parameters
      1. Peak inspiratory pressure (PIP)
      2. Positive end-expiratory pressure (PEEP)
      3. Inspiratory and expiratory tidal volume (V_{TI} and V_{TE}, respectively)
      4. Inspiratory time (T_I)
      5. Expiratory time (T_E)
      6. Flow rate
      7. Synchronization
   B. Evaluation of infant's spontaneous effort
      1. Spontaneous V_T
      2. Minute ventilation (MV)
      3. Respiratory pattern
      4. Readiness for extubation
   C. Therapeutic response to pharmacologic agents
      1. Surfactant
      2. Bronchodilators
      3. Diuretics
      4. Steroids
   D. Evaluation of respiratory waveforms, loops, and mechanics
      1. Waveforms
         a. Pressure
         b. Flow
         c. Volume
      2. Loops
         a. Pressure-volume (P-V) loop
         b. Flow-volume (F-V) loop
      3. Mechanics
         a. Dynamic compliance (C_D) and static compliance (C_{ST})
         b. Inspiratory and expiratory resistance (R_I and R_E, repectively)
         c. Time constants
   E. Disease evaluation
      1. Restrictive
      2. Obstructive
      3. Severity
      4. Recovery

II. Graphical User Interfaces (GUIs)
   A. GUIs provide continuous, real-time feedback of the interaction between the patient and the ventilator.
   B. They are also an excellent teaching tool.
   C. Graphics monitors have been available since the early 1990s as an option that can be added to ventilators; the latest generation of ventilators now has touch screen interfaces with color displays that are integral to the ventilator.
   D. It is important to know where and how data are collected for the graphics. One important consideration is location of the flow sensor.
      1. If the flow sensor is proximal (close to the patient's airway), the waveforms, loops, and data are more reflective of what is actually occurring in the lung.
      2. If the flow sensors are distal (back in the machine), the waveforms, loops, and data include circuit compliance and resistance and may not accurately reflect the pulmonary system.
   E. Types of flow sensors:
      1. Heated wire anemometer: Measures the amount of current required to keep a heated wire at a constant temperature as gas flows past the wire and heat is convected.
      2. Differential pressure pneumotachometer: As gas flows through the sensor across an element, a differential pressure is created between the upstream and downstream sensing ports. The change in pressure across the element is proportional to flow.
   F. Neonatal-capable ventilators with integral GUIs:
      1. Avea (Viasys Healthcare, Yorba Linda, CA)
      2. Draeger Evita XL, Evita 4, and Evita 2 dura (Draeger Medical, Telford, PA, and Luebeck, Germany)
      3. Puritan Bennett 840 (Tyco Healthcare, Pleasanton, CA)
      4. Servo-i (Maquet Critical Care, Bridgewater, NJ)
      5. VIP BIRD/BIRD Graphic Monitor (Viasys Healthcare, Yorba Linda, CA)—Graphics monitoring devices (optional add on) with variable orifice differential pressure transducer flowsensor monitors at the proximal airway:
         a. Waveforms
         b. Loops
         c. Trends
         d. Reference cursor/reference loops
         e. C_D, C_{ST}, peak R_E and static resistance, C20/C_D
         f. Patient monitor and ventilator settings screen
      6. Bear Cub 750 with ventilator graphics monitor (Viasys Healthcare, Yorba Linda, CA)—heated wire flow sensor monitors at the proximal airway:
         a. Waveforms
         b. Loops
         c. C_D, peak R_E

7. Dräger Babylog 8000 Plus (Drager Medical, Telford, PA, and Luebeck, Germany)—heated-wire flow sensor monitors at the proximal airway:
   a. Integrated data
      (1) Single pressure or flow waveform
      (2) Display screens of monitored and set values
      (3) Trends of main ventilation parameters
      (4) Lung function monitoring of C_D, resistance (linear regression, C20/C_D, and time constant)
   b. Babylink (requires computer interface)
      (1) All waveforms displayed
      (2) Loops
      (3) Overlapping reference function
      (4) Trending option (Evitaview)
      (5) Display of all set and measured parameters
8. Servo 300 with 390 Graphics Screen (Maquet Critical Care, Bridgewater, NJ)—pneumotachometer monitors values at the ventilator, not the proximal airway:
   a. Waveforms
   b. Loops
   c. Trends
   d. C_D, C_{ST}, R_E, and R_I
   e. CO_2 analyzer for deadspace (C_D/V_T ratios)
   f. Numerical display of data
   g. Clinical help file

III. Graphic Waveforms
   A. Pressure
      1. Pressure waveforms (shown in Figs. 19-1 and 19-2)
         a. In Figure 19-1, the upsweep of the waveforms represents inspiration and the downsweep represents expiration.
         b. PIP is the maximum pressure point on the curve.
         c. PEEP is the baseline pressure level.
         d. The area under the curve represents the mean airway pressure (Pāw) (shaded).
         e. The shape of the curve represents the breath type—e.g., volume (triangular) or pressure (square).
         f. As shown in Figure 19-2, the presence of a plateau at peak pressure is caused by an inflation hold or prolonged T_I. This may improve distribution of ventilation but is not usually desirable in infants, because it may disrupt synchrony and results in a higher Pāw.

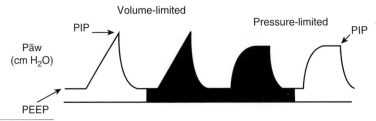

FIGURE 19-1. Pressure waveform for both volume- and pressure-limited breaths.

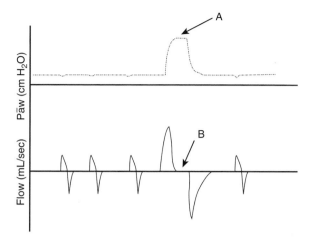

FIGURE **19-2.** Pressure and flow waveforms showing a pressure plateau (A) caused by an inflation hold; note the delay (B) before expiratory flow is seen.

    B. Flow waveforms (shown in Figs. 19-3 to 19-6)
       1. In Figure 19-3, the horizontal line is the zero (no) flow point. Upsweep of the flow waveform above this line is inspiratory flow rate, and downsweep is expiratory flow rate.
       2. Greatest deflection above reference equals peak inspiratory flow rate (PIFR).
       3. Greatest deflection below reference equals peak expiratory flow rate (PEFR).
       4. The shape of the flow waveform is typically square, or constant, as seen in volume ventilation, or a decelerating flow, as seen in pressure ventilation.
       5. T_I is measured from the initial flow delivery until expiratory flow begins.
       6. Inflation time of the lung is measured from initial inspiratory flow delivery to the point at which flow returns to zero.

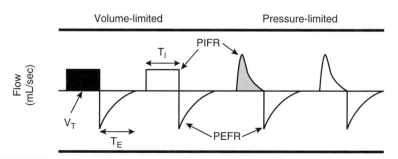

FIGURE **19-3.** Flow waveforms for both volume- and pressure-limited breath types. Inspiratory flow is above the baseline; expiratory flow is below. Peak inspiratory (PIFR) and peak expiratory (PEFR) flow rates are shown.

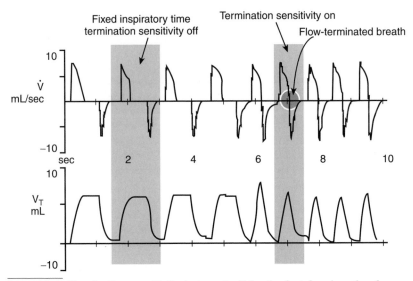

FIGURE 19-4. Termination sensitivity is turned off for the first four breaths, then activated. Note that the breath then ends by a decrease in inspiratory flow rather than at the preset inspiratory time. (From Nicks JJ: Graphics Monitoring in the Neonatal Intensive Care Unit. Palm Springs, CA, Bird Products, 1995, with permission.)

When ventilating newborns, the clinician should evaluate this time interval to set an appropriate T_I.

7. As shown in Figure 19-4, termination sensitivity and flow ($\dot{V}$) cycling allow a mechanical breath to be triggered (cycled) into expiration by a specific algorithm—usually 5% to 25% of peak inspiratory flow. The ability of a patient to control T_I and cycle a

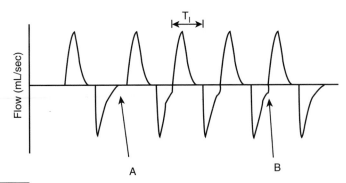

FIGURE 19-5. Demonstration of gas trapping. Note that expiratory flow completely returns to baseline in breath A (zero flow state is achieved), whereas in breath B, there is insufficient expiratory time, and onset of the next breath occurs before zero flow state is achieved.

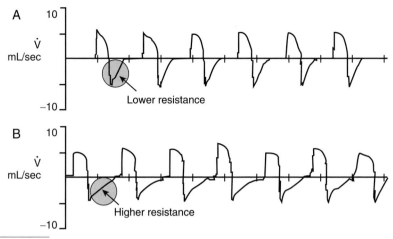

FIGURE 19-6. The shape of a specific waveform can help to identify airway and pulmonary abnormalities. In A, higher airway resistance causes flow to return to baseline more slowly on expiration compared to B, in which resistance is lower. (From Nicks JJ: Graphics Monitoring in the Neonatal Intensive Care Unit. Palm Springs, CA, Bird Products, 1995, with permission.)

breath to expiration may lead to improved synchronization. This feature is available on the newer-generation ventilators and on any ventilator having pressure support).
   8. T_E extends from the point at which expiratory flow begins until the next inspiration begins.
   9. When expiratory flow returns to zero, lung deflation is complete. This is represented as the area from the point where expiration begins to where expiratory flow returns to zero.
   10. If flow has not reached zero before the next breath is delivered, gas trapping may occur, as shown in B in Figure 19-5.
   11. Gas trapping is more likely to occur in airways with increased resistance showing slow emptying time (Figure 19-6).
 C. Volume waveforms (shown in Figs. 19-7 to 19-9)
   1. In Figure 19-7, inspiration (Insp) is represented as the waveform sweeps upward, and expiration (Exp) as the waveform sweeps downward.

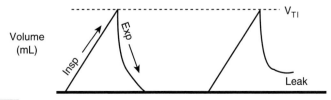

FIGURE 19-7. Volume waveform. Inspiration is represented by the upsweep of the waveform, and expiration by the downward sweep.

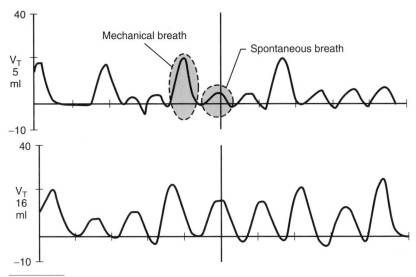

FIGURE **19-8.** The relationship between mechanical V_T and spontaneous V_T in SIMV may be helpful in determining readiness to wean. (From Nicks JJ: Graphics Monitoring in the Neonatal Intensive Care Unit. Palm Springs, CA, Bird Products, 1995, with permission.)

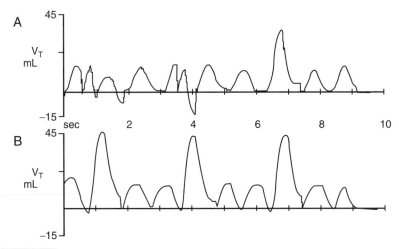

FIGURE **19-9.** Waveforms may be helpful in assessing patient-ventilator interaction (synchrony). In IMV (A), the infant may "fight" the ventilator, resulting in inconsistent tidal volume delivery. In SIMV (B), the synchronized interaction between patient and ventilator results in a more consistent V_T delivery. (From Nicks JJ: Graphics Monitoring in the Neonatal Intensive Care Unit. Palm Springs, CA, Bird Products, 1995, with permission.)

2. The dashed line represents delivered inspiratory tidal volume (V_{TI}).
3. An endotracheal tube leak is observed when the expiratory portion of the waveform fails to return to the zero baseline.
4. In Figure 19-8, the relationship between mechanical breaths and spontaneous breaths in SIMV may be helpful in determining readiness to wean.
5. Asynchronous ventilation may be observed with the volume waveform, as shown in Figure 19-9. In IMV (A), the mechanical breaths delivered are ineffective; however, SIMV (B) is much more effective.

IV. Graphic Loops
   A. Pressure-volume (P-V) loops (shown in Figs. 19-10 to 19-13)
      1. A P-V loop displays the relationship of pressure to volume (compliance).
      2. In Figure 19-10, pressure is displayed along the horizontal axis, and volume is displayed on the vertical axis.
      3. Inspiration (Insp) is represented by the upsweep from the baseline (PEEP) terminating at PIP and V_{TI}. Expiration (Exp) is the downsweep from PIP and V_{TI} back to baseline.
      4. A line drawn from each end point represents compliance ($\Delta V/\Delta P$).
      5. A P-V loop that lies flat indicates poor compliance, and one that stands upright shows improved compliance. Recovery from RDS or response to surfactant therapy demonstrates improvement in compliance (Fig. 19-11).
      6. Graphic monitoring is useful in identifying appropriateness of pressure delivery. A "beaking" of the P-V loop often indicates overdistention. This occurs when pressure continues to rise with minimal change in volume (Fig. 19-12). Note that the compliance of the last 20% of the P-V loop in Figure 19-12C is lower than the C_D of the entire loop. This relationship is often expressed as a mechanics calculation (C20/C_D ratio). A ratio of >1 usually

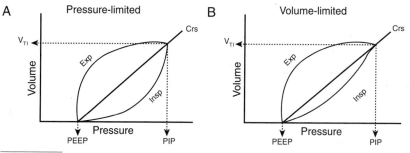

FIGURE 19-10. Pressure-volume loops for both pressure-limited (A) and volume-limited (B) breath types. Note the inspiratory (Insp) and expiratory (Exp) limbs, origin (PEEP), peak inspiratory pressure (PIP), tidal volume (V_T), and compliance line (Crs), drawn by connecting the origin with the point of PIP.

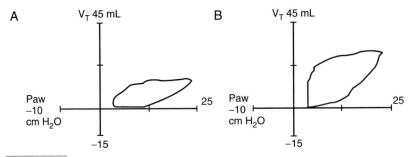

FIGURE 19-11. Compliance is the relationship between volume and pressure. On a pressure-volume loop, pressure is on the horizontal axis, volume is on the vertical axis. A flattened loop (A) indicates poor compliance. A more upright loop (B) indicates improved compliance. This change typically is seen after administration of surfactant to an infant with RDS. (From Nicks JJ: Graphics Monitoring in the Neonatal Intensive Care Unit. Palm Springs, CA, Bird Products, 1995, with permission.)

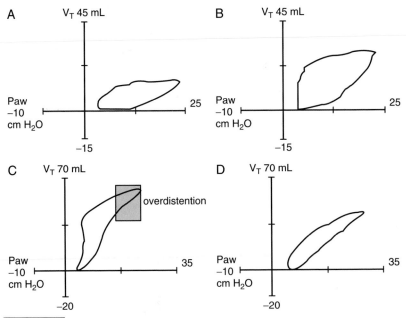

FIGURE 19-12. In pressure-volume monitoring, a pressure change should result in a linear change from the low volume shown in A, as seen in B and D. On the loop in C, however, the last third of the curve is flattened, indicating that pressure continues to be delivered with only a minimal increase in volume. This is a sign of overdistention. (From Nicks JJ: Graphics Monitoring in the Neonatal Intensive Care Unit. Palm Springs, CA, Bird Products, 1995, with permission.)

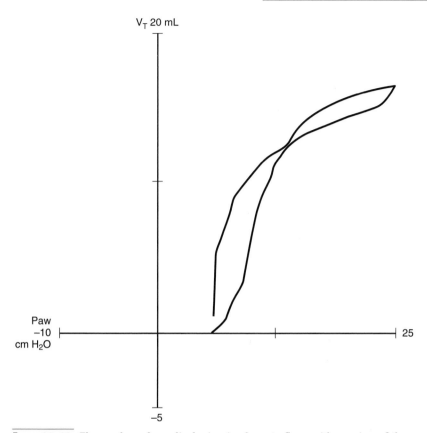

FIGURE **19-13.** Flow-volume loop displaying inadequate flow, with cusping of the inspiratory portion of the loop. This figure-of-eight configuration indicates flow starvation.

indicates overdistention. When this is seen, it is appropriate to evaluate the PIP or V_T and attempt to reduce one of these.

7. P-V loops can help evaluate whether flow delivery from the ventilator is adequate to meet the needs of the patient. Inadequate flow is represented by cusping of the inspiratory portion of the curve. Severe flow limitation may appear as a figure-of-eight (Fig. 19-13). This indicates that volume is increasing more rapidly than pressure (i.e., inadequate flow).

B. Flow-volume ($\dot{V}$-V) loops (shown in Figs. 19-14 and 19-15)

1. In Figure 19-14, a flow-volume loop displays the relationship between volume and flow. Volume (Vol) is plotted on the horizontal axis and flow is plotted on the vertical axis.

2. In this example (may vary with monitor type), the breath starts at the zero axis and moves downward and to the left on inspiration (Insp), terminating at the delivered inspiratory volume and upward, to the right, back to zero on expiration (Exp). Note the

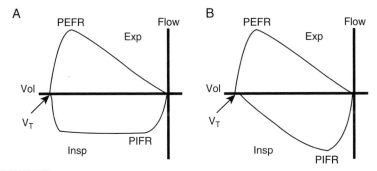

FIGURE **19-14.** Flow-volume loops. **A,** Inspiratory flow limitation is demonstrated by flattening of the loop. The peak inspiratory flow rate (PIFR) is lower for a given volume. **B,** Decreasing the resistance (such as by using a bronchodilator) results in improved PIFR and a more normal appearance of the inspiratory flow-volume loop.

constant flow delivered with a volume breath type (square inspiratory flow on loop in A) versus decelerating inspiratory flow (loop in B) with a pressure breath type.
3. The flow-volume loop is useful in evaluating airway dynamics. During conditions of high airway resistance, peak flow is lower for a given volume. Typically, R_E is higher with airway collapse or bronchospasm.
4. Conditions in the newborn that often result in increased R_E as a result of airway obstruction include MAS and CLD.

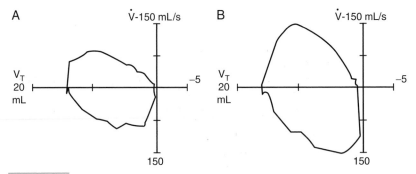

FIGURE **19-15.** Another example of evaluating a treatment using pulmonary graphics: A, Flow-volume loop before administration of a bronchodilator; B, the same loop following treatment. Note the marked improvement in inspiratory and expiratory flow rates in this patient. (From Nicks JJ: Graphics Monitoring in the Neonatal Intensive Care Unit. Palm Springs, CA, Bird Products, 1995, with permission.)

5. The flow-volume loop is useful for evaluating the effectiveness of bronchodilators in treating airway reactivity. In Figure 19-15, increased expiratory flow is seen in the loop shown in A compared to the loop shown in B.

V. Dynamics Measurements/Calculations (shown in Figs. 19-16 to 19-18)

A. V_T is measured on inspiration and expiration. Normal delivered V_T is 4 to 8 mL/kg.

B. MV is the product of V_T and respiratory rate. The normal range is 240 to 360 mL/kg/min.

C. Pressure may be measured as peak P_I or P_{ST}. P_{ST} is obtained by performing an inflation hold maneuver, which measures pressure obtained by closing the exhalation valve and stopping flow delivery during a mechanical breath (Fig. 19-16).

D. Compliance (CD) is the relationship between a change in volume and a change in pressure.

1. C_D is the measurement of compliance based on peak pressure (Fig. 19-17):

$$C_D = \frac{V_{TI}}{PIP - PEEP}$$

2. C_{ST} is the measurement based on static pressure (P_{ST}):

$$C_{ST} = \frac{V_{TI}}{P_{ST} - PEEP}$$

3. C20/C_D is the ratio of compliance of the last 20% to the entire curve. With overdistention, this ratio will be <1.

E. Resistance is the relationship of pressure to flow. The pressure may be dynamic or static, and flow measurements are taken from various measurements (Fig. 19-18).

1. Peak flow is the maximum flow on either inspiration or expiration.

2. Average flow is based on multiple point linear regression.

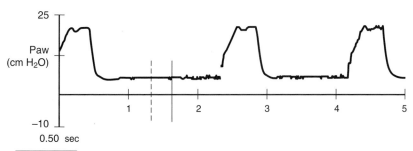

FIGURE 19-16. Static pressure waveform caused by an inflation hold maneuver.

3. Mid-volume flow is based on the flow measured at a point of mid-volume delivery.

$$R_{AW} \text{ (cm } H_2O/L/sec) = \frac{PIP - PEEP}{flow}$$

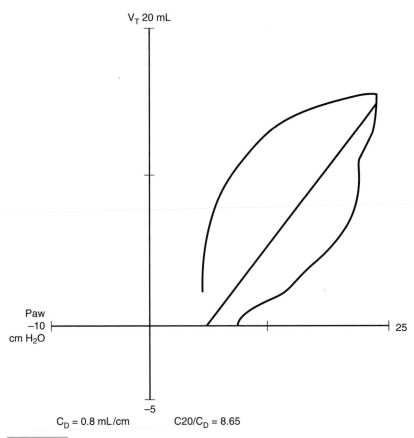

$C_D = 0.8$ mL/cm   C20/C_D = 8.65

FIGURE 19-17. Pressure-volume loop showing a dynamic compliance (C_D) measurement.

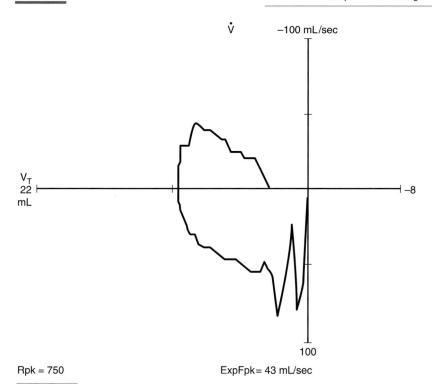

Rpk = 750   ExpFpk= 43 mL/sec

FIGURE 19-18. Flow-volume loop showing peak expiratory flow (ExpFpk) and peak expiratory resistance (Rpk) measurements.

Suggested Reading

Cannon ML, Cornell J, Trip-Hamel D, et al: Tidal volumes for ventilated infants should be determined with a pneumotachometer placed at the endotracheal tube. Am J Respir Crit Care Med 62:2109-2112, 2000.

Cunningham MD, Wood BR: Monitoring of pulmonary function. In Goldsmith JP, Karotkin EH (eds): Assisted Ventilation of the Neonate, 3rd ed. Philadelphia, WB Saunders, 1996, pp 273-289.

Donn SM (ed): Neonatal and Pediatric Pulmonary Graphics: Principles and Clinical Applications. Armonk, NY, Futura Publishing, 1998.

Nicks JJ: Graphics Monitoring in the Neonatal Intensive Care Unit: Maximizing the Effectiveness of Mechanical Ventilation. Palm Springs, CA, Bird Products, 1995.

Sinha SK, Nicks JJ, Donn SM: Graphic analysis of pulmonary mechanics in neonates receiving assisted ventilation. Arch Dis Child 75:F213-F218, 1996.

Wilson BG, Cheifetz IM, Meliones JN: Mechanical Ventilation in Infants and Children with the Use of Airway Graphics. Palm Springs, CA, Bird Products, 1995.

20 Radiography

Gauravi K. Sabharwal and Lawrence R. Kuhns

I. Introduction
   A. Chest radiography is the primary imaging modality for diagnosing respiratory diseases in the neonate.
   B. Other modalities include CT and MRI. Fluoroscopy and ultrasonography are less commonly employed, although they are valuable in certain selected cases.
II. Plain Radiography
   A. The chest radiograph remains the introductory and primary radiographic exam for evaluation of the neonatal chest. An anteroposterior (AP) and sometimes a cross-table lateral view of the chest may be obtained. However, an AP view usually suffices for a routine follow-up study. Digital imaging permits postprocessing without exposing the patient to additional radiation.
   B. Indications
      1. Respiratory distress
      2. Abnormal blood gases
      3. Air leaks
         a. Pneumothorax
         b. Pulmonary interstitial emphysema
         c. Pneumomediastinum
         d. Pneumopericardium
      4. Meconium below the vocal cords
      5. Sepsis/pneumonia
      6. Possible cardiac disease
      7. Chronic lung disease (bronchopulmonary dysplasia)
      8. Suspected thoracic anomaly
         a. Congenital diaphragmatic hernia (Fig. 20-1)
         b. Cystic adenomatoid malformation (Fig. 20-2)
         c. Esophageal atresia/tracheoesophageal fistula
      9. Following procedures
         a. Intubation
         b. Thoracentesis/thoracostomy
         c. Chest tube removal
         d. Vascular catheter placement
   C. Patient Considerations
      1. Postmature newborn
         a. Meconium aspiration syndrome (Fig. 20-3) presents as normal to increased lung volume and irregular aeration with coarse, patchy densities representing atelectasis and consolidation.

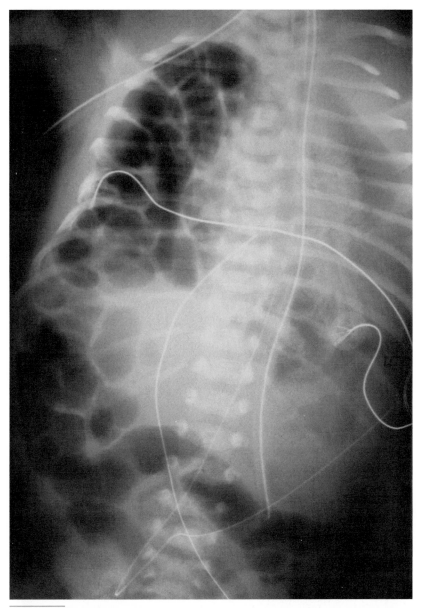

FIGURE **20-1.** Radiograph of the chest and abdomen demonstrates air-filled bowel loops herniating into the right hemithorax. The heart and mediastinum have shifted to the left. The lungs are poorly aerated secondary to passive atelectasis. Congenital diaphragmatic hernia was diagnosed in this patient during a routine prenatal ultrasound examination.

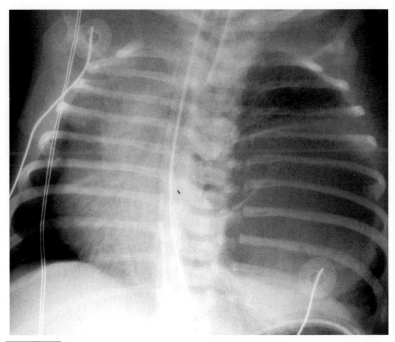

FIGURE 20-2. A large mass is seen occupying the left hemithorax. There is shift of the mediastinum to the right. This mass was cystic on a follow-up CT and consistent with a large congenital cystic adenomatoid malformation.

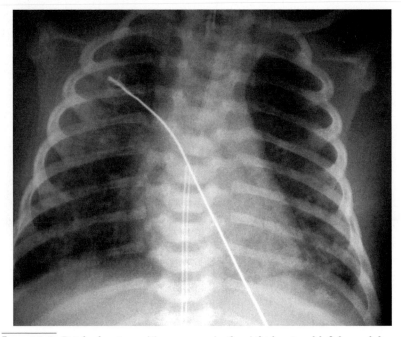

FIGURE 20-3. Patchy lung opacities are seen in the right lung and left lower lobe. The lungs are well expanded. This patient has meconium aspiration syndrome.

Pleural effusions are often present. Air leak and pneumomediastinum are common. Focal areas of overinflation and peripheral air trapping also may be seen.

b. Neonatal pneumonia (Fig. 20-4) may give a picture similar to meconium aspiration or surfactant deficiency. Confluent, asymmetrical opacities are usually noted. The lung volume is normal and some pleural fluid may be present.

2. Term newborn: Mild respiratory distress is often associated with transient tachypnea of the newborn (Fig. 20-5). Coarse, perihilar, streaky densities are seen in well-inflated lungs. Prominent interlobar fissures and pleural stripes representing small effusions are often present. This haziness clears by 24 to 48 hours of age.

3. Premature newborn

a. Respiratory distress and abnormal blood gases are associated with surfactant deficiency (RDS) (Fig. 20-6), which presents with a fine "salt and pepper" or "ground glass" appearance throughout both lungs on the chest radiograph. Radiographic changes usually appear shortly after birth, but can be delayed for 12 to 24 hours. The patient has low lung volumes.

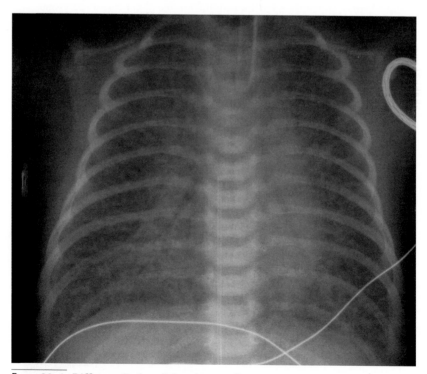

FIGURE 20-4. Diffuse reticulonodular airspace disease throughout both lungs suggest RDS. However, in this term baby (presence of humeral ossification center dates this baby as at least 36 weeks) the findings suggest another etiology—beta streptococcal pneumonia.

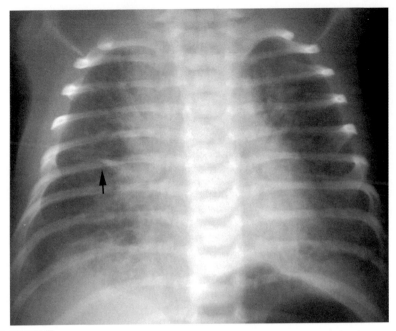

Figure 20-5. This term infant presented with mild dyspnea, which resolved quickly. Diffuse strandlike opacities with fluid in the minor fissure are visible *(arrow)*. The lungs are well expanded. Follow-up radiograph 24 hours later was completely negative. This patient had transient tachypnea of the newborn.

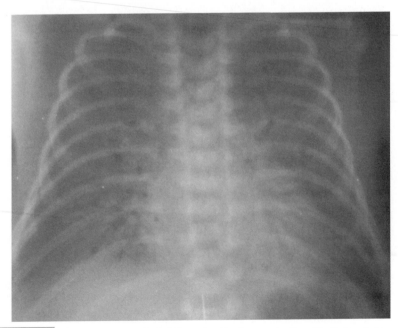

Figure 20-6. There is symmetrical, bilateral reticulogranularity of both lungs in this infant (34-week gestational age), indicating surfactant deficiency and RDS.

   b. As pulmonary opacification increases, the margins of the
      diaphragm and the heart border become obscured. A small
      radiographic focal spot of ≤ 0.3 mm diameter and high-detail
      screen film combination must be used to detect the fine
      reticulogranular appearance of surfactant deficiency (RDS).
4. Very premature newborn
   a. Respiratory distress is associated with immature lungs, which
      presents as a fine hazy appearance on the chest radiograph.
   b. An enlarged heart suggests patent ductus arteriosus.
5. Newborn of any gestational age with sudden onset of severe dyspnea.
   a. Pulmonary interstitial emphysema (PIE) may occur with streaks
      of air seen dissecting toward the pulmonary hilum on either side
      (Fig. 20-7).
   b. PIE may dissect into the mediastinum to produce a
      pneumomediastinum (Fig. 20-8), or the PIE may rupture
      into the pleura to produce a pneumothorax (Fig. 20-9).
      A pneumomediastinum can be detected on a cross-table lateral
      radiograph with the patient supine. A pneumothorax can be
      confirmed using a crosstable radiograph with the patient in
      The decubitus position. Pneumopericardium can also occur
      (Figs. 20-9 and 20-10).

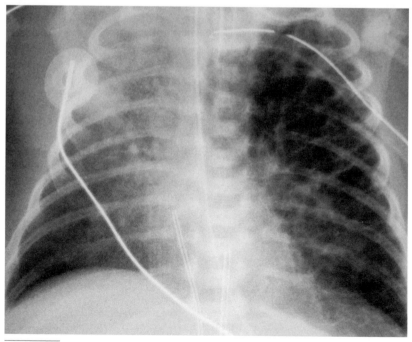

FIGURE 20-7. Small linear and cystic lucencies in the interstitium in the left lung
represents pulmonary interstitial emphysema, which may be the first radiographic
manifestation of barotrauma and air leak.

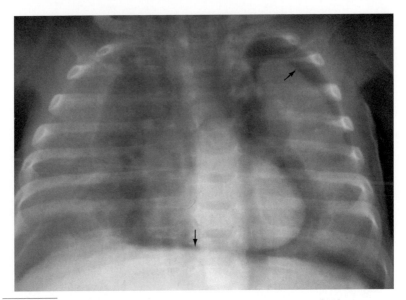

Figure 20-8. Radiograph of infant with bilateral pneumothoraces and subcutaneous emphysema. Pneumomediastinum dissects into the neck and lower chest in the region of the diaphragm. Pneumopericardium (lucency around the heart) is also present. Upper arrow indicates lung margin; lower arrow indicates inferior cardiac margin.

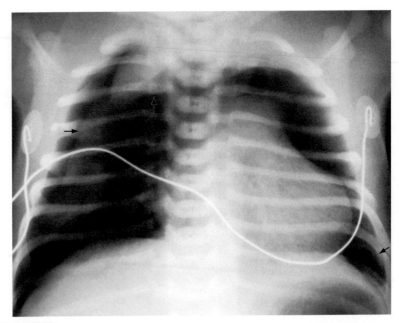

Figure 20-9. Radiograph showing lucency over the right lateral thorax without lung markings *(horizontal arrow)*. Another lucency is seen at the left lateral lung base. These findings are both consistent with a diagnosis of pneumothoraces. Increased lucency over the superior mediastinum displaces the thymus upward *(diagonal arrow)*. This is consistent with a diagnosis of pneumomediastinum.

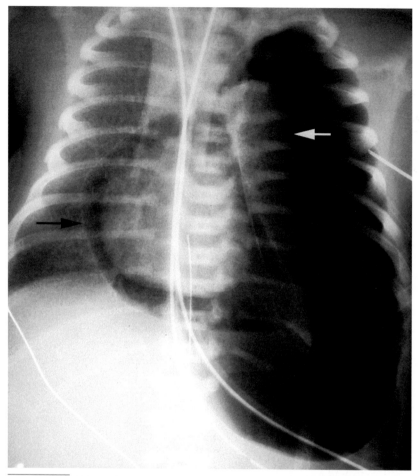

FIGURE 20-10. A large left tension pneumothorax causes shift of the mediastinum to the right and collapse of the left lung *(white arrow)*. Pneumopericardium (lucency around the heart) is also present *(black arrow)*.

6. Infant >2 weeks of age with dyspnea and CO_2 retention
   a. Eventual progression to chronic lung disease should be suspected (Fig. 20-11).
   b. Thick-walled, cystlike areas may eventually be seen in both lungs.

III. Fluoroscopy
   A. Fluoroscopy allows dynamic evaluation of an abnormality in various projections. The examination can be recorded on videotapes for later review and storage.
   B. Indications
      1. Evaluation of cases where there is suspicion of a tracheal, esophageal (Fig. 20-12), or vascular anomaly. A barium swallow is performed and images are obtained in various projections to look for any

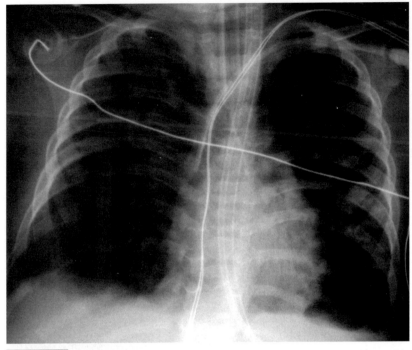

FIGURE 20-11. Diffuse, bilateral, coarse, cystlike changes are seen in this infant with chronic lung disease (bronchopulmonary dysplasia).

fistulas or impressions on the esophagus (Fig. 20-13A and B). Gastroesophageal reflux can also be studied.

    2. Evaluation of swallowing in patients with suspected aspiration pneumonia.

    3. Closer examination of diaphragmatic excursion in suspected paresis or paralysis.

IV. Ultrasound

    A. Ultrasound does not use ionizing radiation, making it a very popular imaging modality in care of the neonate. However, it has limited utility in the diagnosis of respiratory disorders because there is no transmission of sound waves through air. It can be performed at the bedside and carries no morbidity.

    B. Indications

        1. Distinction of solid from cystic intrathoracic masses.

        2. Evaluation of diaphragmatic excursion and position in suspected cases of paresis or paralysis.

        3. Differentiation of pleural effusion from pulmonary consolidation in patients with complete opacification of the hemithorax.

V. Computerized Tomography (CT)

    A. CT is obtained as an adjunct to radiography or ultrasound. The acquisition time has decreased with the advent of newer-generation,

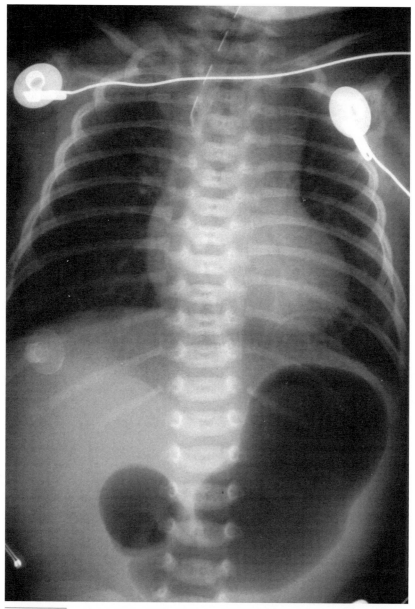

FIGURE 20-12. Radiograph of a term infant born to a 15-year-old mother.
The clinicians were unable to pass a nasogastric (NG) tube. The radiograph
demonstrates the NG tube ending in the proximal atretic esophagus (blind pouch).
Air in the stomach suggests a tracheoesophageal fistula. In addition,
a double-bubble sign of duodenal atresia is present.

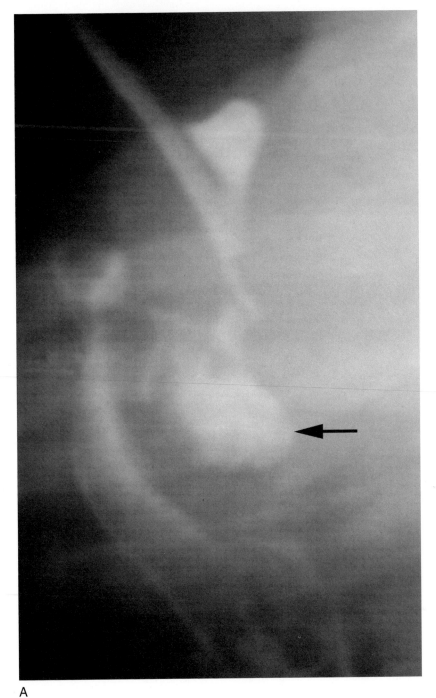

A

FIGURE 20-13. A, A pouchogram performed on the same patient as in Figure 20-12 shows contrast filling the esophageal pouch *(arrow)*.

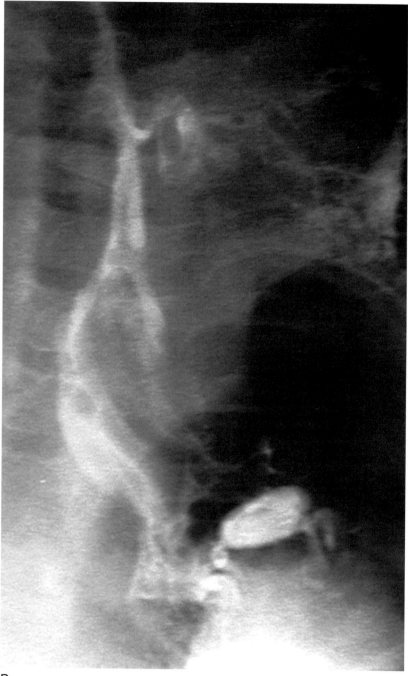

B

Figure 20-13, Cont'd. B, As the pouch fills, contrast is seen flowing through the proximal fistula into the trachea.

multidetector CT scanners. Contiguous axial images of 3- to 5-mm slice thickness at low milliamperage are obtained from the apices of the lungs to the diaphragm following administration of nonionic intravenous contrast. Sagittal and coronal reformatted images from the computerized data can be added when deemed necessary. Sedation or general anesthesia may be required.

B. Indications

1. Lung lesion seen on intrauterine sonography, even if the postnatal chest radiograph is negative (e.g., cystic adenomatoid malformation)

2. Better delineation of an abnormality seen on postnatal chest radiograph (e.g., lobar emphysema or sequestration) (Fig. 20-14)

3. Suspected vascular ring or sling with airway obstruction (Figs. 20-15 and 20-16)

VI. Magnetic Resonance Imaging (MRI)

A. MRI does not require ionizing radiations. It makes use of the ability of protons of different tissues to resonate at a specific frequency when subjected to an electromagnetic field. Its advantages include multiplanar imaging and exquisite soft tissue detail. Sedation or general anesthesia is required.

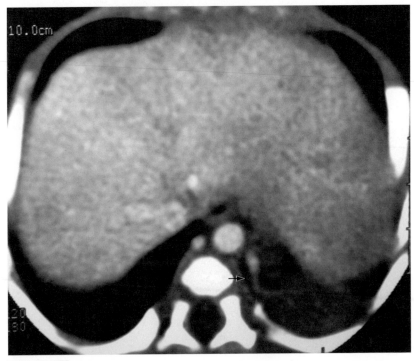

FIGURE 20-14. Infant with a mass demonstrated on a chest radiograph. This CT scan demonstrates a left intrathoracic mass receiving its vascular supply from an anomalous vessel arising from the aorta (arrow). This is characteristic of a pulmonary sequestration.

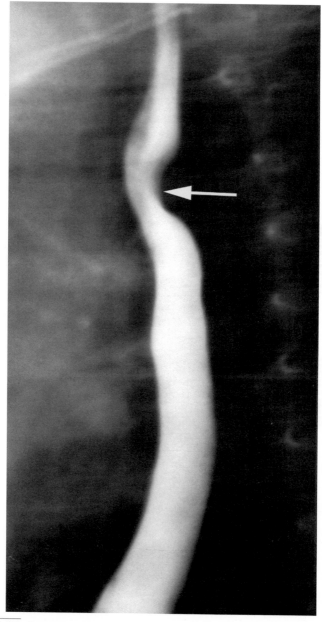

Figure 20-15. An upper gastrointestinal barium examination was performed on a 3-month-old infant who presented with noisy breathing. The scout view of the chest showed a right-sided aortic arch. There is an indentation on the posterior esophagus *(arrow)*, suggestive of a vascular ring.

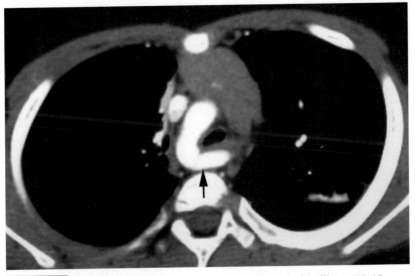

FIGURE **20-16.** This follow-up CT of the same infant described in Figure 20-15 demonstrated a vessel coursing posterior to the esophagus (*arrow*) and was consistent with the diagnosis of an aberrant left subclavian artery in the presence of a right aortic arch.

  B. Indications
      1. Pulmonary sequestration (to show the vascular supply from below the diaphragm, as well as the relationship of the sequestration to the diaphragm).
      2. Complex congenital heart disease when there is insufficient information from echocardiography (e.g., anomalous pulmonary venous return).
      3. Evaluation of presence and size of the pulmonary arteries when they cannot be delineated by cardiac catheterization or echocardiography.

Suggested Reading

DiPietro MA: A radiological atlas of neonatal emergencies. In Donn SM, Faix RG (eds): Neonatal Emergencies. Mount Kisco, NY, Futura Publishing, 1991, pp 123-206.

Transillumination

21

Steven M. Donn

I. Description: Use of a high-intensity light to help define normal from abnormal structures or functions. Using transillumination, the density and composition of tissue is assessed by its diffusion of light.
II. Clinical Applications
   A. Diagnosis of air leaks
   B. Distinguishing cystic from solid masses
   C. Finding veins or arteries for blood sampling or catheter insertion
   D. Initial diagnosis of CNS abnormalities that involve formation of fluid collections
III. Technique
   A. Prepare light source:
      1. Check power supply.
      2. Connect fiberoptic cable if necessary.
      3. Practice good infection control by disinfecting light probe with antiseptic solution.
   B. Darken room as much as possible. Allow some time for dark adaption.
   C. Apply light probe to infant's skin surface in area to be examined; contralateral side can be used as control.
   D. Normally, extent of visible light corona around probe tip is 2 to 3 cm; presence of air (or fluid) in light path will substantially increase the degree of lucency. A significant collection of air will cause the entire hemithorax to "glow."
   E. Pneumomediastinum
      1. Suggested if cardiac pulsations are clearly evident in lucent area.
      2. Best seen if light probe is placed next to costal margin.
      3. Has a high predictive value (94%) if >20 mL air.
   F. Pneumothorax
      1. Generally expands uniformly in anterior direction.
      2. Best demonstrated if light probe is placed on anterior chest wall.
      3. Can be diagnosed with >95% accuracy under favorable conditions.
   G. Pneumopericardium
      1. Place light probe in third or fourth intercostal space in left mid-clavicular line.
      2. Angle light probe toward xiphoid process.
      3. When probe is moved over thorax, corona will appear brightest over the pericardial sac, and silhouette of heartbeat may be seen.
   H. All three collections (pneumomediastinum, pneumothorax, and pneumopericardium) may be aspirated under transillumination guidance.

IV. Special Considerations

A. Care must be taken to avoid burning the patient with the high-intensity light. This is prevented by using a red filter inserted in front of the light source and limiting contact of the light with skin.

B. Cross-contamination of patients is avoided by covering the light with cellophane.

Suggested Reading

Cabatu EE, Brown EG: Thoracic transillumination: aid in the diagnosis and treatment of pneumopericardium. Pediatrics 64:958-960, 1979.

Donn SM: Transillumination. In Donn SM (ed): The Michigan Manual: A Guide to Neonatal Intensive Care, 2nd ed. Armonk, NY, Future Publishing, 1997, pp 27-28.

Donn SM, Kuhns LR: Pediatric Transillumination. Chicago, Year Book Medical Publishers, 1983.

Wyman ML, Kuhns LR: Accuracy of transillumination in the recognition of pneumothorax and pneumomediastinum in the neonate. Clin Pediatr 16:323-324, 1997.

Echocardiography

<big>**22**</big>

Jonathan P. Wyllie

I. Background
   A. Until the advent of echocardiography, cardiac function in the ventilated baby was monitored by clinical assessment and invasive monitoring, which is limited by the size of the patient.
   B. Tissue perfusion is the most relevant parameter in assessing cardiovascular function. This depends upon peripheral vascular resistance and cardiac output.
   C. Previously, heart rate and blood pressure had been utilized as indicators of these parameters.
   D. Echocardiography now offers a number of different modalities that can be used to assess cardiac function in the ventilated infant.
II. Influences on Newborn Cardiovascular Adaptation
   A. Preterm delivery
   B. Surfactant deficiency
   C. Ventilation
   D. Hypoxia
   E. Acidosis
III. Effects of Prematurity and Respiratory Disease on Cardiovascular Adaptation
   A. Delayed fall in pulmonary vascular resistance
   B. Myocardial dysfunction
   C. Ductal patency
   D. Ventilation effects on venous return and diminished venous return
   E. Hypovolemia
IV. Ideal Cardiac Assessment
   A. Cardiac output
   B. Cardiac function
   C. Pulmonary resistance
   D. Tissue perfusion
   E. Systemic vascular resistance
V. Echocardiographic Assessment
   A. Echocardiographic principles
      1. Cross-sectional echocardiography is used to assess anatomy, to allow accurate positioning of an M-mode continuous wave Doppler or pulsed wave Doppler beam, and to obtain a subjective impression of function. Views used include:
         a. Long-axis parasternal (Fig. 22-1)
         b. Short-axis parasternal mitral (Fig. 22-2)
         c. Short-axis parasternal pulmonary (Fig. 22-3)

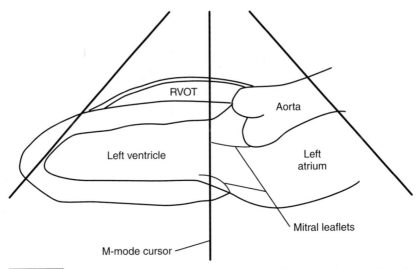

FIGURE 22-1. Long-axis parasternal view. Positioning of the M-mode cursor for left ventricular measurements is shown. RVOT, right ventricular outflow tract.

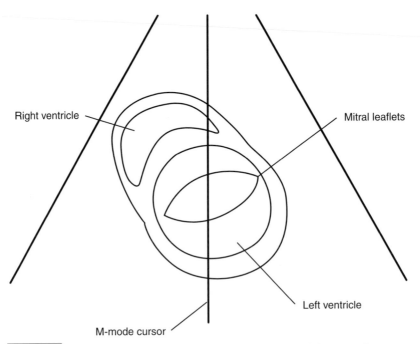

FIGURE 22-2. Short-axis parasternal mitral view. Positioning of the M-mode cursor for left ventricular measurements is shown.

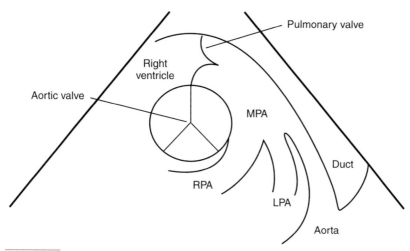

FIGURE 22-3. Short axis parasternal pulmonary view. MPA, main pulmonary artery; RPA, right pulmonary artery; LPA, left pulmonary artery.

       d. Four-chamber apical (Fig. 22-4)
       e. Subcostal
       f. Suprasternal view of aortic arch or ductal arch
       g. Subcostal short-axis pulmonary (Fig. 22-5) (useful if lungs are overdistended)
  B. M-mode assessment obtains detailed echocardiographic information along a thin beam. It is simplest to position initially using a cross-sectional image (see Fig. 22-1) and then switch to M-mode. It is used

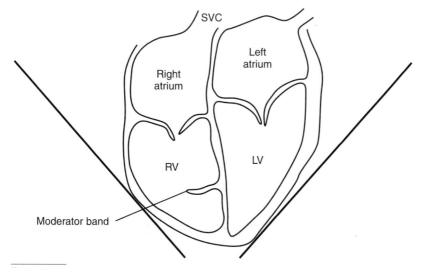

FIGURE 22-4. Four-chamber apical view. Offset of tricuspid and mitral valves is seen. SVC, superior vena cava; RV, right ventricle; LV, left ventricle.

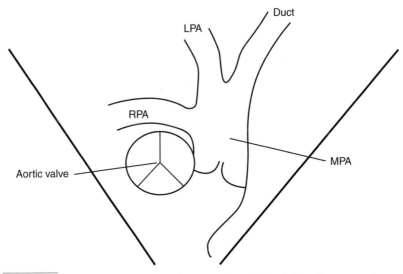

FIGURE 22-5. Subcostal short-axis pulmonary view. RPA, right pulmonary artery; LPA, left pulmonary artery; MPA, main pulmonary artery.

to obtain views of the left ventricle at the level of the mitral leaflets (Fig. 22-6), in assessment of left ventricular function, and in measurement of left ventricular dimensions. It is also used in measurement of the left atrium and aorta (Fig. 22-7).

C. Pulsed wave Doppler echocardiography uses Doppler shift of sound waves from moving red blood cells to assess flow velocity. It can sample the velocity at a point specified on a cross-sectional image

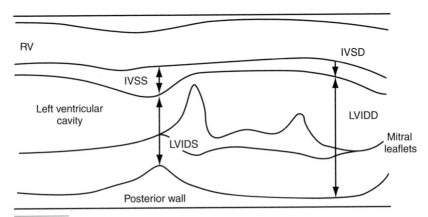

FIGURE 22-6. M-mode view showing measurements of left ventricle. RV, right ventricle; IVSS, intraventricular septum systole; LVIDS, left ventricular internal diameter systole; IVSD, intraventricular septum diastole; LVIDD, left ventricular internal diameter diastole.

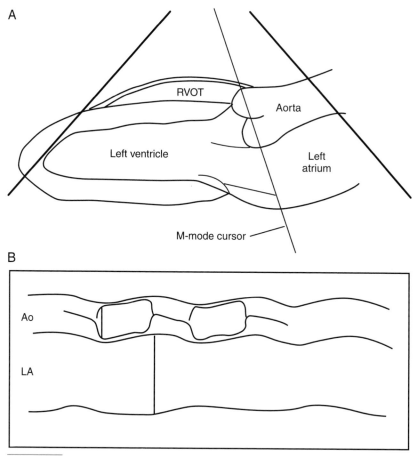

FIGURE 22-7. A, Long-axis parasternal view with M-mode cursor across aorta and left atrium. RVOT, right ventricular outflow tract. B, M-mode view of aorta (Ao) and left atrium (LA), showing measurements of each.

(range-gated) but often is only useful for relatively low velocities. It is useful for velocity measurement in the pulmonary artery, ductus arteriosus (Fig. 22-8), foramen ovale, celiac axis, and superior vena cava.

D. Continuous wave Doppler echocardiography also uses Doppler shift of sound waves from moving red blood cells to assess flow velocity but is not range-gated; it samples velocities along the cursor line. It can be used in line with cross-sectional views or using a stand-alone "pencil" probe. To be accurate, both continuous and pulsed wave Doppler beams must be within 15 degrees of the direction of flow.

E. Color Doppler echocardiography simplifies accurate diagnosis and delineation of ductal patency. It also enables identification of

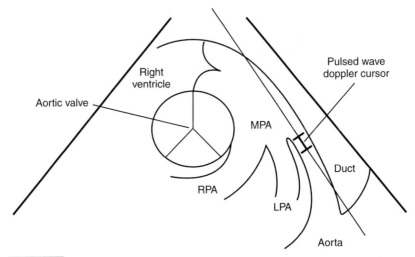

FIGURE 22-8. Short-axis parasternal pulmonary view showing the position of the pulsed wave Doppler cursor for sampling ductal flow velocity. LPA, left pulmonary artery; MPA, main pulmonary artery; RPA, right pulmonary artery.

tricuspid regurgitation and patency of the foramen ovale as well as the direction of flow. Flow velocity measurement is possible when it is used in conjunction with continuous or pulsed wave Doppler. It is used to measure ductal diameter.

VI. Indications for Echocardiographic Assessment
  A. Suspected congenital heart disease
  B. Suspected persistent pulmonary hypertension
  C. Suspected patent ductus arteriosus
  D. Hypotension or shock
  E. Asphyxia
  F. Suspected cardiac dysfunction
  G. Use of high positive end-expiratory pressure (PEEP)
  H. High-frequency oscillatory ventilation

VII. Cardiac Function
  A. Depressed ventricular function may occur in neonatal disease processes such as hypoxia, sepsis, hemolytic disease, hyaline membrane disease (RDS), persistent pulmonary hypertension, and transient tachypnea.
  B. A dysfunctional heart may be tachycardic, bradycardic, or have a normal rate. In hypotensive newborns, cardiac function may be depressed, normal, or even hyperdynamic.

VIII. Left Ventricular Assessment
  A. Cross-sectional and M-mode assessment
  B. Cross-sectional echocardiography permits accurate positioning of the M-mode beam just at the mitral leaflet tips in the long-axis (parasternal; see Fig. 22-1) or centered in the short-axis parasternal

views (see Fig. 22-2) of the left ventricle. Measurements must be taken from standard and reproducible positions; otherwise, increased variability will obscure the results.

C. On the M-mode picture (see Fig. 22-6), the interventricular septum (IVS), left ventricular internal diameter (LVID), and posterior wall dimensions are measured at end-systole (S) and end-diastole (D). From these measurements, several parameters of ventricular function can be calculated.

1. Fractional shortening characterizes left ventricular contractility, although it is also affected by preload and afterload.

$$\text{Fractional shortening (\%)} = \frac{\text{LVIDD} - \text{LVIDS}}{\text{LVIDD}} \times 100\%$$

Normal Ranges
25-45% in adults
25-41% in term babies
23-40% in preterm babies

Errors in estimation of fractional shortening may occur in early preterm life from distortion of the left ventricle and abnormal septal motion.

2. Circumferential fiber shortening: Mean velocity of circumferential fiber shortening (VCF) has been suggested as a simple alternative measurement of left ventricular contractility. It is less sensitive to minor dimensional discrepancies and involves no assumptions about ventricular shape, offering a reproducible measurement of neonatal ventricular contractility.

To calculate VCF, LVIDD and LVIDS are measured as above, but ejection time is measured from the time of mitral valve closure to the onset of mitral valve opening:

$$\text{VCF} = \frac{\text{LVIDD} - \text{LVIDS}}{\text{LVIDD} \times \text{ejection time}}$$

(Units are circumferences per second)

3. Stroke volume

a. Stroke volume measurement assumes an ellipsoidal ventricle. This is a reasonable assumption in adults but less so in neonates. Using measurements of left ventricular internal diameter in diastole (LVIDD) and systole (LVIDS), the stroke volume (SV) can be calculated:

$$\text{SV} = \text{LVIDD}^3 - \text{LVIDS}^3$$

b. Similarly, a proportion of ventricular contents or ejection fraction (EF) can be calculated:

$$EF = \text{stroke volume/end-diastolic volume}$$

$$= \frac{LVIDD^3 - LVIDS^3}{LVIDD^3}$$

4. Volume load assessment
   a. M-mode assessment of the left ventricle and atrial size provides information about changes in ventricular preload. The ratio of these chambers to the aorta is used to assess the effect of shunts on the heart, especially the ductus arteriosus.
   b. Normal left atrial–aortic ratio is 0.84:1.39 in preterm infants and 0.95:1.38 in term infants.
   c. Left atrial:aortic ratio >1.5 suggests volume loading.
   d. Left ventricular diastolic:aortic internal diameter ratio >2:1 suggests ventricular volume loading.
   e. It is important to realize that apparant volume loading actually may be due to poor contractility in a normovolemic neonate.

IX. Doppler Assessment of Systolic Function
   A. Stroke volume: Stroke volume is calculated from the product of the integral of the Doppler velocity-time curve (VTi, also known as stroke distance) (Fig. 22-9) and the cross-sectional area of the aorta (A = πd) derived from the M-mode diameter:

$$SV = VTi \times \Pi(\text{aortic diameter/2})^2$$

   B. Cardiac output: Multiplying SV by the heart rate (HR) produces the left ventricular cardiac output (CO):

$$CO = VTi \times \Pi(\text{aortic diameter/2})^2 \times HR$$

Note: Minute distance (MD = VTI × HR) is directly related to CO but removes the aortic diameter from the calculation, which is the major source of error. This can be used to assess changes in therapy in an individual.

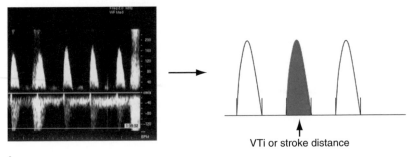

VTi or stroke distance

A

FIGURE 22-9. Aortic Doppler trace showing measurement of the integral of the velocity time curve (VTi), or stroke distance. A, Calculating the stroke distance (velocity time integral [Vti]) from Doppler trace.

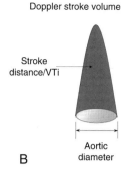

Doppler stroke volume

FIGURE 22-9, Cont'd. B, Calculating the stroke volume from stroke distance and aortic diameter.

Normal Ranges

Preterm	221 ± 56 mL/kg/min
Term	236 ± 47 mL/kg/min
Range	158-325 mL/kg/min

X. Right Ventricular Assessment
   A. The normal shape of the right ventricle is more complex than that of the left. It consists of inflow, outflow, and apical segments and is wrapped around the left ventricle.
   B. This makes quantitative evaluation by M-mode difficult in patients of any age and not useful in the newborn. However, qualitative information about right ventricular systolic function can be obtained by the experienced operator from cross-sectional views.
   C. Paradoxical movement of the intraventricular septum is seen in right ventricular dysfunction. Such movement prevents any assessment of left ventricular fractional shortening.
XI. Doppler Assessment of Systolic Function: One of the most important determinants of right ventricular systolic function in newborns is pulmonary arterial pressure. This can be estimated in several ways.
   A. Tricuspid regurgitation: If present, the most accurate assessment of right ventricular (and therefore pulmonary) pressure is obtained by measuring the velocity of the regurgitant jet (V). Then, assuming right atrial pressure is low,

$$\text{Pulmonary pressure} = 4V^2$$

   B. Ratio of pre-ejection period to right ventricular ejection time is related to pulmonary pressure and requires ECG monitoring while performing echoardiography. It is useful for assessment of babies with chronic lung disease but difficult to interpret acutely.
   C. Ratio of time to peak velocity to right ventricular ejection time is inversely related to pulmonary pressure, and measurement does not require ECG monitoring. A ratio of >0.3 indicates normal pulmonary pressures, and a ratio of <0.2 indicates pulmonary

hypertension. If the ratio is between these two, it is likely that the pulmonary pressure is mildly elevated.

   D. Ductal flow: If the ductus arteriosus is patent, the direction of flow (as well as the pattern) gives an indication of pulmonary pressure (i.e., right-to-left flow = pulmonary > systemic) (Fig. 22-10A-D). However, the velocity of flow cannot accurately predict pulmonary pressure.

   E. Foramen ovale: Right-to-left flow suggests high right-sided pressures or dysfunction. It is seen best in the subcostal view.

   F. Diastolic function

      1. Few studies of diastolic function have been carried out in children and infants.

      2. Right ventricular filling is modified by positive pressure ventilation and especially by high PEEP and oscillatory ventilation.

  XII. Assessment of the Patent Ductus Arteriosus (see Chapter 67)

   A. The ductus arteriosus is best seen in the parasternal short-axis view (see Fig. 22-3), although the suprasternal and subcostal approaches may be needed in babies with overdistended lungs. Color Doppler assessment simplifies identification and allows subjective assessment of flow and velocity. Doppler interrogation of the ductus arteriosus (Fig. 22-8) demonstrates the pattern of flow and the velocity profile. Velocity depends on both the size of the vessel and the pressure difference between the aorta and the pulmonary artery. The classic flow pattern associated with a large shunt is high in systole and low in diastole. The size can be estimated in cross-sectional view in relation to the branch pulmonary arteries or aorta.

   B. Ductal diameter can be assessed by measuring the narrowest waist of the ductal color flow when the view is frozen. Ensure maximal color Doppler scale, optimize the color gain, and then measure. In some units, this modality is used to predict which ducts are likely to be significant and require treatment. A diameter of >1.5 mm in the first 30 hours has 83% sensitivity and 90% specificity for ducts needing treatment.

   C. Measurement of the left atrium–aortic ratio (see preceding discussion) gives some indication of flow but may not be accurate if the left atrium decompresses through the foramen ovale. A ratio of >1.5 after the first day of life has sensitivity of 88% and specificity of 95% for ductus.

   D. A 60% increase in left ventricular output predicts development of significant ductus arteriosus.

   E. Echocardiographic evidence of a significant ductus arteriosus precedes clinical evidence. On day 3 of life it can predict significance with 100% sensitivity and 85% specificity.

   F. Assessment of descending aortic or celiac axis diastolic flow beyond ductal insertion:

      1. Normal: Continuous antegrade flow

      2. Abnormal: Absent or reversed diastolic flow

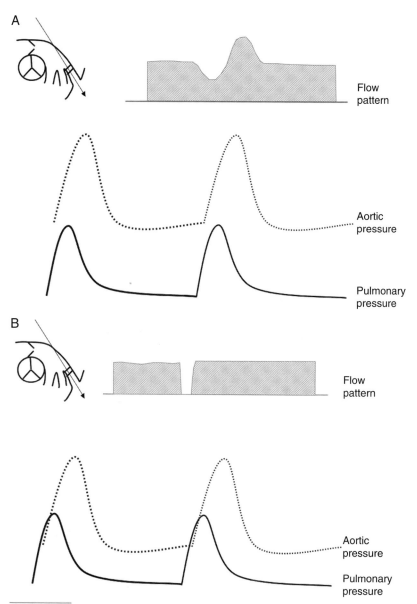

FiGURE 22-10. Ductal flow patterns associated with differing systemic and pulmonary pressures. A, Pulmonary pressure < aortic pressure; B, pulmonary pressure = aortic pressure in early systole; C, bidirectional flow, with pulmonary pressure > aortic pressure in early systole; D, pulmonary pressure > aortic pressure.

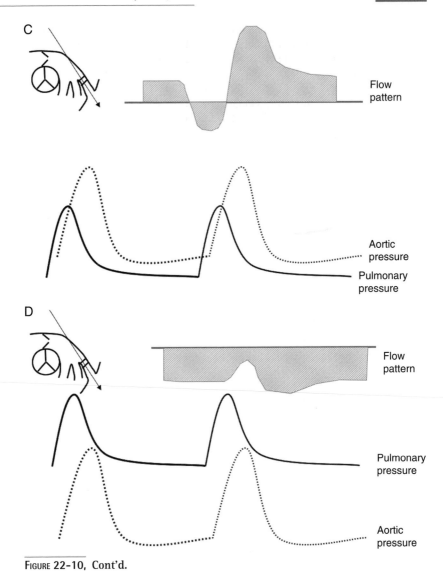

FIGURE 22-10, Cont'd.

XIII. Accuracy and Reproducibility
    A. M-mode measurements have been made using leading and trailing
        edges. In measurements of the left ventricle, both leading and
        trailing edges are used. Intraobserver variability for these
        measurements range from 5% for distances to 10% for calculated
        volumes. Interobserver variability is greater, ranging from 7% to
        25% for volume measurements.

B. Measurement of the aorta and left atrium by M-mode is more reproducible in newborns if it is made from trailing-to-leading echo edge (i.e., internal aortic diameter). Accuracy is vital, because an error of 1 mm in the measurement of an aorta with a 10-mm diameter will produce a 17% error in CO.

C. The main sources of errors in Doppler measurement are from the site of sampling and the angle of incidence of the Doppler wave. If the angle is >15 degrees, the error will be <3%. A further source of error in calculating cardiac output is coronary artery flow, which may cause an underestimate of 10% to 15% in flow.

Suggested Reading

Evans N, Kluckow M: Early determinants of right and left ventricular output in ventilated preterm infants. Arch Dis Child 74:F88-F94, 1996.

Gill AB, Weinding AM: Echocardiographic assessment of cardiac function in shocked very low birthweight infants. Arch Dis Child 68:17-21, 1993.

Hudson I, Houston A, Aitchison T, et al: Reproducibility of measurements of cardiac output in newborn infants by Doppler ultrasound. Arch Dis Child 65:15-19, 1990.

Skinner J, Alverson D, Hunter S (eds): Echocardiography for the Neonatologist. London, Churchill Livingstone, 2000.

Skinner JR, Boys RJ, Hunter S, Hey EN: Pulmonary and systemic arterial pressure in hyaline membrane disease. Arch Dis Child 67:366-373, 1992.

23 Bronchoscopy

Neil N. Finer

I. Equipment
  A. Flexible 2.2-mm or 2.7-mm bronchoscope
    1. Bronchoscope should be able to pass through a 2.5-mm or 3.0-mm endotracheal tube (ETT).
    2. Note that a 2.2-mm bronchoscope does not have suction channel.
  B. Appropriate light source (preferably xenon)
  C. Optional videocamera and recorder, as well as a microphone (allows determination of phase of respiration)
II. Patient Preparation
  A. Suction airway thoroughly.
  B. Medications
    1. Atropine (0.01 mg/kg) can be used to decrease secretions and block vagal-mediated bradycardia.
    2. Morphine (0.05 to 0.1 mg/kg) or meperidine (0.5 to 1.5 mg/kg) may be given for analgesia at least 10 to 15 minutes prior to procedure.
    3. For unintubated patients, apply topical lidocaine (Xylocaine) to one naris.
    4. For intubated infants, utilize a bronchoscopic adapter attached on the ETT connector to maintain FiO_2 and airway pressure during procedure.
    5. Inject lidocaine (4 to 7 mg/kg) at tip of ETT, using a feeding catheter, 3 minutes prior to procedure. Suction again just prior to procedure.
  C. Follow principles of conscious sedation; continuously monitor:
    1. Pulse oximetry
    2. Blood pressure if possible
    3. Heart rate
    4. Respiratory rate
III. Indications: Emergent*
  A. Acute/subacute suspected airway obstruction or misplacement
    1. Mucus
    2. Blood
    3. Dislodged ETT, tube in main bronchus (usually right-sided), esophageal intubation
    4. Check ETT position after intubation if infant is unstable.

---

*Emergent bronchoscopy can be done in <2 min by an experienced operator.

B. Evaluation of airway obstruction in recently extubated infant

C. Performance of fiberoptic nasotracheal intubation in conditions with associated airway anomalies, including:

    1. Pierre Robin syndrome

    2. Goldenhar syndrome

IV. Procedure

    A. Premedicate—use only topical lidocaine and smallest dose of narcotic for fiberoptic intubation; initially, try with patient awake following atropine administration.

    B. Provide oxygen using a single nasal cannula or a laryngeal mask.

    C. Monitor as discussed earlier.

    D. Slide proper-size nasotracheal tube with proximal connector removed over bronchoscope and lodge at proximal end of bronchoscope.

    E. Visualize larynx via nares.

    F. Pass bronchoscope during inspiration through vocal cords to carina.

    G. Have assistant hold bronchoscope as straight as possible without pulling back.

    H. Slide ETT over bronchoscope until it is in trachea; check position as bronchoscope is being withdrawn, remove bronchoscope, and tape ETT in place.

    I. After taping, recheck position of ETT; it should be approximately 1 cm above carina in a 3-kg infant.

V. Indications: Elective

    A. Confirm ETT placement

    B. Stridor

    C. Persistent or recurrent atelectasis or wheezing in an intubated patient

    D. Evaluation of known or suspected tracheoesophageal fistula

    E. Placement of ETT for unilateral lung ventilation

    F. Placement of Fogarty catheter for unilateral ventilation for pulmonary interstitial emphysema

VI. Practical Clinical Hints

    A. Take the time to properly identify patient and ensure that consent form is signed.

    B. Examine patient and review procedure with staff.

    C. Always preoxygenate the patient and provide continuous oxygen during procedure, using a single nasal cannula.

    D. Use either oximeter audible tone or heart rate monitor audible tone to be aware of patient status during procedure.

    E. Videocamera recording can decrease procedure time.

    F. Consult with pediatric otolaryngologist when findings are in doubt, and whenever there is a suspicion of vocal cord lesions or other laryngeal abnormalities.

VII. Common Neonatal Diagnoses Amenable to Bronchoscopy (Table 23-1)

TABLE 23-1. Common Neonatal Diagnoses Amenable to Bronchoscopy

Upper Airway Lesions	Lower Airway Lesions
Unilateral and bilateral choanal atresia	Tracheomalacia
Laryngomalacia	Bronchomalacia
Laryngeal dyskinesia	Tracheal or bronchial granulations, mucus plugs, blood clots (especially in ECMO patients)
Subglottic narrowing, secondary to edema, web, stenosis	Obstructed, malpositioned, or dislodged endotracheal or tracheotomy tube
Vocal cord paralysis, unilateral or bilateral	Tracheoesophageal fistula
Laryngeal hemangioma, cystic hygroma	Tracheal stenosis or web
Laryngeal edema and/or inflammation	Abnormal tracheal anatomy, tracheal bronchus
Gastroesophageal reflux	
Laryngotracheoesophageal cleft	

ECMO, extracorporeal membrane oxygenation.

Suggested Reading

Berkowitz RG: Neonatal upper airway assessment by awake flexible laryngoscopy. Ann Otol Rhinol Larngol 107:75-80, 1998.

Bloch ED, Filston HC: A thin fiberoptic bronchoscope as an aid to occlusion of the fistula in infants with tracheoesophageal fistula. Anesth Analg 67:791-793, 1988.

Ellis DS, Potluri PK, O'Flaherty JE, Baum VC: Difficult airway management in the neonate: A simple method of intubating through a laryngeal mask airway. Paediatr Anaesth 9:460-462, 1999.

Etches PC, Finer NN: Use of an ultrathin fiberoptic catheter for neonatal endotracheal tube problem diagnosis. Crit Care Med 17:202, 1989.

Finer NN, Etches PC: Fibreoptic bronchoscopy in the neonate. Pediatra Pulmonol 7:116-120, 1989.

Finer NN, Muzyka D: Flexible endoscopic intubation of the neonate. Pediatr Pulmonol 1992; 1248-1251.

Lee YS, Soong WJ, Jeng MJ, et al: Endotracheal tube position in pediatrics and neonates: Comparison between flexible fiberoptic bronchoscopy and chest radiograph. Zhonghua Yi Xue Za Zhi 2002;65:341-344.

Reeves ST, Burt N, Smith CD: Is it time to reevaluate the airway management of tracheoesophageal fistula? Anesth Analg 1995;81:866-869.

Rotschild A, Chitayat D, Puterman ML, et al: Optimal positioning of endotracheal tubes for ventilation of preterm infants. Am J Dis Child. 1991;145:1007-1017.

Shinwell ES, Higgins RD, Auten RL, Shapiro DL: Fiberoptic bronchoscopy in the treatment of intubated neonates. Am J Dis Child 1989;143:1064-1065.

Vauthy PA, Reddy R: Acute upper airway obstruction in infants and children. Evaluation by the fiberoptic bronchoscope. Ann Otol Rhinol Laryngol 1980;89:417-418.

Noninvasive and Invasive Ventilatory Techniques

Continuous Positive Airway Pressure

24

Colin J. Morley

I. Definition
   A. Continuous positive airway pressure (CPAP) is positive pressure applied to the airways of a spontaneously breathing baby throughout the respiratory cycle.
   B. Positive end-expiratory pressure (PEEP) is pressure applied to the airways through an endotracheal tube using positive pressure mechanical ventilation during the expiratory phase of ventilation.
   C. CPAP and PEEP are used to treat babies with acute respiratory difficulty, mainly premature infants with respiratory distress syndrome (RDS). In particular, they are used to maintain lung volume and improve oxygenation. CPAP is also used to treat premature infants with apnea or airway obstruction.
II. Rationale for Use: CPAP and PEEP are needed to support the airways and avoid alveolar collapse to a level below functional residual capacity (FRC) for the following reasons:
   A. The newborn infant normally maintains a small PEEP in the airways in the first few hours and possibly days after birth.
   B. The newborn infant with lung disease and a low lung volume has two mechanisms to maintain FRC. First, the baby may breathe fast, which may shorten the expiratory time to stop the lung from emptying completely. Second, the baby may "grunt" during expiration. During these breaths the baby inspires as much as possible, closes the larynx to maintain the lung volume that has been achieved, and then contracts the abdominal muscles to increase intrathoracic pressure and prevent the alveoli and airways from collapsing. The baby then opens the larynx slightly and exhales through a narrowed larynx, maintaining pressure in the airway and creating the grunting expiration. If the baby tires and cannot maintain adequate laryngeal tone, or if the larynx is by-passed by an endotracheal tube, lung volume may decrease rapidly and hypoxia may result.
   C. Fluid is secreted by the alveolar epithelium before birth, and there is as much fluid in the lungs before birth as there is gas after birth. During labor, adrenergic hormones inhibit secretion and promote absorption. In term infants, the lung fluid leaves the air spaces during birth. Inflation of the lungs moves the liquid from the lung lumen into distensible perivascular spaces and away from the sites of

gas exchange. Postnatal clearance of lung liquid is much slower after premature birth and after cesarean section delivery.

The premature lung may even continue to secrete fluid into the alveoli, adding to the problems of maintaining alveolar patency. Elevated left atrial pressure and low plasma protein concentrations also slow the rate at which lung liquid is removed from potential air spaces. This means that the very premature infant has considerable difficulty producing and maintaining FRC. This is helped by CPAP/PEEP.

D. The FRC of a newborn lung is close to airway closing volume. Premature babies may have to work hard with each breath to maintain lung volume. This is helped by CPAP/PEEP.

E. Term infants generate large positive pressures (up to 100 cm H_2O) with the first few breaths in order to open the lung. Very premature infants are not able to do this because they are not strong enough to expand their stiff, surfactant-deficient, fluid-filled lungs, and the chest wall retracts with each inspiration.

F. The upper airway in the term infant is supported by a fat-laden superficial fascia and also actively held open by the pharyngeal muscles. In the premature infant, the pharynx is not so well stabilized and is more likely to collapse. Pharyngeal closure or narrowing can occur with relatively small changes in airway pressure. If there are large, negative pharyngeal pressures during inspiration, this may collapse the extrathoracic airway. Infants with periodic breathing easily develop obstruction of the pharynx, which is reversible by CPAP.

G. The premature infant has an immature lung structure with a relatively undeveloped internal architecture to maintain lung volume, so that it is not held open by internal support. The immature lung also has thicker and fewer alveolar septa. This reduces gas exchange.

H. The newborn's chest wall is very compliant—probably five times more than the normal lung tissue. The chest wall of the premature baby is so soft and flexible that it is incapable of holding the lung open during excessive inspiratory efforts, and the pull of the diaphragm and negative pressure generated distorts the chest wall and reduces the tidal volume.

I. The round shape of the premature infant's chest wall, with horizontal ribs, also reduces the potential for lung expansion. The diaphragm of the preterm infant is relatively flat and potentially less effective. During rapid eye movement (REM) sleep, there is loss of intercostal muscle activity. This destabilizes the chest wall, so that rib cage and abdominal respiratory movements are out of phase. This results in a further loss of end-expiratory lung volume. Atelectasis and airway closure develop easily, especially considering the relative paucity of collateral ventilation channels in the newborn.

J. Premature babies often have a patent ductus arteriosus. If there is a high pulmonary artery pressure, this shunts blood away from the lungs. As the pulmonary artery pressure falls, it shunts blood from the aorta to the pulmonary arteries and lungs. This increases the fluid in the lungs, making them less compliant, and predisposes to pulmonary edema.

K. Surfactant in normal lungs has two important functions:
1. It lowers the surface tension and facilitates lung expansion at birth.
2. It "solidifies" on the alveolar surface, increasing the surface pressure, and helps hold the lung open during expiration. Very immature lungs lack adequate surfactant so there is a tendency toward low lung volume or airway collapse during expiration. This results in a further loss of surfactant from the alveolar surface as the surface area falls and surfactant is extruded.

L. The epithelium of the collapsing lung is easily damaged, and plasma proteins exude onto the surface. This compounds the problem of inadequate surfactant by inhibiting its function.

M. A decrease in lung volume is associated with inadequate oxygenation, a persistently elevated alveolar-arterial oxygen gradient, and ventilation/perfusion mismatch, with increased arterial carbon dioxide levels. Oxygenation is related to the surface area of the lung. If this is reduced, oxygenation is compromised. Carbon dioxide diffuses more easily and elimination is primarily related to minute volume. This can be compromised by low lung volume and atelectasis.

N. Reduced arterial oxygen availability impairs the respiratory pump, including the diaphragm.

III. How CPAP or PEEP Improves Respiratory Function
A. CPAP reduces the chance of upper airway occlusion and decreases upper airway resistance by mechanically splinting it open. It increases the pharyngeal cross-sectional area and decreases genioglossus activity.
B. CPAP/PEEP alters the shape of the diaphragm and increases diaphragmatic activity.
C. CPAP/PEEP improves lung compliance and decreases airway resistance in the infant with unstable lung mechanics in whom the lungs are stiff and the FRC is low. This allows a greater tidal volume for a given negative pressure, with subsequent reduction in the work of breathing.
D. In a baby with stiff lungs, CPAP/PEEP increases the mean airway pressure. The associated increase in FRC improves lung surface area and ventilation-perfusion mismatch, and reduces oxygen requirements.
E. CPAP/PEEP conserves surfactant on the alveolar surface.
F. PEEP helps overcome the resistance of the endotracheal tube.
G. Successful extubation may be more likely to succeed if the baby is treated with nasal CPAP.

IV. Indications for CPAP or PEEP
A. PEEP must always be used if a baby is intubated. Zero PEEP is associated with a serious loss of lung volume.

B. Increased work of breathing:
1. Increased respiratory rate, usually more than 60 breaths/min, results when the baby tries to maintain lung volume by shortening the expiratory time.
2. Retractions of the lower ribs and sternum where the diaphragm inserts result from strong diaphragmatic contractions and a compliant chest wall.
3. Grunting results when the baby tries to maintain positive pressure in the lungs during expiration.
C. Need for increased inspired oxygen
D. Chest radiograph showing inadequately expanded or infiltrated lung fields, atelectasis, or pulmonary edema
E. Apnea of prematurity
F. Recent extubation
G. Tracheomalacia or abnormalities of the airways predisposing to airway collapse
V. How CPAP Can Be Given
A. The following devices have been used but are unsatisfactory.
1. Face mask
a. This can provide positive pressure throughout the respiratory cycle and has the benefit of no loss of pressure through the mouth.
b. It has several problems, including:
(1) It is difficult to get a good seal without excessive pressure on the baby's face.
(2) The mask has to be removed, and the pressure is lost when the mouth and nose are cleared by suction.
(3) It is difficult to pass a nasogastric or orogastric tube because of problems with forming a seal.
2. Head box with a neck seal
a. This was the original method devised by Gregory (1971).
b. Design included a seal around the neck with preset blow-off valves to control the pressure.
c. It had many problems, including:
(1) Difficult to get a good neck seal
(2) Poor access to baby's face
(3) Loss of pressure caused by any attention to baby's face
(4) High flow of gas cooling baby's head
(5) Very noisy
3. Negative pressure box
a. Various types have been designed.
b. It is a cuirass that encircles the chest and abdomen and maintains a negative pressure outside the lung to help resist the forces causing collapse.
c. Although effective, it has many practical problems.
(1) Difficult to get a good seal
(2) Poor access to baby's body
(3) Loss of pressure caused by any attention to baby's body
(4) High flow of gas cooling baby

B. The following devices are now used because they are more satisfactory.
   1. Nasal mask. This can be effective but is difficult to attach and get a good seal without undue pressure.
   2. Endotracheal tube (ETT)
      a. Whenever an ETT is used in an infant and the larynx is by-passed, PEEP should be applied to prevent loss of lung volume.
      b. An ETT should not be used solely for the purpose of delivering CPAP because the resistance makes it difficult for the baby to breathe effectively for more than a short while.
      c. Endotracheal CPAP may be used for a short while, just before extubation, to ensure that the baby does not become apneic as soon as inflations are stopped.
   3. Nasal prong(s)
      a. This is the most satisfactory (or least unsatisfactory) method of delivering CPAP.
      b. For the most part, newborns are obligatory nose breathers; therefore nasal CPAP is easily facilitated.
      c. This is accomplished by inserting nasopharyngeal tubes or nasal prongs.
         (1) One or two prongs are inserted into one or both nostrils and attached to a ventilator or other device for delivering CPAP. Binasal (double) prongs are more effective than a single long prong. A binasal device that is claimed to have a "fluidic flip" when the baby expires through the device is said to reduce the work of breathing, but there are few clinical data to substantiate any superiority over other devices, and there is no evidence that babies on binasal CPAP actually breathe out through the device unless the mouth and nose are held closed.
         (2) A single prong can be short, inserted into the nostril about 1.5 cm or inserted deep into the pharynx. Long nasal prongs have a higher resistance than short prongs and lose some of the applied pressure. They are more likely to become blocked by secretions.
VI. Which Levels of CPAP or PEEP Can Be Used?
   A. Because each baby's respiratory problems are unique, the level of CPAP/PEEP required needs to be individualized and should be altered to suit each baby's problems as they change. Using one pressure for all babies with different problems is not appropriate.
      1. If an infant has stiff lungs or a low lung volume, increasing CPAP/PEEP improves oxygenation. Some babies with very stiff lungs may need a higher pressure. However, if the pressure is too high, overdistention occurs, and the oxygenation may be compromised. The maximum pressure is not known but is probably at least 10 cm H_2O for a baby with stiff lungs.

2. Increasing CPAP/PEEP may increase $PaCO_2$ if the pressure is too high when the lung compliance is also high. A trade-off may be necessary between improving the oxygenation and increasing the $PaCO_2$. Conversely, if a baby with highly compliant lungs is treated with CPAP/PEEP and the $PaCO_2$ levels are high, reducing the pressure may improve the $PaCO_2$.

B. Ways to determine the appropriate level of CPAP or PEEP for a baby:

1. Look at the chest radiograph. Do the lungs look consolidated, atelectatic, or edematous, or are they well- or overexpanded? Higher or lower pressures may be required, depending on the problem seen.

2. Observe the baby—if retracting, tachypneic, or grunting, a higher pressure is needed to improve lung volume.

3. If oxygenation is the main problem, it will probably improve if the pressure is increased.

4. If CO_2 retention is the main problem, this may be secondary to overinflation from pressure that is too high. Consider reducing the pressure, but look at a chest radiograph first.

5. Increased hypoxia can also occur if the pressure is too high because the pulmonary blood vessels may be compressed.

6. Start CPAP at 4 to 5 cm H_2O and gradually increase up to 10 cm H_2O, as required, to improve oxygenation and stabilize the chest wall while maintaining appropriate gas exchange (pH > 7.25 and $PaCO_2$ < 60 mm Hg [8 kPa]).

7. For PEEP, applied through an ETT, the same criteria apply.

VII. Use of CPAP Post Extubation

A. Several studies have shown that very premature babies breathe and oxygenate better and are less likely to need reintubation, particularly if they were ventilated for RDS, if they are treated with nasal CPAP immediately after extubation. This may occur because the larynx has been stretched, is edematous, and is not functioning properly during the first few hours after extubation. Alternatively, CPAP helps to maintain airway patency and alveolar distention and lower the work of breathing.

VIII. When CPAP Should Not Be Used

A. A baby who is apneic should be intubated and ventilated

B. The need for intubation or ventilation because the baby has ventilatory failure—inability to maintain oxygenation with an FiO_2 >0.6, a $PaCO_2$ >60 mm Hg (8 kPa), and pH <7.25

C. Upper airway abnormalities (cleft palate, choanal atresia, tracheoesophageal fistula)

D. Severe cardiovascular instability

E. Unstable respiratory drive with frequent apneas and or bradycardias

IX. Hazards/Complications of CPAP and PEEP

A. Obstruction of the nose or nasal tubes with secretions so that the baby mouth breathes and gets less oxygen and pressure than expected

  B. CPAP applied to a compliant lung may cause overdistention of the lung and reduce the tidal volume. It may also lead to:
    1. Air leaks
    2. CO_2 retention
    3. Hypoxia
    4. Increased work of breathing
    5. Impedance of pulmonary blood flow with subsequent increased pulmonary vascular resistance and decreased cardiac output
    6. Gastric distention (This is not a big problem as long as the baby has an orogastric tube, left open to atmosphere, and any residual gas is aspirated regularly. Concern about gastric distention from gas is not a reason to withhold enteral feeding.)
    7. Nasal irritation, damage to the septum, and mucosal damage
    8. Skin irritation and necrosis or infection of the face from the fixation devices
    9. Failure of the disconnect alarms because of the increased resistance in the tube or obstruction in the tubes continuing to measure a high pressure
    10. Inadvertent decannulation of the CPAP device from the nose

X. Inadvertent PEEP
  A. The development of inadvertent PEEP may be a problem in ventilated babies in whom the expiratory time is so short that there is inadequate time for full expiration.
  B. This can be a problem in several situations:
    1. Term babies with "normal" lungs (i.e., babies undergoing surgery).
    2. Babies with normally expanded lungs on the chest radiograph.
    3. Babies with gas trapping (e.g. meconium aspiration syndrome or chronic lung disease).
  C. Clinically, this can be recognized from the chest radiograph and because oxygenation deteriorates as the pressure is increased.
  D. Except in babies with chronic lung disease, an expiratory time of 0.5 seconds will usually be sufficient.
  E. It must be recognized that babies frequently shorten their own expiratory time by increasing the respiratory rate in order to create their own intrinsic PEEP.

XI. Weaning Babies from CPAP
  A. There is no good evidence for how long CPAP should be used.
  B. The pressure required and the length of time that CPAP is used has to be determined by personal observation of the baby, the observations of attending nurses, and clinical experience.
    1. In babies who are not having apneic or bradycardic episodes and require a low inspired oxygen concentration, management without CPAP can be tried. It is a matter of trial and error to see how they manage.
    2. Conversely, babies who require a high level of inspired oxygen and are clinically unstable will probably benefit from continuing with CPAP.
  C. Some babies appear to be able to breathe well without CPAP but then tire after a few hours; their FiO_2 increases, and apnea and bradycardia occur.

Suggested Reading

AARC Clinical Practice Guideline: Application of continuous positive airway pressure to neonates via nasal prongs or nasopharyngeal tube. Respir Care 39:817-823, 1994.

Alex CG, Aronson RM, Onal E, Lopata M: Effects of continuous positive airway pressure on upper airway and respiratory muscle activity. J Appl Physiol 62:2026-2030, 1987.

Bartholomew KM, Brownlee KG, Snowden S, Dear PRF: To PEEP or not too PEEP. Arch Dis Child 70:F209-F212, 1994.

Da Silva WJ, Abbasi S, Pereira G, Bhutani VK: Role of positive end-expiratory pressure changes on functional residual capacity in surfactant treated preterm infants. Pediatr Pulmonol 18:89-92, 1994.

De Paoli A, Lau R, Davis PG, Morley CJ: Pharyngeal pressure in preterm infants receiving nasal continuous positive airway pressure. Arch Dis Child Fetal Neonatal Ed 90:F79-F81, 2005.

De Paoli AG, Morley C, Davis PG: Nasal CPAP for neonates: What do we know in 2003? Arch Dis Child Fetal Neonatal Ed 88:F168-F172, 2003.

De Paoli AG, Morley CJ, Davis PG, et al: In vitro comparison of nasal continuous positive airway pressure devices for neonates. Arch Dis Child Fetal Neonatal Ed 87:F42-F45, 2002.

Gregory GA, Kitterman JA, Phibbs RH, et al: Treatment of the idiopathic respiratory distress syndrome with continuous positive airway pressure. N Engl J Med 284:1333-1340, 1971.

Klausner JF, Lee AY, Hutchinson AA: Decreased imposed work with a new nasal continuous positive airway pressure device. Pediatr Pulmonol 22:188-194, 1996.

Kosch PC, Stark AR: Dynamic maintenance of end-expiratory lung volume in full term infants. J Appl Physiol 57:1126-1133, 1984.

Morley C: Continuous distending pressure. Arch Dis Child Fetal Neonatal Ed 81:F152-F156, 1999.

Robertson NJ, McCarthy LS, Hamilton PA, Moss ALH: Nasal deformities resulting from flow driver continuous positive airway pressure. Arch Dis Child 75:F209-F212, 1996.

So B, Tamura M, Mishina J, et al: Application of nasal continuous positive airway pressure to early extubation in very low birthweight infants. Arch Dis Child 72:F191-F193, 1995.

Verder H, Robertson B, Griesen G, et al: Surfactant therapy and nasal continuous positive airway pressure for newborns with respiratory distress syndrome. N Engl J Med 331:1051-1055, 1994.

Vilstrup CT, Bjorklund LJ, Larsson A, et al: Functional residual capacity and ventilation homogeneity in mechanically ventilated small neonates. J Appl Physiol 73:276-283, 1992.

Noninvasive Ventilation

25

Eugene M. Dempsey and Keith J. Barrington

I. Definition
   A. A mode of assisted ventilation that delivers positive pressure throughout the respiratory cycle with additional phasic increases in airway pressure, without the presence of an endotracheal tube (ETT) in the trachea. These additional phasic increases in airway pressure can be either synchronized or nonsynchronized, depending on the delivery system used.
   B. The terminology in the area of noninvasive ventilation is confusing. Some of the more common terms include:
      1. NV (nasal ventilation)
      2. NIMV (nasal intermittent mandatory ventilation)
      3. SNIMV (synchronized nasal intermittent mandatory ventilation)
      4. NPSIMV (nasopharyngeal synchronized intermittent mandatory ventilation)
      5. NPPV (noninvasive positive pressure ventilation)
      6. BiPAP (bilevel positive airway pressure) systems used in older patients have a similar underlying rationale, with a system allowing spontaneous breathing throughout the respiratory cycle and patient triggering of the inspiratory phase.
II. Mode of Action
   A. Nasal ventilation provides the benefits of continuous positive airway pressure (CPAP) and also additional positive pressure breaths. CPAP splints the airway throughout the respiratory cycle, increases functional residual capacity, provides effective chest wall stabilization, and improves ventilation-perfusion mismatch and thereby improves oxygenation.
   B. Compared to CPAP, synchronized NIMV delivers larger tidal volumes by enhancing transpulmonary pressure during inspiration, and also probably secondary to augmented inspiratory reflexes and sigh breaths.
      1. Synchronized NIMV leads to a reduction in respiratory rate and respiratory effort and at the same time leads to a reduction in $PaCO_2$.
      2. It also provides enhanced chest wall stabilization, as evidenced by decreased asynchronous thoracoabdominal motion.
      3. The physiologic effects of nonsynchronized NIMV have not been studied in detail, but this modality may actually trigger respiratory efforts owing to Head's paradoxical reflex and may provide assisted ventilation during apneic spells, as long as the airway is patent.

III. How Noninvasive Ventilation Can Be Delivered

    A. Airflow can be delivered via binasal prongs, or a by single prong placed with the tip in the nose or nasopharynx. Nasal ventilation can be delivered in either a synchronized or nonsynchronized mode. Use of a face mask held in place by a device or netting around the head is not recommended because it has been associated with cerebellar hemorrhage.

    B. Nonsynchronized nasal ventilation can be delivered from any ventilator type. Synchronized nasal ventilation can be delivered only by respirators with specific triggering devices. These triggering devices include abdominal pressure capsules (Infant Star with Star Sync mode) and flow sensors (Ginevri MOG 2000). The latter system analyzes the flow from the sensor to eliminate flow from leaks from the mouth and nose, thereby the variation in the signal is related only to the patient's inspiration. Use of flow sensors has not been successful in extubated infants, as the leaks are huge and very variable, leading to major difficulty in synchronization.

    C. The Infant Flow Advance system is a variation of the variable flow CPAP systems that can deliver synchronized pressure support breaths triggered by an abdominal wall sensor of the same type as that used in the Infant Star.

IV. Indications for Use

    A. Postextubation: Four randomized, controlled trials demonstrated the efficacy of NIMV (all synchronized devices) compared to CPAP in the reduction of the need for reintubation following extubation. A meta-analysis of these studies revealed that three patients treated with NIPPV, prevent one extubation failure compared to post-extubation CPAP.

    B. Apnea of prematurity: Two studies compared CPAP with NIMV (both nonsynchronized) specifically for the treatment of apnea of prematurity. Both of these were short-term studies (over 4 to 6 hours) and results were conflicting. It is not clear whether NIMV will reduce the frequency of apnea more effectively than NCPAP. The postextubatiion studies noted above do seem to show a reduction in apnea with NIMV compared to CPAP.

    C. Primary mode of ventilation for respiratory distress syndrome (RDS): There are no studies addressing this mode of ventilation as a primary therapeutic intervention for the treatment of mild RDS, and therefore the routine use of NIMV for the treatment of RDS cannot be recommended at present. However future studies addressing this use are warranted.

V. Settings

    A. The settings chosen depend on the indication for assisted ventilation. One study (postextubation) commenced with a PEEP of 6 cm H_2O and a peak inspiratory pressure to a maximum of 16 cm H_2O. With these settings, there was no increase in abdominal distention or feeding intolerance compared to CPAP alone.

Individual patients may require higher PEEP (up to 7 to 8 cm H_2O on occasion). A respiratory rate of 15 breaths/min with an inspiratory time of 0.4 seconds is usually sufficient.

B. The settings chosen for apnea of prematurity are generally lower for this subgroup of patients, at least in the absence of significant lung disease. When the pulmonary status is normal, it may be effective with a peak inspiratory pressure of 10 to 12 cm H_2O, and a PEEP between 4 and 6 cm H_2O, the higher PEEP being used to prevent airway closure during apnea in some infants.

VI. Benefits

A. Avoidance of ETT placement and a reduction in the duration of endotracheal intubation, resulting in a decreased risk of airway problems and nosocomial respiratory infections

B. Reduction in need for reintubation following extubation

C. Reduction in apnea frequency following extubation

D. Possible reduction in chronic lung disease (CLD). There was a trend toward a reduction in the incidence of CLD in the two studies included in a meta-analysis of postextubation NIMV. This important possibility needs to be addressed in an adequately powered study with CLD as a primary end point.

VII. Potential Complications

A. Abdominal distention secondary to flow delivered preferentially to the stomach. This risk is higher with nonsynchronized breaths because flow cannot enter the upper airway against a closed glottis. An orogastric tube in situ may attenuate this risk.

B. Gastric perforation was associated with the use of NIMV in a case control study of 15 patients, in whom NIMV was being used as primary therapy for severe RDS. However, five subsequent randomized trials totaling over 230 patients have not reported a single case of gastric perforation.

C. Tube displacement or blockage secondary to secretions can result in impaired ventilation or oxygenation.

D. Pneumothorax and other air leaks may occur (although none have been reported in randomized studies to date).

E. Nasal erosion may result from the prongs, face mask, or ETT.

F. Skin necrosis may occur secondary to securing of nasal prongs, face mask, or ETT.

VIII. Unanswered Questions

A. A number of key areas remain that need to be addressed.
1. Is synchronization a necessary requirement for this mode of ventilation? If so, can we improve these systems to deliver synchronous breaths?
2. Can NIMV be used as a safe mode for primary treatment of RDS and so prevent intubation?
3. Are clinically important outcome variables (mortality and CLD rates) improved?

B. Future studies of NIMV will need to address these important issues.

Suggested Reading

Barrington KJ, Bull D, Finer NN: Randomized trial of nasal synchronized intermittent mandatory ventilation compared with continuous positive airway pressure after extubation of very low birth weight infants. Pediatrics 107:638-641, 2001.

Davis PG, Lemyre B, de Paoli AG: Nasal intermittent positive pressure ventilation (NIPPV) versus nasal continuous positive airway pressure (NCPAP) for preterm neonates after extubation. Cochrane Database Syst Rev (3):CD003212, 2001.

De Paoli AG, Davis PG, Lemyre B: Nasal continuous positive airway pressure versus nasal intermittent positive pressure ventilation for preterm neonates: A systematic review and meta-analysis. Acta Paediatr 92:70-75, 2003.

Friedlich P, Lecart C, Posen R, et al: A randomized trial of nasopharyngeal-synchronized intermittent mandatory ventilation versus nasopharyngeal continuous positive airway pressure in very low birth weight infants after extubation. J Perinatol 19:413-418, 1999.

Garland JS, Nelson DB, Rice T, Neu J: Increased risk of gastrointestinal perforations in neonates mechanically ventilated with either face mask or nasal prongs. Pediatrics 76:406-410, 1985.

Khalaf MN, Brodsky N, Hurley J, Bhandari V: A prospective randomized, controlled trial comparing synchronized nasal intermittent positive pressure ventilation versus nasal continuous positive airway pressure as modes of extubation. Pediatrics 108:13-17, 2001.

Kiciman NM, Andreasson B, Bernstein G, et al: Thoracoabdominal motion in newborns during ventilation delivered by endotracheal tube or nasal prongs. Pediatr Pulmonol 25:175-181, 1998.

Lemyre B, Davis PG, de Paoli AG: Nasal intermittent positive pressure ventilation (NIPPV) versus nasal continuous positive airway pressure (NCPAP) for apnea of prematurity. Cochrane Database Syst Rev (1):CD002272, 2002.

Lin CH, Wang ST, Lin YJ, Yeh TF: Efficacy of nasal intermittent positive pressure ventilation in treating apnea of prematurity. Pediatr Pulmonol 26:349-53, 1998.

Moretti C, Gizzi C, Papoff P, et al: Comparing the effects of nasal synchronized intermittent positive pressure ventilation (nSIPPV) and nasal continuous positive airway pressure (nCPAP) after extubation in very low birth weight infants. Early Hum Dev 56:167-177, 1999.

Moretti C, Marzetti G, Agostino R, et al: Prolonged intermittent positive pressure ventilation by nasal prongs in intractable apnea of prematurity. Acta Paediatr Scand 70:211-216, 1981.

Ryan CA, Finer NN, Peters KL: Nasal intermittent positive-pressure ventilation offers no advantages over nasal continuous positive airway pressure in apnea of prematurity. Am J Dis Child 143:1196-1198, 1989.

Intermittent Mandatory Ventilation

26

Steven M. Donn and Sunil K. Sinha

I. Description
   A. Definition: Intermittent mandatory ventilation (IMV) provides a fixed rate of mechanical ventilation, determined by the clinician, and allows spontaneous breathing between mechanical breaths. This mode may be utilized in the acute care phase (high rates) or the weaning phase (low rates). This mode historically has been called time-cycled, pressure-limited ventilation (TCPLV).
   B. Characteristics
      1. Mandatory breaths occur at fixed intervals determined by the preset breath rate (BR), or breaths per minute (BPM). Total cycle time is the BR divided by 60 sec/min.
      2. The mandatory tidal volume (V_T) from breath to breath is determined by the preset pressure limit (PL), flow, and inspiratory time (T_I), as well as by the patient's compliance (C_L) and airway resistance (R_{AW}).
      3. V_T may not be stable from breath to breath, particularly if the patient is breathing asynchronously with the ventilator.
      4. The patient may breath spontaneously between mandatory breaths from a flow of gas, with a preset oxygen fraction (FiO_2), provided by the ventilator (continuous and/or demand flow).
      5. The spontaneous BR, V_T, peak flow, and T_I are determined by the patient.
      6. The baseline pressure (positive end-expiratory pressure [PEEP]) may be increased to a preset level to enhance the patient's oxygenation.
   C. Indications
      1. Hypoxemic respiratory failure—PaO_2 <50 mm Hg (6.7 kPa) while receiving FiO_2 of 0.5
      2. Hypercapnic respiratory failure—$PaCO_2$ >60 mm Hg (8 kPa)
      3. Unstable cardiovascular status (bradycardia, hypotension)
      4. Impaired respiratory drive (apnea, neurologic impairment)
      5. Excessive work of breathing (impaired pulmonary function, airway obstruction)
   D. Management of potential complications
      1. Overdistention/barotrauma/volutrauma
         a. If possible, avoid PL settings >35 cm H_2O. Wean pressure aggressively.

    b. The risk of barotraumas as well as intraventricular hemorrhage in preterm infants increases when the infant is breathing asynchronously with the ventilator. Consider use of sedation and/or paralytics.

  2. Cardiovascular compromise

    a. The risk increases at mean airway pressures >15 cm H_2O. Avoid excessive ventilator settings whenever possible.

    b. Additional medical management of hypotension and/or hypovolemia may be required.

  3. Airway complications include upper airway trauma, endotracheal tube malpositioning, and tube obstruction from plugging or kinking

    a. Endotracheal tubes and ventilator circuits should be firmly secured to avoid excessive movement.

    b. Lavage and suction should be performed when the physical assessment indicates the need for these procedures and is most safely accomplished by two people.

  4. Oxygen toxicity

    a. Utilize optimal mean airway pressure and PEEP to improve oxygenation.

    b. Wean from oxygen as quickly as possible.

  5. Ventilator-acquired infection

    a. Infection control policies and procedures should be strictly followed.

    b. Prophylactic use of antibiotics is a common practice, although of unproved efficacy and is potentially risky.

II. Controls, Monitors, and Alarms

  A. Controls

    1. Breath rate (BR)

      a. BR adjusts the number of mandatory (i.e., ventilator-controlled breaths) delivered each minute.

      b. Conventional ventilators typically have a range of zero (continuous positive airway pressure [CPAP]) to 150 BPM.

      c. The initial BR generally will be between 30 and 40 BPM; however, rates up to 60 BPM may be necessary.

    2. Pressure limit (PL)

      a. The PL adjusts the peak inspiratory pressure applied to the airway during the inspiratory phase. It is the primary determinant of the delivered V_T (i.e., the depth of inspiration).

      b. Typically, the adjustable range will be 3 to 80 cm H_2O.

      c. The PL is usually started at the lowest level (e.g., 15 to 20 cm H_2O) necessary to produce adequate breath sounds and chest excursions and adjusted upward in increments of 1 to 2 cm H_2O.

      d. If the ventilator system in use has a V_T monitor, the PL may be set to achieve a desired V_T based on the infant's weight. General standards are 4 to 6 mL/kg for very-low-birth-weight (VLBW) infants, 5 to 7 mL/kg for low-birth-weight (LBW) infants , and 6 to 8 mL/kg for term infants.

    3. Inspiratory time (T_I)

     a. T_I adjusts the length of time that pressure is applied to the airway during inspiration (i.e., the length of the inspiratory phase).

     b. The adjustable range typically is 0.1 to 3.0 seconds.

     c. Initial T_I generally ranges from 0.3 to 0.5 seconds. A shorter T_I may be required if BR is >60 BPM.

  4. Flow rate

     a. This control generally has a dual purpose. First, it adjusts the magnitude of flow directed to the airway during the inspiratory phase of each breath. It also determines the flow available for spontaneous breathing between mandatory breaths. Some ventilators automatically adjust the flow available for spontaneous breathing to a value lower than the preset inspiratory flow to reduce expiratory resistance (R_E).

     b. The range of flow varies among ventilators. The low end is usually 2 to 3 liters per minute (L/min) with the high end 20 to 30 L/min and, in some cases, up to 40 L/min.

     c. To avoid excessive R_E, the flow rate should be set to the lowest value that will generate the desired inspiratory pressure and pressure or flow waveforms. The preset flow rate typically will be 5 to 8 LPM for preterm infants and up 10 to 12 L/min for term infants.

B. Monitors and alarms

  1. The peak inspiratory pressure (PIP) monitor reflects the highest pressure recorded during the inspiratory phase of mandatory breaths. It reflects the PL control setting and, therefore, it usually does not vary from breath to breath. Ventilators also have an airway pressure gauge which reflects the dynamic increase and decrease in pressure between the PL and PEEP (ΔP or amplitude).

     a. The High Pressure alarm, usually set 5 to 10 cm H_2O above the PL setting, is activated audibly and visually by an increase in airway pressure.

     b. The Low Pressure alarm, usually set 5 to 10 cm H_2O below the peak pressure, is activated audibly by a patient circuit leak or disconnection.

     c. The Low PEEP alarm is set 2 to 3 cm H_2O below the PEEP setting. It also is activated by a patient circuit leak or disconnect.

  2. The Mean Airway Pressure monitor reflects the average pressure applied over time (i.e., a moving average). This monitor responds to changes in the PL, BR, T_I, flow, and PEEP settings.

  3. In IMV, the BR and T_I monitors reflect the control settings for these parameters. The Expiratory Time (T_E) and I:E Ratio monitors reflect calculated values based on the T_I and BR settings. I:E ratio and T_E are valuable in assessing the risks of air trapping and inadvertent or auto-PEEP.

  4. The Apnea alarm reflects decreases in respiratory rate. Often the Apnea alarm is factory-preset at 20 seconds but may be adjustable from 10 seconds to 2 minutes on some ventilators.

  5. Neonatal ventilators do not always include an oxygen analyzer. However, a stand-alone monitor may be added externally.

Most monitors include high and low FiO_2 alarms that are usually set 0.05 above and below the preset level.

6. Most present-generation ventilators include V_T and minute volume monitors, either built in or as external options. Inspiratory/expiratory V_T is the volume (in milliliters) inspired or expired per breath. When both are provided, the degree of airway leak can be assessed. Minute volume is the volume exhaled during a 1-minute time frame.

    a. The V_T monitor is a valuable tool for titrating the PL setting to achieve an optimal V_T based on patient weight (see preceding discussion).

    b. The Low Minute Volume alarm can be activated by a significant drop in V_T or BR or by a leak/disconnection in the patient circuit. It may be set 20% to 25% below the prevailing minute volume.

7. An early sign of failure to wean from mechanical ventilation may be tachypnea. Some ventilator monitoring systems may include a High Breath Rate alarm or a High Minute Volume alarm that is activated by this situation.

8. Most ventilators include alarms for loss of air and/or oxygen gas pressure, loss of electrical power, and ventilator inoperative conditions. These alarm conditions should be addressed immediately because patient compromise is highly likely.

III. Positive End-Expiratory Pressure (PEEP)

   A. PEEP enhances lung volume (functional residual capacity [FRC]) by preventing the collapse of alveoli at end-expiration. Increases in PEEP increase mean airway pressure, which correlates with improvement in oxygenation.

   B. The range of PEEP available on most ventilators is 1.0 to 25 cm H_2O.

   C. PEEP should be started at moderate levels (4 to 6 cm H_2O) and changed in increments of 1 cm H_2O until the desired effect is achieved. In newborns, PEEP levels higher than 10 cm H_2O are rarely utilized.

IV. Patient Management

   A. Ventilation

   1. The primary controls that adjust the level of ventilation are the amplitude ($\Delta P = PL - PEEP$) and BR.

   2. The PL should be adjusted to achieve adequate lung inflation and discourage atelectasis. Assessment of bilateral breath sounds, chest excursion, exhaled V_T, and chest radiography can guide subsequent adjustments.

   3. Once adequate lung inflation has been achieved, BR should be adjusted for $PaCO_2$ and pH within target ranges.

   B. Oxygenation

   1. The primary parameters that affect oxygenation are FiO_2 and P_{AW}.

   2. FiO_2 should be maintained below 0.6, if possible, to avoid an increased risk of oxygen toxicity.

   3. Excessive PEEP levels should be avoided to reduce the risk of cardiovascular compromise.

4. Mean airway pressure correlates with oxygenation. Increases in T_I may improve oxygenation, without changes in FiO_2 or PEEP and without significantly changing the patient's ventilation status.

C. Weaning (see Chapter 58)

1. As the patient's C_L increases, delivered V_T will increase. To avoid overinflation, the PL should be decreased 1 to 2 cm H_2O for minor adjustments and 3 to 5 cm H_2O for moderate adjustments, to a minimum of 12 to 15 cm H_2O.

2. BR should be decreased in increments of 3 to 5 BPM for slight adjustments in $PaCO_2$ and 5 to 10 BPM for moderate adjustments, to a minimum of 5 to 10 BPM.

3. PEEP should be reduced in increments of 1 to 2 cm H_2O, to a minimum of 2 to 3 cm H_2O.

4. FiO_2 should be reduced aggressively to less than 0.4.

5. Once ventilator parameters have been weaned to minimum values, readiness for extubation may be assessed. Evaluation of respiratory parameters, chest radiography, airway clearance, and hemodynamics can aid the decision process.

Suggested Reading

Aloan CA, Hill TV: Respiratory Care of the Newborn, 2nd ed. Philadelphia, Lippincott, 1997.
Chatburn RL: Fundamentals of Mechanical Ventilation: A Short Course in the Theory and Application of Mechanical Ventilators. Cleveland Heights, OH, Mandu Press, 2003.
Donn SM (ed): Neonatal and Pediatric Pulmonary Graphics: Principles and Clinical Applications. Armonk, NY, Futura Publishing, 1998.
Goldsmith JP, Karatokin EH (eds): Assisted Ventilation of the Neonate, 4th ed. Philadelphia, WB Saunders, 2003.
Koff PB, Eitzman D, Neu J: Neonatal and Pediatric Respiratory Care. St. Louis, Mosby, 1993.
Whitaker KB: Comprehensive Perinatal and Pediatric Respiratory Care, 3rd ed. Albany, NY, Delmar Publishers, 2001.

27 Synchronized Intermittent Mandatory Ventilation

Steven M. Donn and Sunil K. Sinha

I. Description
   A. Synchronized intermittent mandatory ventilation (SIMV) is a ventilatory mode in which mechanical breaths are synchronized to the onset of a spontaneous patient breath (if trigger threshold is met) or are delivered at a fixed rate if patient effort is inadequate or absent. Spontaneous patient breaths between mechanically assisted breaths are supported by baseline pressure only.
   B. SIMV is a type of patient-triggered ventilation (PTV).
II. Cycling Mechanisms
   A. Time
   B. Flow
   C. Volume
III. Trigger Mechanisms
   A. Airway flow
      1. Differential pressure transducer
      2. Heated-wire anemometer
   B. Airway pressure
   C. Abdominal impedance
IV. SIMV Breath
   A. In SIMV, breathing time is divided into "breath periods" or "assist windows," based on the selected ventilatory rate.
   B. The first time a patient attempts to initiate a breath during an assist window (which begins immediately after a mechanically delivered breath), the ventilator delivers an assisted breath, provided that patient effort exceeds trigger threshold.
   C. Further attempts to breathe during the same assist window result only in spontaneous breaths, supported only by the baseline pressure.
   D. Mechanical breaths are delivered only if there is insufficient patient effort or apnea during the preceding assist window.
   E. Patient-controlled variables
      1. Spontaneous respiratory rate
      2. Inspiratory time (if flow-cycled)
   F. Clinician-controlled variables
      1. Peak inspiratory pressure (if pressure-targeted)
      2. Tidal volume delivery (if volume-targeted)

3. Inspiratory time (if time-cycled)
4. Flow
5. SIMV rate
  G. Flow-cycling
1. Inspiration is terminated at a percentage of peak flow rather than time.
2. Flow-cycling synchronizes the expiratory as well as the inspiratory phase, and thus total patient/ventilator synchrony can be achieved for assisted breaths.
V. Spontaneous Breath
  A. Supported by baseline pressure (positive end-expiratory pressure [PEEP]) only.
  B. Work of breathing is greater than for assist/control or pressure support ventilation.
  C. Observation of spontaneous tidal volume is a useful indicator of suitability for weaning.
VI. Patient Management
  A. Indications
1. Works best as a weaning mode, although many clinicians prefer using it to assist/control as a primary management mode.
2. Flow-triggering is especially useful in extremely-low-birth-weight infants.
3. Provides partial ventilatory support, because patient can breathe between mechanical breaths.
4. Synchrony can decrease need for sedatives/paralytics.
  B. Initiation
1. Use minimal assist sensitivity.
2. Set SIMV rate at a reasonable level to maintain adequate minute ventilation.
3. For flow-cycling, termination at 5% of peak flow generally works best, but check to see that the patient is receiving adequate tidal volume.
4. Other parameters are set as for IMV.
  C. Weaning
1. Primary weaning parameters include SIMV rate, peak inspiratory pressure (for time or flow cycling), and tidal volume (for volume cycling).
2. If $PaCO_2$ is too low, it is most likely the result of overventilation. Decrease the rate, pressure, or volume, depending on lung mechanics.
3. As patient status improves, spontaneous tidal volumes will increase, enabling lowering of the SIMV rate.
4. Can extubate directly from SIMV, or add or switch to pressure support ventilation (PSV).
5. Can also wean by increasing assist sensitivity, thus increasing patient work to increase tolerance.
VII. Problems
  A. Autocycling and false triggering
1. Leaks anywhere in the system (e.g., around the endotracheal tube, in circuit) can cause flow and pressure-triggered devices to misread this as patient effort, resulting in delivery of a mechanical breath.

    2. Abdominal impedance device may trigger as a result of artifactual motion.
- B. Failure to trigger
  1. Assist sensitivity too high
  2. Patient unable to reach trigger threshold
  3. Patient fatigue
- C. Inadequate inspiratory time (flow-cycling) results in inadequate tidal volume delivery. Patient may compensate by breathing rapidly.

Suggested Reading

Donn SM, Becker MA: Special ventilator techniques and modalities I: Patient-triggered ventilation. In Goldsmith JP, Karotkin EH (eds): Assisted Ventilation of the Neonate, 4th ed. Philadelphia, WB Saunders, 2003, pp 203-218.

Donn SM, Nicks JJ, Becker MA: Flow-synchronized ventilation of preterm infants with respiratory distress syndrome. J Perinatol 14:90-94, 1994.

Donn SM, Sinha SK: Controversies in patient-triggered ventilation. Clin Perinatol 25:49-62, 1998.

Sinha SK, Donn SM: Advances in neonatal conventional ventilation. Arch Dis Child 75: F135-F140, 1996.

Assist/Control Ventilation

28

Steven M. Donn and Sunil K. Sinha

I. Description
   A. Assist/control ventilation is a ventilatory mode in which mechanical breaths are either patient- (assist) or ventilator- (control) initiated.
   B. It is also referred to as patient-triggered ventilation (PTV).
II. Cycling Mechanisms
   A. Time
   B. Flow
   C. Volume
III. Trigger Mechanisms
   A. Airway flow
      1. Differential pressure transducer
      2. Heated-wire anemometer
   B. Airway pressure
   C. Thoracic impedance
   D. Abdominal impedance
IV. Assist Breath
   A. If patient effort exceeds trigger threshold, a mechanical breath is initiated.
      1. Trigger delay (response time) is the time from signal detection to rise in proximal airway pressure.
      2. A long trigger delay increases work of breathing because the patient may complete own inspiratory cycle before receiving mechanical breath.
   B. Patient-controlled variables
      1. Respiratory rate
      2. Inspiratory time (if flow-cycled)
   C. Clinician-controlled variables
      1. Peak inspiratory pressure (if pressure-limited)
      2. Tidal volume delivery (if volume-cycled)
      3. Inspiratory time (if time-cycled)
      4. Flow
      5. Control rate
   D. Flow-cycling
      1. Inspiration is terminated at a percentage of peak flow rather than time.
      2. Fully synchronizes patient and ventilator.
      3. Prevents inversion of inspiratory to expiratory ratio and minimizes gas trapping.

      4. May result in insufficient inspiratory time and tidal volume delivery.

V. Control Breath

    A. This is essentially back-up intermittent mandatory ventilation (IMV) in case of insufficient patient effort or apnea.

    B. Provides minimal minute ventilation if the patient is unable to trigger the ventilator or fails to breathe.

    C. If rate set too high, the patient may "ride" the ventilator and not breathe spontaneously.

    D. If the patient is consistently breathing above the control rate, lowering it has no effect on the mechanical ventilatory rate.

VI. Patient Management

    A. Indications

        1. Works well for virtually all patients.

        2. Flow-triggering is especially useful in extremely-low-birth-weight infants.

        3. Provides full ventilatory support.

        4. Synchrony can decrease need for sedatives/paralytics.

    B. Initiation

        1. Use minimal assist sensitivity.

        2. Set control rate at reasonable level until patient demonstrates reliable respiratory drive.

        3. For flow-cycling, termination at 5% of peak flow generally works best, but check to see that patient is receiving adequate tidal volume.

        4. Set other parameters as for IMV.

    C. Weaning

        1. Because reduction in ventilator rate will have no impact on minute ventilation if patient breathes above the control rate, the primary weaning parameter is peak inspiratory pressure.

        2. If $PaCO_2$ is too low, it is most likely the result of overventilation (too high a peak inspiratory pressure), as infant is unlikely to spontaneously hyperventilate. Lower the pressure.

        3. As soon as the patient demonstrates reliable respiratory drive, lower the control rate (20-30 breaths/min).

        4. Can extubate directly from assist/control or switch to synchronized intermittent mandatory ventilation (SIMV).

        5. Can also wean by increasing assist sensitivity, thus increasing patient work to increase tolerance.

VII. Problems

    A. Autocycling and false triggering

        1. Leaks anywhere in the system (e.g., around the endotracheal tube, in circuit.) can cause flow and pressure-triggered devices to misread this as patient effort, resulting in delivery of a mechanical breath.

        2. Thoracic impedance triggering may result in mechanical breaths secondary to cardiac impulses rather than respiratory motion.

        3. Abdominal impedance device may trigger as a result of artifactual motion.

B. Failure to trigger
  1. Assist sensitivity too high
  2. Patient unable to reach trigger threshold
  3. Patient fatigue
  4. Sedative drugs
C. Inadequate inspiratory time (flow-cycling) results in inadequate tidal volume delivery. Patient may compensate by breathing rapidly.

Suggested Reading

Donn SM, Nicks JJ: Special ventilator techniques and modalities I: Patient-triggered ventilation. In Goldsmith JP, Karotkin EH (eds): Assisted Ventilation of the Neonate, 3rd ed. Philadelphia, WB Saunders, 1996, pp 215-228.

Donn SM, Nicks JJ, Becker MA: Flow-synchronized ventilation of preterm infants with respiratory distress syndrome. J Perinatol 14:90-94, 1994.

Donn SM, Sinha SK: Controversies in patient-triggered ventilation. Clin Perinatol 25:49-62, 1998.

Sinha SK, Donn SM: Advances in neonatal conventional ventilation. Arch Dis Child 75: F135-F140, 1996.

29 Volume–Controlled Ventilation

Steven M. Donn and Kenneth P. Bandy

I. Description
  A. Volume-controlled ventilation (VCV) is a form of mechanical ventilation in which the inspiratory phase ends when a preset volume of gas has been delivered.
  B. Tidal volume may be monitored at the ventilator or (more accurately) at the patient airway.
  C. Because uncuffed endotracheal tubes are used in newborns, there may be a variable loss of delivered gas volume from leaks. It is thus more appropriate to describe this form of ventilation as volume-controlled, volume-limited, or volume-targeted, rather than volume-cycled ventilation.
II. Modes That Use VCV
  A. Intermittent mandatory ventilation (IMV)
  B. Synchronized intermittent mandatory ventilation (SIMV)
    1. Alone
    2. With pressure support ventilation (PSV)
  C. Assist/Control (A/C)
  D. Pressure-regulated volume control (PRVC)
  E. Volume-assured pressure support (VAPS)
  F. Mandatory minute ventilation (MMV)
  G. Volume guarantee (VG)
III. Characteristics of Volume-Controlled Breaths
  A. May be patient-triggered or machine-initiated.
    1. Pressure or flow trigger.
    2. May be at proximal airway or within ventilator.
  B. Flow-limited (fixed flow rate).
    1. Determines inspiratory time.
    2. Square flow waveform; some ventilators allow choice of decelerating flow.
    3. Some newer ventilators offer variable flow, but data regarding use in newborns are unavailable.
  C. Dependent variable is pressure.
    1. Low compliance will result in higher pressure delivery.
    2. As compliance improves, pressure will be auto-weaned.
    3. May be influenced by inspiratory flow setting.
  D. Tidal volume is guaranteed.
  E. Maximum alveolar distention depends on end-alveolar pressure.

IV. Advantages of VCV
   A. Consistent tidal volume delivery even in the face of changing compliance.
   B. Volume-limited breaths; avoidance of volutrauma.
   C. Combination with other modes to facilitate weaning.
      1. PSV
      2. VAPS
      3. MMV
V. Clinical Limitations-Minimal Tidal Volume Delivery
   A. Must know smallest tidal volume machine is capable of delivering.
   B. Should not exceed patient's physiologic tidal volume.
      1. <1000 g: 4 to 7 mL/kg
      2. >1000 g: 5 to 8 mL/kg
   C. Ventilator circuit should be of reasonable rigidity (compliance) so as not to cause excessive compressible volume loss in circuit if pulmonary compliance is low.
   D. Patients with smaller endotracheal tube (2.5 to 3.0 mm) may have difficulty triggering (especially if device is pressure-triggered).
   E. Flow-limitation may result in inadequate inspiratory time in smaller patients.
   F. Leaks
      1. May cause loss in baseline pressure.
      2. May result in autocycling.
VI. Clinical Indications
   A. Respiratory failure
      1. Persistent pulmonary hypertension of the newborn
      2. Meconium aspiration syndrome
      3. Sepsis/pneumonia
      4. Respiratory distress syndrome
      5. Congenital diaphragmatic hernia
      6. Pulmonary hypoplasia
      7. Congenital cystic adenomatoid malformation
   B. Ventilator-dependent cardiac disease with normal lungs
   C. Weaning infants recovering from respiratory illness
   D. Chronic lung disease (bronchopulmonary dysplasia)
VII. Initiating Volume Ventilation
   A. Select desired mode.
      1. SIMV or A/C is recommended for acute illness.
      2. SIMV and/or PSV is recommended for weaning.
   B. Select desired delivered tidal volume.
      1. <1000 g: 4 to 7 mL/kg
      2. >1000 g: 5 to 8 mL/kg
      3. Confirm that patient is receiving appropriate tidal volume.
         a. Volume monitoring
         b. Pulmonary graphics
            (1) Tidal volume waveform
            (2) Pressure-volume loop
   C. Set flow rate to achieve desired inspiratory time.
   D. Set mechanical ventilatory rate.

E. Set trigger sensitivity if using patient-triggered mode.
  1. Generally use minimal setting unless autocycling.
  2. Make sure that the patient is able to trigger the ventilator.
F. Some clinicians prefer to set a pressure limit; do not set this too close to peak pressure, or desired tidal volume may not be delivered.
G. Some ventilators have a leak compensation system. Although this is beneficial in maintaining a stable baseline in the presence of a leak, it may increase the work of breathing and possibly expiratory resistance.
H. Assessment of patient includes:
  1. Adequacy of breath sounds
  2. Adequacy of chest excursions
  3. Patient-ventilator synchrony
  4. Patient comfort
  5. Blood gases
  6. Pulmonary mechanics
VIII. Weaning Infants from VCV
A. As pulmonary compliance improves, inspiratory pressure will be automatically decreased to maintain set tidal volume delivery.
B. Adjustments in set tidal volume should be made to maintain desired tidal volume delivery.
C. Adjustments in flow rate may need to be made to maintain the same inspiratory time or I:E ratio.
D. If using A/C:
  1. Decrease control rate (allow patient to assume greater percentage of work of breathing).
  2. May also increase assist (trigger) sensitivity.
E. If using SIMV:
  1. Decrease SIMV rate, but remember that the patient receives no support for spontaneous breaths other than positive end-expiratory pressure.
  2. Consider adding pressure support (see Chapter 31), or even switching to it completely if the baby has consistently reliable respiratory drive.
F. Newer modes (VAPS, MMV) may prove more beneficial for weaning, but clinical experience using these modes in newborn infants has been limited.

Suggested Reading

Bandy KP, Nicks JJ, Donn SM: Volume-controlled ventilation for severe neonatal respiratory failure. Neonatal Intensive Care 5:70-73, 1992.

Donn SM: Alternatives to ECMO. Arch Dis Child 70:F81-84, 1994.

Donn SM, Becker MA: Baby in control: Neonatal pressure support ventilation. Neonatal Intensive Care 11:16-20, 1998.

Donn SM, Becker MA: Mandatory minute ventilation: A neonatal mode of the future. Neonatal Intensive Care 11:22-24, 1998.

Nicks JJ, Becker MA, Donn SM: Neonatal respiratory failure: Response to volume ventilation. J Perinatol 13:72-75, 1993.

Sinha SK, Donn SM: Volume-controlled ventilation. In Goldsmith JP, Karotkin EH (eds):
    Assisted Ventilation of the Neonate, 4th ed. Philadelphia, WB Saunders, 2003, pp 171-183.
Sinha SK, Donn SM, Gavey J, McCarty M: Randomized trial of volume controlled versus time
    cycled, pressure limited ventilation in preterm infants with respiratory distress syndrome.
    Arch Dis Child 77:F202-F205, 1997.
Tsai WC, Bandy KP, Donn SM: Volume-controlled ventilation of the newborn. In Donn SM (ed):
    Neonatal and Pediatric Pulmonary Graphic Analysis: Principles and Clinical Applications.
    Armonk, NY, Futura Publishing, 1998, pp 279-300.

30 Pressure Control Ventilation

Steven M. Donn

I. Description
   A. Pressure control (PC) was developed in the 1980s for the treatment of ARDS. It is now included in several neonatal ventilators.
   B. Mechanical breaths are delivered at a preset peak inspiratory pressure, but with a fixed inspiratory time and variable inspiratory flow, which distinguishes PC ventilation from traditional time-cycled, pressure-limited ventilation.
   C. It may be applied as intermittent mandatory ventilation (IMV), synchronized intermittent mandatory ventilation (SIMV) (with or without pressure support), or asssist/control (A/C).

II. Features
   A. Constant peak inspiratory pressure
   B. Variable tidal volume depending on patient lung mechanics
   C. Square or plateau pressure waveform
   D. Decelerating flow waveform
   E. Variable pressure rise time
      1. Rise time refers to the slope of the inspiratory pressure waveform.
      2. Rise time is a qualitative number.
      3. If slope is excessive, pressure overshoot may occur. This may be observed as a notch on the inspiratory limb of the pressure-volume loop.
      4. If slope is inadequate, there may be inadequate hysteresis on the pressure-volume loop.
   F. High flow rapidly pressurizes the ventilator circuit, resulting in rapid gas delivery and alveolar filling.

III. Clinical Applications
   A. Patients at risk for barotrauma but in need of high peak pressure
      1. Respiratory distress syndrome (RDS)
      2. Bronchopulmonary dysplasia (BPD)
      3. Meconium aspiration syndrome (MAS)
   B. Patients with large endotracheal tube leaks
   C. Patients with airway obstruction or high airway resistance

IV. Clinician-Set Parameters
   A. Peak inspiratory pressure
   B. Positive end-expiratory pressure (PEEP)
   C. Inspiratory time

TABLE **30-1.** Comparison of Pressure-Targeted Modalities

Parameter	Pressure-Limited	Pressure Control	Pressure Support
Limit	Pressure	Pressure	Pressure
Flow	Continuous, fixed	Variable	Variable
Cycle	Time or flow	Time	Flow
Breath type	Mechanical	Mechanical	Spontaneous

     D. Mode
     E. Rate
     F. FiO_2
     G. Trigger sensitivity
     H. Rise time
     I. Alarm limits
  V. Advantages
     A. Variable flow capability to meet patient demand
     B. Reduced inspiratory muscle workload
     C. Lower peak inspiratory pressures
     D. Adjustable inspiratory time
     E. Rapid filling of alveoli
     F. Improved gas distribution, V/Q matching, and oxygenation
 VI. Disadvantages
     A. Delivered tidal volume is variable and depends on the patient's lung mechanics, including changes in airway resistance and lung compliance.
     B. May have adverse effects on tidal volume delivery.
     C. Pressure overshoot may occur.
     D. Data are limited on use in newborns.
VII. Comparison with Other Pressure-Targeted Modalities (Table 30-1)

Suggested Reading

Donn SM, Sinha SK: Invasive and noninvasive neonatal mechanical ventilation. Respir Care 48:426-441, 2003.
Donn SM, Sinha SK: Newer techniques of mechanical ventilation: An overview. Semin Neonatol 7:401-408, 2002.

31 Pressure Support Ventilation

Sunil K. Sinha and Steven M. Donn

I. Description
   A. Pressure support ventilation (PSV) is a ventilatory mode in which spontaneous breaths are partially or fully supported by an inspiratory pressure assist above baseline pressure to decrease the imposed work of breathing created by the narrow lumen ETT, ventilator circuit, and demand valve.
   B. PSV is a form of patient-triggered ventilation (PTV); it may be used alone in patients with reliable respiratory drive, or in conjunction with synchronized intermittent mandatory ventilation (SIMV).
II. Cycling Mechanisms
   A. Time: Inspiratory time limit is chosen by the clinician.
   B. Flow: Termination of inspiratory cycle based on a percentage of peak flow. This varies according to both delivered tidal volume and specific algorithm of the ventilator in use. For most neonatal ventilators, this occurs at 5% of peak inspiratory flow.
III. Trigger Mechanisms
   A. Airway pressure change (minimum 1.0 cm H_2O)
   B. Airway flow change (minimum 0.2 L/min)
IV. Pressure Support Breath
   A. Pressure support breath is a spontaneous inspiratory effort that exceeds the trigger threshold initiates delivery of a mechanically generated pressure support breath.
   B. There is a rapid delivery of flow to the patient, which peaks and then decelerates.
   C. The airway pressure will rise to the pressure support level, set by the clinician as a value above baseline (positive end-expiratory pressure [PEEP]).
   D. When the flow-cycling criterion is met (decline to the termination level), the breath will ended and flow will cease. If this has not occurred by the end of the set inspiratory time limit, the inspiratory phase of the mechanical breath will be stopped.
   E. The amount of flow delivered to the patient during inspiration is variable and is proportional to patient effort.
   F. Patient-controlled variables
   1. Respiratory rate

2. Inspiratory time
3. Peak inspiratory flow
G. Clinician-controlled variables
   1. Pressure support level
   2. Inspiratory time limit
   3. Baseline flow
   4. Baseline pressure (PEEP)
   5. SIMV rate, flow, inspiratory time, and tidal volume or pressure limit (if SIMV is used)
V. Patient Management
   A. Indications
      1. PSV is designed primarily as a weaning mode to enable full or partial unloading of respiratory musculature during mechanical ventilation.
      2. PSV is fully synchronized with spontaneous breathing and can decrease the need for sedatives/paralytics.
   B. Initiation
      1. Use minimal assist sensitivity.
      2. The pressure support level can be adjusted to provide either full support (PS_{max}), delivering a full tidal volume, or at a lower level to provide partial support. Remember that the pressure support level is the pressure applied above baseline (i.e., a patient receiving 4 cm H_2O PEEP and 16 cm H_2O pressure support actually gets 20 cm H_2O peak inspiratory pressure).
      3. Set the inspiratory time limit for the pressure support breath.
      4. Set parameters for the SIMV breaths if they are to be used.
         a. These can be used analogously to control breaths during assist/control ventilation, providing a "safety net" of background ventilation in the event of inadequate effort (triggering) or apnea.
         b. If the SIMV rate is set too high, and the majority of minute ventilation is provided by SIMV, the patient may have no impetus to breathe, thus defeating the purpose of PSV.
   C. Weaning
      1. Weaning may be accomplished in a variety of ways:
         a. Decrease the SIMV rate to as low a level as possible, thus increasing spontaneous effort.
         b. Decrease the pressure support level, thus increasing the percentage of the work of breathing assumed by the patient.
         c. Consider the use of pressure support alone in patients with a reliable respiratory drive who have no difficulty triggering.
      2. Consider extubation when the pressure support level has been reduced to the point where it delivers about 4 mL/kg tidal volume, if the patient appears comfortable and is not tachypneic at this level.
VI. Problems
   A. Failure to trigger (may occur with small endotracheal tubes and inadequate patient effort)
   B. Pressure overshoot
   C. Premature termination

    D. A common error is using a high SIMV rate with PSV. This interrupts the synchrony of PSV and subjects the patient to a possibly unnecessary mandatory breath. If a high SIMV rate is needed, the patient may not be ready for PSV.

VII. Clinical Applications
    A. Weaning mode
    B. Chronic lung disease (CLD)
       1. Infants with CLD exhibit reactive airways with elevated inspiratory resistance.
       2. Pulmonary mechanics in most modes display a flattened inspiratory flow-volume loop.
       3. Variable inspiratory flow during PSV enables the patient to overcome increased inspiratory resistance and decreases ventilatory work.

VIII. Advantages of PSV
    A. Complete patient-ventilator synchrony.
    B. Decreased work of breathing compared to other modes:
       1. Same tidal volume is delivered at lower work of breathing.
       2. Larger tidal volume is delivered at same work of breathing.
    C. Adults treated with PSV have described increased comfort and endurance compared to other weaning modes.

IX. Additional Applications and Variations
    A. Volume-assured pressure support (VAPS)
       1. Has been used primarily in adults but is now available for use in infants.
       2. Combines features of volume-controlled ventilation and PSV.
       3. The clinician determines the minimum tidal volume.
       4. As long as spontaneous patient effort results in delivery of desired tidal volume, breath "behaves" like a pressure support breath.
       5. If breath delivers a tidal volume below the desired minimum, it is transitioned to a volume-controlled breath by prolonging inspiration at the minimal set flow and slightly ramping up the pressure, assuring delivery of the desired tidal volume.
    B. Mandatory minute ventilation (MMV)
       1. This mode combines PSV with SIMV.
       2. The clinician chooses the minute ventilation rate the patient is to receive by selecting a desired tidal volume and frequency.
       3. As long as spontaneous breathing results in minute ventilation that exceeds the minimum, all breaths are pressure support breaths.
       4. If minute ventilation falls below the set minimum, the ventilator will provide sufficient SIMV breaths to allow the patient to "catch up" to the desired level of minute ventilation. This is based on a moving average.

Suggested Reading

Donn SM, Becker MA: Baby in control: Neonatal pressure support ventilation. Neonatal Intensive Care 11:16-20, 1998.

Donn SM, Becker MA: Mandatory minute ventilation: A neonatal mode of the future. Neonatal Intensive Care 11:20-22, 1998.

Donn SM, Becker MA: Special ventilator techniques and modalities I: Patient-triggered ventilation. In Goldsmith JP, Karotkin EH (eds): Assisted Ventilation of the Neonate, 4th ed. Philadelphia, WB Saunders, 2003, pp 203-218.

Donn SM, Sinha SK: Pressure support ventilation of the newborn. Acta Neonat Jap 33:472-478, 1997.

Donn SM, Sinha SK: Controversies in patient-triggered ventilation. Clin Perinatol 25:49-62, 1998.

Nicks JJ, Becker MA, Donn SM: Bronchopulmonary dysplasia: Response to pressure support ventilation. J Perinatol 11:374-376, 1994.

Sinha SK, Donn SM: Advances in neonatal conventional ventilation. Arch Dis Child 75: F135-F140, 1996.

Sinha SK, Donn SM: Pressure support ventilation. In Donn SM (ed): Neonatal and Pediatric Pulmonary Graphics: Principles and Clinical Applications. Armonk, NY, Futura Publishing, 1998, pp 301-312.

32

Proportional Assist Ventilation and Respiratory Mechanical Unloading in Infants

Andreas Schulze

I. Introduction
  A. Patient-triggered ventilation (PTV) attempts to synchronize the upstroke in ventilator pressure with the onset of spontaneous inspiration. Other parameters of the mechanical cycle, such as peak inspiratory pressure (PIP), pressure rise time, and duration of lung inflation are preset by the clinician. They will be imposed on the infant without adapting to the course of spontaneous inspiratory activity.
  B. In addition to the features of conventional PTV, pressure support ventilation (PSV) (flow-cycling) terminates inflation toward the end of spontaneous inspiration. PSV, by allowing variability in inflation time and preventing inflation from extending into spontaneous expiration, can reduce asynchrony between spontaneous inspiratory activity and cycling of the respirator.
  C. Proportional assist ventilation (PAV) does not couple a more or less preset cycling profile of the ventilator to a single time point event, such as the onset and the end of inspiration. In the PAV modalities, the ventilator is continuously sensitive to the instantaneous respiratory effort, adjusting the assist pressure in a proportionate and ongoing fashion. This may achieve near-perfect synchrony between the ventilator and spontaneous breathing, with relief from disease-related increased mechanical work of breathing.
II. The Concept of PAV
  A. PAV Servo-controls the applied ventilator pressure, based on continuous input from the patient. This input signal alone controls the instantaneous ventilator pressure, which is adjusted continuously according to the input signal waveform contour, virtually without a time lag.
  B. The input signal is derived from the infant's spontaneous respiratory activity. It ultimately reflects the output of the respiratory center. Therefore, theoretically it can be obtained anywhere along the pathway from the respiratory center to the end organ (i.e., recorded as phrenic nerve activity, diaphragmatic EMG activity), but also as tidal volume

and airflow signals from probes inside the airway or from plethysmography.

C. The pressure output of the ventilator, being proportional to the input signal in a PAV mode, will enhance the effect on ventilation of the respiratory center activity. This implies the following:

1. The PAV mode increases the amount of ventilation per unit of spontaneous respiratory activity—that is, proportionately to the instantaneous magnitude of the effort. In contrast, patient-triggered ventilation adds a given amount of tidal volume to the spontaneous breath whenever a breath is detected, regardless of the magnitude of the inspiratory effort and its time course.

2. The ventilator becomes fully enslaved, allowing the infant to control timing, depth, and the entire tidal volume and airflow contours of the breath.

3. The clinician sets the "gain" of this enhancement.
   a. The gain is the ratio of applied ventilator pressure per "unit of respiratory center output" (i.e., pressure per input-signal unit).
   b. The higher the gain, the less mechanical work of breathing needs to be performed by the infant for a given amount of ventilation.

4. The PAV mode relies on a largely intact functioning of the biologic control of breathing. The mode does not by itself initiate breaths. It cannot revert a waning respiratory drive.
   a. During episodes of cessation of spontaneous breathing or hypoventilation, back-up conventional mechanical ventilation needs to be started automatically.
   b. When the infant resumes spontaneous breathing, the ventilator must automatically withdraw back-up ventilation.

III. Ventilator Settings for PAV when Based on Airflow and Tidal Volume Signals of Spontaneous Breathing (Respiratory Mechanical Unloading Modes).

A. The positive end-expiratory pressure (PEEP) level affects the functional residual capacity, as with any other assist modality.

B. The gain of the volume-proportional assist (elastic unloading gain) (Fig. 32-1):
   1. Sets the ratio of delivered ventilator pressure per tidal volume in units of cm H_2O/mL. (The control of the volume-proportional assist is located on the ventilator front panel with a continuous scale.)
   2. Rises in proportion to the inspired tidal volume and thus specifically opposes the increase in lung elastic recoil pressure that develops during each inspiration.
   3. Exerts an elastic unloading effect that specifically reduces the elastic work of breathing.

C. The gain of the flow-proportional assist (resistance unloading gain) (Fig. 32-2):
   1. Sets the ratio of delivered ventilator pressure per tidal airflow in units of cm H_2O/L/sec. (The control of the volume-proportional assist is located on the ventilator front panel with a continuous scale.)

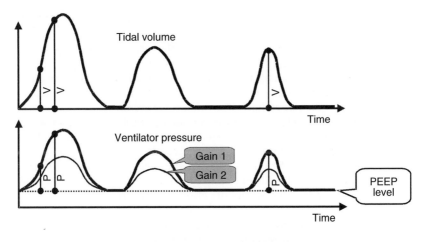

$$\text{Gain} = \frac{\text{Ventilator pressure (P, cm H}_2\text{O)}}{\text{Tidal volume (V, mL)}}$$

FIGURE 32-1. Schematic representation of spontaneous breathing during volume-proportional assist (elastic unloading) at two different settings (gain 1 and gain 2) of the assist gain level. *Vertical lines* demonstrate that the gain (ratio of change in ventilator pressure per unit of change in tidal volume) is maintained constant over time while the tidal breathing pattern varies. Gain 2 represents a lower level of the assist.

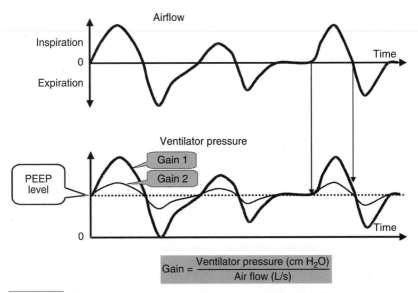

$$\text{Gain} = \frac{\text{Ventilator pressure (cm H}_2\text{O)}}{\text{Air flow (L/s)}}$$

FIGURE 32-2. Schematic representation of spontaneous breathing during flow-proportional assist (full-cycle resistive unloading) at two different settings (gain 1 and gain 2) of the assist gain level. *Vertical lines* indicate that ventilator pressure changes occur virtually without a time lag to the airflow signal. The gain (ratio of change in ventilator pressure per unit of airflow) is maintained constant over time while the tidal breathing pattern varies. Gain 2 represents a lower level of the assist.

2. Specifically opposes airflow resistive forces because it changes in proportion to the inspiratory airflow signal.

3. Exerts a resistive unloading effect that reduces the resistive work of breathing. If this feature is activated during both inspiration and expiration (full-cycle resistive unloading), it will also facilitate exhalation, shorten the expiratory time constant, and help to avoid inadvertent PEEP in infants with high airway resistance.

D. Safety limits on ventilator pressure.

E. Back-up conventional ventilation for episodes of hypoventilation or apnea.

IV. Patient Management

A. Indications

1. Preserved spontaneous breathing activity, but impending respiratory failure from an imbalance between the ability of the respiratory pump and the mechanical workload of breathing.

2. Elastic unloading (volume-proportional assist), primarily for conditions of reduced lung compliance (restrictive disease types).

3. Resistive unloading (flow-proportional assist), primarily for conditions of increased airway resistance (obstructive disease types), including resistance imposed by the ETT.

4. Combined elastic and resistive unloading for conditions with combined derangements of lung mechanics. Separate and independent gain settings for the elastic and resistive unloading components allow customization of the ventilatory waveform contour to the relative severity of lung compliance and airway resistance problems.

5. Proportional assist ventilation has not been studied in preterm infants with acute severe pulmonary parenchymal disease before the application of exogenous surfactant; air leak syndromes; meconium aspiration syndrome; or other types of severe respiratory disease in the term newborn.

B. Initiation of PAV in infants

1. Set the controls before enabling the mode on the infant.

   a. Set elastic unloading gain and resistive unloading gain to zero and choose the PEEP level as for intermittent mandatory ventilation (IMV).

   b. Set the upper airway pressure safety limit.

   c. Choose settings for back-up conventional ventilation to provide appropriate full ventilatory support while avoiding hyperventilation.

   d. PAV can be set up as "pure" PAV, which essentially is modulated continuous positive airway pressure (CPAP) with back-up control. It can also be applied in tandem with low-rate IMV or sychronized intermittent mandatory ventilation (SIMV) to mechanically unload spontaneous breathing between the mandatory inflations. In addition, optional settings allow provision of a minimum guaranteed tidal volume during PAV-supported breathing.

2. Start the mode while observing the patient.
   a. Gradually increase the elastic unloading gain from zero to an appropriate level. Ventilator pressure remains constant at zero gain (CPAP); it will be modulated to track the tidal volume signal with elastic unloading gain settings above zero.
   b. A suitable elastic unloading gain can be identified by clinical criteria. It will reduce chest wall distortion and establish physiologic tidal volumes of about 3 to 5 mL/kg. Smaller infants will need higher gains of elastic unloading (in absolute terms— i.e., in cm H_2O/mL) because tidal volume and compliance are related to body weight. As a general rule, infants <1000 g body weight usually need about 1 cm H_2O/mL or more of elastic unloading gain, while larger infants need less.
   c. If the gain is turned up above an appropriate level (stronger then current elastic recoil of the lung), ventilator pressure will rise to the set upper pressure limit with each inspiration. The ventilator pressure subsequently will always be automatically returned to the PEEP level. Levels of unloading that are too high thereby convert the mode into the cycling pattern of patient-triggered ventilation—that is, cycling between set PEEP and PIP levels with each onset of spontaneous inspiration. This occurrence identifies an excessive gain and helps to find the range of appropriate gain levels.
   d. Increase the gain of resistive unloading to compensate at least for the resistance imposed by the endotracheal tube (ETT). This is about 20 to 30 cm H_2O/L/sec of resistive unloading for a 2.5-mm ID ETT. Higher gains may be required when pulmonary resistance is elevated.
   e. Preterm infants on PAV typically adopt a fast, shallow breathing pattern.
C. Weaning
   1. Reduce gain levels gradually with improvement in pulmonary mechanics.
   2. Try to be specific in lowering resistive versus elastic support levels, depending on how pulmonary pathophysiology develops. Compared to other assist modes, reduction in ventilator pressure "cost" with proportional assist is likely related to the quality of matching of the unloading settings to the specific type and the degree of lung mechanics derangement.
   3. Improvement in pulmonary mechanics can be recognized during PAV when a previously suitable gain turns into overassist with repetitive cycling of airway pressure to the set upper pressure limit. This indicates the possibility of further weaning the assist by reducing the gain.
   4. With gains weaned to near zero levels, the patient has to shoulder the entire work of breathing near the CPAP level and is probably ready to be extubated.

D. Problems
  1. ETT leaks
     a. An ETT leak flow mimics inspiratory airflow to a flow sensor mounted at the Y adapter. This may cause the ventilator pressure to increase out of proportion to the inspiratory airflow and/or volume that is truly entering the lung.
     b. Current devices use software algorithms to estimate and adjust for leak flows. This allows PAV to function in infants in the presence of variable leak flows of up to about 20% to 30% of tidal volume.
     c. Major leaks will have effects similar to those of inappropriately high gain settings and preclude the use of PAV based on direct airflow measurements.
  2. Sensor malfunction
     a. When the flow signal serves as driving input to the closed-loop PAV system, any flow sensor malfunction will inevitably lead to a derangement of the applied ventilator pressure pattern.
     b. Distortions of the driving signal and the ventilator pressure waveforms that result from such sensor artifacts can be recognized on the ventilator's monitor display.

Suggested Reading

Musante G, Schulze A, Gerhardt T, et al: Respiratory mechanical unloading decreases thoraco-abdominal asynchrony and chest wall distortion in preterm infants. Pediatr Res 49:175-180, 2001.

Schulze A, Bancalari E: Proportional assist ventilation in infants. Clin Perinatol 28:561-578, 2001.

Schulze A, Gerhardt T, Musante G, et al: Proportional assist ventilation in low birth weight infants with acute respiratory disease: A comparison to assist/control and conventional mechanical ventilation. J Pediatr 135:339-344. 1999.

Schulze A, Rich W, Schellenberg L, Heldt GP: Effects of different gain settings during assisted mechanical ventilation using respiratory unloading in rabbits. Pediatr Res 44:132-138, 1998.

Schulze A, Schaller P, Töpfer A, et al: Resistive and elastic unloading to assist spontaneous breathing does not change functional residual capacity. Pediatr Pulmonol 16:170-176, 1993.

Younes M: Proportional assist ventilation: A new approach to ventilatory support. Am Rev Respir Dis 145:114-120, 1992.

33 High-Frequency Ventilation: General Concepts

J. Bert Bunnell

I. Why Use High-Frequency Ventilation (HFV)?
   A. HFV is very gentle; tidal volumes can be smaller than anatomic dead space.
      1. It has proved effective in preventing lung injury.
      2. It has proved effective in treating lung injury.
   B. HFV can ventilate patients that are impossible to ventilate any other way.
      1. Examples include patients with upper airway leaks (e.g., tracheoesophageal fistula, bronchopleural fistula) and postcardiac surgery patients in respiratory failure.
      2. Its combination of characteristics—small tidal volume (V_T), clear separation of ventilation and oxygenation control, and in some devices, the ability to accommodate concomitant intermittent mandatory ventilation (IMV) and ventilate using a wide range of Paw—offers a broad range of capabilities.
   C. HFV enables safe use of positive end-expiratory pressure (PEEP) higher than that used during conventional ventilation (CV).
      1. Higher PEEP and Paw better stabilize surfactant-deficient alveoli.
      2. Lung injury is caused by V_T size on top of PEEP; small-V_T HFV enables higher mean airway pressures and better oxygenation without increasing risk of lung injury.
      3. Limiting factor: Cardiac output (if PEEP is too high, it impedes venous return to the heart).
   D. Safe and reliable devices are available.
      1. HFV devices were the first and are still the only type of mechanical ventilator required to be proven safe and effective before they can be marketed in the United States.
         a. The FDA administers this premarket approval (PMA) process.
         b. All other ventilators are approved via the 510(k) process, whereby new equipment must be shown to be "substantially equivalent" to devices that are currently being legally sold in the U.S. (Products legally marketed in the United States before May 28, 1976, are the bases for comparison.)
      2. Three HFV devices have been FDA-approved via the PMA process for use on neonates in the United States.
      3. Several other devices are in use outside the United States.

II. How HFV Works
  A. HFV does not try to mimic normal breathing.
    1. HFV is similar to panting without hyperventilation, as seen in some animals.
    2. HFV provides a different distribution of gas within lungs.
      a. Airway resistance is the primary determinant of gas distribution.
      b. Unlike in CV, lung compliance is not an important factor.
  B. Resonant Frequency Phenomena
    1. Forced oscillations pulmonary-function experiments revealed that lungs have a natural or "resonant" frequency (e.g., 4 to 8 Hz [cycles per second] in adult humans).
    2. At resonance:
      a. Gas momentum supplies the energy to overcome lung compliance, and lung recoil supplies the energy to send gas back out of the lungs.
      b. Timing and energies are perfectly matched to conserve energy.
      c. Outside force is required *only* to overcome airway resistance.
    3. Therefore, less pressure is required to move gas in and out of the lungs at resonant frequency.
  C. Asymmetric gas flow-streaming, dead space reduction, and direct alveolar ventilation
    1. High-velocity HFV inspiratory gas flows into the lungs down the central core of airways or along one wall of some airways, as it passes bifurcations in short, abrupt bursts.
      a. The higher the velocity, the sharper the point on the bullet-shaped velocity profile of the inrushing gas.
      b. Effective dead space volume is reduced because only portions of the anatomic dead space (V_D) are used.
      c. Fresh gas penetrates some alveoli directly even when

$$V_T < \text{anatomic } V_D$$

    2. In high-frequency oscillatory ventilation (HFOV), gas is sucked from many airways into one (the trachea), causing a turbulent, flat expiratory wave front (velocity profile).
    3. In high-frequency jet ventilation (HFJV), gas flows out passively, seeking the path of least resistance in the annular or "unused" spaces around the highly accelerated inspired gas.
    4. The net effect of several oscillations or HFJV cycles: Fresh gas advances down the core of airways while exhaled gas moves out along the airway walls.
  D. Increased bulk flow (convection) and enhanced diffusion.
    1. Abundant fresh gas of high-frequency inspirations washes expired gas from the airways.
    2. Increased washout of expired gases increases O_2 and decreases CO_2 partial pressures at the intra-airway/alveolar gas exchange boundary, thereby increasing diffusion.

3. Examples of enhanced intrapulmonary gas exchange in nature occur in running and panting animals and in birds during vigorous flight.
E. Ventilator Design Varieties
  1. HFJV
    a. Inspired gas is injected down the endotracheal tube through a jet nozzle (typical frequency range is 240 to 660 breaths/min or 4 to 11 Hz).
    b. The jet nozzle is built into a special 15-mm endotracheal tube (ETT) adapter (Bunnell LifePort) with two side ports for:
      (1) Gas injection
      (2) Distal airway pressure monitoring
    c. Spontaneous breathing, concomitant IMV, and HFV expirations occur via the main ETT lumen.
  2. HFOV
    a. HFOV provides sinusoidal, push-pull, piston-type ventilation from ~180 to 900 breaths/min (3 to 15 Hz).
    b. Some devices allow the I:E ratio, or T_I, to be adjusted from 1:1 to approximately 1:2.33.
  3. Hybrids (high-frequency positive pressure ventilation [HFPPV] devices, "flow-interrupters," and combined HFV/IMV devices) may provide jet, oscillatory, or conventional ventilation over similar frequency ranges.
III. How HFV Devices Differ from Conventional Ventilators and Each Other
A. Airway pressure monitoring is somewhat misleading during HFV compared to CV.
  1. High-velocity HFV gas flows create large pressure drops across the ETT.
  2. Thus, proximal pressure amplitude (i.e., $\Delta P = PIP - PEEP$) is misleadingly large compared to CV.
  3. Meaningful proximal pressure monitoring during HFV is limited to Paw.
  4. However, if airways collapse or exhalation time is inadequate, mean *alveolar* pressure can be greater than mean *airway* pressure.
B. Active versus passive exhalation
  1. HFOV devices actively "suck" gas back from the patient's lungs during exhalation.
    a. In cases in which high Paw is useful, active exhalation allows higher frequencies to be used with fewer gas-trapping problems.
    b. When lower Paw is used, the sucking action may promote airway collapse ("choke points") and gas trapping, causing mean *alveolar* pressure to exceed mean *airway* pressure.
  2. All other types of HFV devices rely on the patient's passive exhalation.
    a. Inspiration time must be minimized and rate limited to allow sufficient time for exhalation.

      b. They work well when lower Paw is desired (e.g., some pulmonary air leaks, postcardiac surgery).

  C. Efficiency

    1. HFOV uses 15 to 20 L/min to ventilate infants.

    2. HFJV uses 1 to 2 L/min for neonatal ventilation.

  D. Interdependency of controls, fixed I:E ratio, and their effects

    1. Some devices, particularly HFOV devices, exhibit direct interdependency between rate and delivered V_T when I:E ratios are held constant.

      a. As rate is increased, T_I decreases, and therefore less V_T is delivered (and vice versa).

      b. Because V_T is much more important for ventilation compared to rate (see later), $PaCO_2$ rises when rate is increased, which is counterintuitive.

    2. Other HFV devices maintain constant V_T when the rate is changed.

      a. T_I is held constant.

      b. $PaCO_2$ rises and falls intuitively as the rate is lowered and raised, respectively.

 IV. Similarities of HFV Devices

  A. Effective high-frequency rate is ~10 times the normal rate

    1. Optimal frequency produces the best ventilation with the lowest ΔP and V_T and no gas trapping.

    2. Primary determinant of appropriate frequency is patient size.

    3. Venegas and Fredberg (1994) recommend finding and using the "corner frequency" (Fig. 33-1).

      a. Plot peak pressure or pressure amplitude measured at the carina versus frequency.

      b. The "corner" occurs where pressure changes from falling rapidly to flattening out or rising.

      c. At this frequency, the lowest pressure for ventilation is required while avoiding gas trapping.

      d. The analysis by Venegas and Fredberg indicates that the optimal frequency for the smallest premature infant with the stiffest lungs and high airway resistance is 10 to 12 Hz or 600 to 720 breaths/min.

      e. As compliance goes up, optimal frequency goes down. Thus, a frequency of <600 to 720 breaths/min would be required for anyone larger than the smallest premature infant.

      f. As airway resistance improves (decreases), optimal frequency increases because it is easier for the insufflated gas to be eliminated quickly.

  B. Determinants of ventilation

    1. Several investigators of HFV have found CO_2 elimination to be proportional to frequency times V_T^2.

    2. Thus, choose a frequency consistent with patient's size and condition (i.e., lung impedance), and adjust ΔP or V_T to produce the desired $PaCO_2$.

  C. Determinants of oxygenation

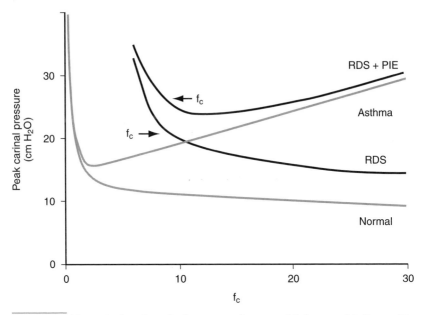

FIGURE 33-1. Theoretical peak carinal pressures for normal infants and infants with decreased compliance (RDS), increased airway resistance (asthma), and both low compliance (C_L) and high resistance (R_{AW}) (RDS + PIE) with PEEP = 10 cm H_2O. Note how increased resistance reduces optimal frequency; however, most infants with RDS are well served using the corner frequency (f_c) of ~10 Hz in these examples. Using higher frequencies increases the risk of gas trapping. PEEP, positive end-expiratory pressure; PIE, pulmonary interstitial emphysema; RDS, respiratory distress syndrome. (Modified with permission from Venegas JG, Fredberg JJ: Understanding the pressure cost of high frequency ventilation: Why does high-frequency ventilation work? Crit Care Med 22:S49-S57, 1994. ©1994 Williams and Wilkins.)

1. As in every form of mechanical ventilation, Paw and appropriate management of functional residual capacity (FRC) are the primary determinants of oxygenation.
2. Because HFV offers the opportunity to use higher PEEP, it is helpful to separate alveolar recruitment from alveolar stabilization maneuvers.
   a. To recruit collapsed alveoli, raise Paw with HFOV or add concomitant IMV with HFJV at rates up to 10 breaths/min.
   b. Once alveolar recruitment is evidenced by improved O_2 saturation, discontinue the recruitment maneuver (i.e., decrease Paw on HFOV or discontinue concomitant IMV on HFJV) and rely on lower Paw on HFOV or PEEP, with HFJV for maintenance of adequate alveolar volume.
   c. If arterial oxygen saturation subsequently falls, PEEP or Paw is evidently too low, so raise it immediately. (You may also have

to re-recruit collapsed alveoli with higher Paw on HFOV, or concomitant IMV with HFJV if you have waited too long.)
3. To increase lung volume in the absence of frank atelectasis, just raise Paw or PEEP.
   a. Many neonatologists are reluctant to use PEEP >6 cm H_2O.
   b. Most premature infants need PEEP >6 cm H_2O (~7 to 10 cm H_2O) to establish normal FRC. (This level of PEEP should not interfere with cardiac output.)
4. With nonhomogeneous lung disease, in which spotty atelectasis may be present, or in cases in which cardiac output is impeded with higher PEEP levels, using HFJV with low rate IMV at lower PEEP (4 to 6 cm H_2O) may improve ventilation-perfusion matching.

V. Delivering HFV in the NICU
   A. What clinical disorders are theoretically amenable to HFV treatment?
      1. Restrictive lung diseases (conditions accompanied by low lung compliance), such as pneumonia, tension pulmonary interstitial emphysema, diaphragmatic hernia, and pulmonary hypoplasia
      2. Atelectatic lung diseases, such as respiratory distress syndrome, in which collapsed alveoli can be opened safely through the use of high mean airway pressure HFOV or HFJV in conjunction with conservative IMV and optimal PEEP
      3. Some obstructive lung disorders, such as airway stenoses and aspiration pneumonia, in which the HFV modality applied facilitates removal of aspirated material and mucus and improves ventilation-perfusion matching (e.g., HFJV using lower rate and longer expiratory time for MAS)
      4. Patients with pulmonary air leak syndromes and cardiac surgery patients in whom lower mean airway pressure HFJV, with its small V_T, short T_I, and low intrapulmonary pressure amplitudes, matches the pathophysiology
      5. Upper airway leaks and fistulas, in which abrupt, high-velocity HFJV insufflations "shoot" inspired gas right past disruptions, enabling ventilation downstream and airway injuries to heal
   B. In what clinical conditions might HFV treatment be contraindicated?
      1. Disorders such as asthma wherein airway resistance is uniformly increased. Very low rates and long expiration times should be more effective here.
      2. Some nonhomogeneous lung disorders may not respond well to HFOV because of its active exhalation, which can further aggravate an already unfortunate distribution of ventilation.

VI. How to Initiate, Optimize, and Minimize the Risks of HFV
   A. Learn when to start HFV without hesitation when indicated by pathophysiology, experience, and worsening patient condition.
   B. Match ventilator strategy to pathophysiology and the availability of an appropriate device.

C. Using appropriate ventilator strategies for specific lung disorders is more important than which ventilator you use, but know the limitations of the devices you have available. (See later.)

D. Choose HFV rate based on patient size and lung time-constant (10× normal rate is a good starting point).

E. Use minimum T_I or I:E ratio to maximize inspired gas penetration and minimize gas trapping.

1. Shorter T_I allows more time for passive exhalation with HFJV.

2. Greater % expiration with HFOV means that less force is required to suck gas back out, which means there is less chance of creating choke points.

F. Find and use optimal PEEP or Paw, paying particular attention to whether you need to recruit more lung volume or you need to stabilize the volume already available.

1. Recruit collapsed alveoli by *temporarily* increasing the concomitant IMV rate with HFJV or Paw with HFOV.

2. If recruitment is successful, as indicated by improved oxygenation, the IMV rate should be reduced and PEEP should be optimized with HFJV, or Paw should be optimized with HFOV to support open alveoli without compromising cardiac output.

G. Keep $PaCO_2$ in the proper range using ΔP or V_T.

H. Adjust settings rationally as patient's condition changes.

I. Do not stop prematurely.

1. If you get a bad blood gas result, reassess and adjust strategy.

2. If you get a good blood gas reading, wean appropriately.

a. Do not change back to conventional ventilation too soon. (Injured lungs take time to heal!)

b. Do not drop PEEP or Paw when FiO_2 is >0.30.

VII. HFV Device Limitations, Risks, and Benefits

A. HFJV Limitations

1. Passive exhalation

a. Pay attention to lung time constants: More compliant lungs require lower rates.

b. Keep frequency tuned to patient size: Bigger patients require lower rates.

2. Be ready to suction right after initiation of HFJV.

a. HFJV very effectively facilitates mucociliary clearance; be ready to take advantage of it!

b. Do *not* suction as often after initial airway clearance; it just collapses alveoli.

B. HFOV limitations

1. Active exhalation

a. Watch out for "choke point" gas trapping (airway collapse caused by sucking action).

(1) Is evident when you cannot reduce high $PaCO_2$.

(2) Must increase Paw.

b. Select HFOV patients who will benefit from higher Paw.

2. May not work well with nonhomogeneous lung disorders.

3. Watch out for mucus impaction.

a. HFOV with an I:E ratio of 1:1 to 1:2 may hamper mucociliary clearance.

b. Do *not* suction unless necessary; it just collapses alveoli.

C. Hybrids and combined HFV and CV

1. Compressible volume of conventional-style circuits limits ventilator power and effectiveness.

2. Concomitant IMV must be managed appropriately.

a. Increase IMV rate to actively recruit collapsed alveoli (5 to 10 breaths/min).

b. Decrease rate (0 to 3 breaths/min) when atelectasis resolves.

c. Cease IMV (i.e., use continuous positive airway pressure) when air leaks are present.

D. Primary risk of HFV: Cerebral injury (intraventricular hemorrhage, periventricular leukomalacia)

1. Risk is associated with hyperventilation and hypocarbia.

2. Use of transcutaneous PCO_2 monitoring is highly recommended.

3. Hyperventilation is easier to avoid when proper lung volume is attained.

E. Secondary risks: Air leaks, mucous plugs

1. Risks of air leaks are mitigated by minimizing concomitant IMV and optimizing Paw.

2. Risk of mucous plugs is mitigated by proper humidification and use of short T_I and much longer expiratory time (i.e., I:E ratios favoring exhalation, such as 1:6).

F. Proper alveolar-volume recruitment and stabilization are critical for good oxygenation

1. Judicious use of concomitant IMV can aid alveolar recruitment.

2. Optimizing PEEP and Paw is essential for alveolar stability.

VIII. Conclusions

A. HFV is not for every patient, but it can provide incredible benefits if the appropriate device is used on the appropriate patient in the appropriate way at the appropriate time.

B. Let common sense and solid knowledge of pulmonary pathophysiology and respiratory therapy be your guides.

Suggested Reading

Bandy DP, Donn SM, Nicks JJ, Naglie RA: A comparison of proximal and distal high-frequency jet ventilation in an animal model. Pediatr Pulmonol 2:225-229, 1986.

Boros SJ, Mammel MC, Coleman JM, et al: A comparison of high-frequency oscillatory ventilation and high-frequency jet ventilation in cats with normal lungs. Pediatr Pulmonol 7:35-41, 1989.

Boynton BR, Villanueva D, Hammond MD, et al: Effect of mean airway pressure on gas exchange during high-frequency oscillatory ventilation. J Appl Physiol 70:701-707, 1991.

Clark RH: High-frequency ventilation. J Pediatr 124:661-670, 1994.

Donn SM, Zak LK, Bozynski MEA, et al: Use of high-frequency jet ventilation in the management of congenital tracheoesophageal fistula associated with respiratory distress syndrome. J Pediatr Surg 25:1219-1221, 1990.

Harris TR, Bunnell JB: High-frequency jet ventilation in clinical neonatology. In Pomerance JJ, Richardson CJ (eds): Neonatology for the Clinician. Norwalk, CT, Appleton & Lange, 1993, pp 311-324.

Haselton FR, Scherer PW: Bronchial bifurcations and respiratory mass transport. Science 208: 69-71, 1980.

Henderson Y, Chillingworth FP, Whitney JL: The respiratory dead space. Am J Physiol 38:1-19, 1915.

Kocis KC, Meliones JN, Dekeon MK, et al: High-frequency jet ventilation for respiratory failure after congenital heart surgery. Circulation 86(Suppl II): II127-II132, 1992.

Perez Fontan JJ, Heldt GP, Gregory GA: Mean airway pressure and mean alveolar pressure during high-frequency jet ventilation in rabbits. J Appl Physiol 61:456-463, 1986.

Venegas JG, Fredberg JJ: Understanding the pressure cost of high-frequency ventilation: Why does high-frequency ventilation work? Crit Care Med 22:S49-S57, 1994.

High-Frequency Jet Ventilation

34

Martin Keszler

I. Mechanism of Gas Exchange
   A. Pulses of high-velocity gas (jet stream) move down the center of the airway, penetrating through the dead space gas, which simultaneously moves outward along the periphery of the airway. The kinetic energy of the gas emerging from the jet nozzle at high velocity, rather than the pressure gradient, drives gas movement in the large airways.
   B. Enhanced molecular diffusion probably plays an important role in the distal airways.
   C. Gas exchange is achieved with smaller tidal volumes and pressure amplitude than with conventional ventilation (CV).
II. Indications
   A. *Late rescue treatment:* High-frequency jet ventilation (HFJV) has been used extensively for the treatment of refractory respiratory failure unresponsive to CV. Air leak syndrome has been the most commonly treated underlying disorder, but infants with pulmonary hypoplasia from diaphragmatic hernia, respiratory distress syndrome (RDS), meconium aspiration syndrome (MAS), and pneumonia are also routinely treated with HFJV, with considerable success in a rescue mode.
   B. *Early rescue treatment:* HFJV has documented efficacy (and extensive clinical experience) in the treatment of moderate to severe RDS, pulmonary interstitial emphysema (PIE), large leaks through a bronchopleural fistula (intractable pneumothorax) and tracheoesophageal fistula, abdominal distention with poor chest wall compliance, congenital diaphragmatic hernia, and selected cases of MAS with or without pulmonary hypertension.
   C. *Prophylactic use:* Despite evidence of the effectiveness of HFJV in lowering the incidence of chronic lung disease (CLD) in one large multicenter study, first-line treatment of infants with RDS at high risk for developing CLD is not yet widely practiced.
III. Benefits of HFJV
   A. Lower pressure amplitude (change in pressure = peak inspiratory pressure – positive end-expiratory pressure [$\Delta P = P_I - PEEP$]), compared to conventional ventilation
   B. Very effective CO_2 elimination
   C. Ability to use low mean airway pressure (Pāw) when indicated

    D. More rapid resolution of air leaks

    E. Decrease in airflow through points of airway disruption

    F. Capability to use high PEEP safely when indicated

    G. Effective recruitment and maintenance of lung volume

    H. Improved hemodynamics because of less interference with venous return

    I. Mobilization of secretions and aspirated material

    J. Decreased risk of CLD

IV. Possible Complications of HFJV

    A. Mucosal damage to the trachea and large bronchi was reported in some early studies when inadequate humidification was used. This is no longer a problem.

    B. Increased incidence of periventricular leukomalacia (PVL) and intraventricular hemorrhage (IVH) was reported in one study—likely related to inadvertent hyperventilation. Similar findings were seen in some oscillatory ventilation studies and with CV. Risk of inadvertent hyperventilation can be minimized by using transcutaneous PCO_2 monitoring, especially when initiating HFJV.

    C. Air trapping is possible if an inappropriately high ventilator rate is used. This is a phenomenon that can occur with all ventilators.

V. Clinical Use

    A. Patient selection

       1. Risks and benefits should be carefully considered before initiating HFJV.

       2. Early rather than late initiation is preferable in most situations.

       3. Patient selection should be based on clinical experience and published evidence of efficacy.

    B. Basic control of blood gases

       1. Oxygenation is determined by FiO_2 and Pāw (increased Pāw = improved oxygenation).

       2. Pāw is determined by peak inspiratory pressure (PIP), PEEP, and inspiratory time (T_I).

       3. Ventilation (CO_2 elimination) is primarily determined by pressure amplitude ($\Delta P = PIP - PEEP$).

       4. Rate has a relatively minor effect on ventilation. the usual range is 360 to 500 breaths/min, depending on the baby's size and on time constants. A rate that is too fast may increase $PaCO_2$ because of gas trapping.

       5. T_I should almost always remain at the lowest possible value of 0.02 second.

       6. Background intermittent mandatory ventilation (IMV) rate of 2 to 5 breaths/min is superimposed on the HFJV pulses to maintain lung volume (periodic sigh). The PIP should be the same as the HFJV PIP or slightly lower so as not to interrupt the jet ventilator. T_I of the sigh breaths should be 0.3 to 0.5 second. Background IMV should be omitted in the presence of overexpansion or air leak.

       7. Note that sighs recruit lung volume, but adequate Paw (PEEP) is needed to maintain it.

8. Weaning from HFJV is accomplished primarily by weaning PIP, leaving rate unchanged, except as dictated by changes in time constants (see below).
9. Note that decreasing amplitude by lowering PIP also lowers P̄aw and thus affects oxygenation. This problem can be avoided by increasing PEEP to compensate.

C. Matching ventilator strategy to disease pathophysiology
1. Choosing appropriate ventilator strategy is critical—a wrong strategy may lead to lack of response and/or complications.
2. Ventilator settings should be selected according to the patient's specific needs.
3. The underlying disease, postnatal age, and patient size must all be considered in choosing an appropriate strategy and settings.

D. Low pressure strategy
1. This approach is appropriate when air leak is a major problem (e.g., PIE, pneumothorax), and the imperative is to reduce peak and mean airway pressures in an effort to resolve the air leak.
2. PIP should be set 10% to 15% below the current levels on CV.
3. PEEP should be 3 to 6 cm H_2O, depending on the severity of the air leak and the presence of coexisting lung disease (may need to be higher if severe atelectasis coexists with PIE).
4. Remember that oxygenation is related to P̄aw and that it may deteriorate with the drop in pressure. Marginal PaO_2 may have to be accepted, and generous FiO_2 is often needed.
5. T_I should be kept at the minimum value of 0.02 second.
6. Background IMV should be omitted if the lungs are overexpanded and severe PIE is present.
7. Optimal HFJV rate depends on an estimation of the patient's time constants (usual range, 360 to 420 breaths/min to allow adequate expiratory time).
8. If marginal oxygenation prevents further decrease in PIP, but $PaCO_2$ is low, decrease the pressure amplitude by increasing PEEP to avoid hypocarbia and to maintain oxygenation.
9. If diffuse atelectasis develops and oxygenation is inadequate, an increase in Paw, usually by increasing PEEP, is indicated, provided ventilation is adequate. The background IMV may be (re)started at this time.
10. If ventilation is also inadequate, PIP should be increased.
11. When the air leak resolves and atelectasis becomes the dominant problem, switch to the optimal volume strategy (see later).

E. Optimal volume strategy
1. This strategy is appropriate in most situations, especially in RDS.
2. The goal is to optimize lung volume, thereby improving V/Q matching and to avoid the recruitment/de-recruitment cycle typical of conventional large V_T ventilation.
3. When switching from CV, P̄aw should be increased by 10% to 15% by increasing PEEP.
4. The following rule of thumb can be used for initial PEEP settings:
   a. Set PEEP at 5 cm H_2O if FiO_2 is <0.30.

     b. Set PEEP at 6 to 7 cm H_2O if FiO_2 is 0.30 to 0.50.

     c. Set PEEP at 8 to 10 cm H_2O if FiO_2 is >0.50.

5. PIP initially should remain the same as on CV. If starting HFJV without prior CV, choose a pressure that results in adequate chest wall movement.

6. Background sigh rate is set at 5 breaths/min with T_I of 0.3 to 0.5 second and PIP set as high as possible without interrupting the jet ventilator.

7. Rate of 420 to 500 breaths/min with T_I of 0.02 second is appropriate early in the course of RDS, because time constants are short. Later, as compliance improves, rate should be lowered to avoid air trapping.

8. Optimization of lung volume is reflected by marked improvement in oxygenation. If the initial settings do not allow weaning of FiO_2 to <0.35, PEEP should be increased further.

9. When adequate lung volume recruitment has been achieved, as evidenced by improved oxygenation, turn the background IMV rate down to 2 breaths/min and observe for possible deterioration of oxygenation. If oxygenation remains good, the PEEP is adequate. If oxygenation is deteriorating, return to a rate of 5/min to re-recruit lung volume and increase PEEP by 1 to 2 cm H_2O. Repeat the process, if necessary. When oxygenation remains stable, with a background rate of 2 breaths/min, leave the settings there.

10. *Rarely,* when severe atelectasis is present and not resolving with the above approach, conventional PIP may need to be increased above the jet PIP for a *brief* period and may be allowed to interrupt the jet ventilator in order to re-expand the lungs. Remember that without sufficient PEEP to maintain lung volume, this will be ineffective and potentially damaging.

11. The background sigh rate or PIP should *not* be increased as a primary means of increasing mean Paw. This is more safely accomplished by raising PEEP. Remember that the large V_T of CV is the very thing you are trying to avoid.

12. Once lung volume is optimized, compliance will improve rapidly. This will be reflected in improved chest wall movement and CO_2 elimination. *PIP must be lowered promptly to avoid hypocarbia.* Follow $PaCO_2$ closely.

13. Paw should not be weaned until the FiO_2 is = 0.30 to 0.40. Remember to compensate for decreasing PIP by raising PEEP.

14. Periodic chest radiographs are helpful in verifying adequate lung expansion or detecting overexpansion.

F. Treatment of MAS and persistent pulmonary hypertension of the newborn (PPHN)

1. MAS is a heterogeneous disorder and evolves rapidly over time. The effectiveness of HFJV patients with this syndrome is variable, ranging from poor to dramatic.

2. In the acute phase, when large airways are obstructed with particulate meconium, HFJV may be ineffective, because the jet stream is broken up by the obstructing debris.

3. When the surfactant inactivation or inflammatory effect predominates, HFJV is usually quite effective and the high volume strategy is appropriate. However, beware of overexpansion and gas trapping. Remember: Larger infants need slower rates; higher airway resistance requires slower rates. Typical range is 300 to 360 breaths/min.

4. HFJV provides a type of internal vibration that helps to mobilize secretions/aspirated material. The expiratory flow along the periphery of the large airways moves the secretions proximally. Be ready to suction when initiating HFJV.

5. HFJV is an effective and relatively gentle means of hyperventilation, if this is desired to as treatment of PPHN. Avoid extremes of $PaCO_2$ and pH, which are easily achieved with HFJV but may be dangerous.

G. Miscellaneous conditions responsive to HFJV

1. When diaphragmatic excursion is impaired by increased intra-abdominal pressure, the small V_T of HFJV with sufficiently high PEEP to apply counterpressure on the diaphragm and maintain lung volume is advantageous. Babies with acute abdominal distention from necrotizing enterocolitis or similar conditions and infants following repair of gastroschisis, diaphragmatic hernia, or omphalocele often respond dramatically, with improved gas exchange and hemodynamics.

2. Infants with airway disruption such as intractable pneumothorax with constant large flow through chest tubes, tracheoesophageal fistula, or tracheal tear respond with improved gas exchange and decreased flow through the point of airway disruption. This is because the jet stream moves down the center of the airway with virtually no lateral pressure on the airway walls. The gas that does escape is probably expiratory gas. The low-pressure strategy is indicated in these situations.

3. Infants with lung hypoplasia appear to benefit from the more gentle, small V_T ventilation possible with HFJV. Gentle hyperventilation is easily achieved in most cases when PPHN is present. An intermediate approach between the optimal volume and low pressure strategy works best. Be aware that overexpansion of the lungs will exacerbate pulmonary hypertension.

4. Limited clinical experience and small studies suggest that HFJV may be useful in extremely immature preterm infants with evolving or established CLD. These infants have distended, "floppy" airways and are prone to gas trapping as the airways collapse during expiration. HFJV may benefit these infants by splinting these airways open with fairly high PEEP (7 to 9 cm H_2O), and allowing more efficient gas exchange and more even aeration of the lungs.

H. Weaning from HFJV

1. Weaning is accomplished by lowering FiO_2 first and PEEP second, once the FiO_2 is 0.30.

2. PIP is lowered in response to low normal $PaCO_2$ or excessive chest wall movement. Remember to compensate for decreasing PIP by increasing PEEP, if necessary, to maintain Paw.

3. The ventilator rate is not decreased as a means of weaning. However, if initially it is >420 breaths/min, it may need to be lowered to accommodate lengthening time constants because of increasing compliance and/or increasing airway resistance as RDS evolves.

4. Infants can be weaned from HFJV directly to continuous positive airway pressure (CPAP). This is usually possible, once PIP is 10 to 12 cm H_2O and PEEP is 6 cm H_2O.

5. Alternately, once the pressure is 14 to 18 cm H_2O and PEEP is 6 cm H_2O, the infant can be switched to CV Usually PIP higher than 10% to 15% is needed after the change.

I. Miscellaneous

1. A combination of high PaO_2 and high $PaCO_2$ may reflect "super-PEEP" secondary to obstruction. This requires immediate suctioning.

2. Servo pressure may be used to monitor the infant. A sudden drop may indicate a sudden decrease in compliance (e.g., pneumothorax), whereas a sudden increase may indicate a sudden improvement (e.g., following surfactant).

Suggested Reading

Donn SM, Zak LK, Bozynski MEA, et al: Use of high-frequency jet ventilation in the management of congenital tracheo-esophageal fistula associated with respiratory distress syndrome. J Pediatri Surg 25:1219-1222, 1990.

Gonzalez F, Harris T, Black P, et al: Decreased gas flow through pneumothoraces in neonates receiving high-frequency jet versus conventional ventilation. J Pediatr 110:464-466, 1987.

Harris TR, Bunnell JB: High-frequency jet ventilation in clinical neonatology. In Pomerance JJ, Richardson CJ, (eds): Neonatology for the Clinician. Norwalk, CT, Appleton & Lange, 1993, pp 311-324.

Keszler M, Donn S, Bucciarelli R, et al: Multi-center controlled trial of high-frequency jet ventilation and conventional ventilation in newborn infants with pulmonary interstitial emphysema. J Pediatr 119:85-93, 1991.

Keszler M, Durand D: High-frequency ventilation: Past, present, and future. Clin Perinatol 28:579-607, 2001.

Keszler M, Modanlou HD, Brudno DS, et al: Multi-center controlled clinical trial of high-frequency jet ventilation in preterm infants with uncomplicated respiratory distress syndrome. Pediatrics 100:593-599, 1997.

Sugiura M, Nakabayashi H, Vaclavik S, Froese AB: Lung volume maintenance during high-frequency jet ventilation improves physiological and biochemical outcome of lavaged rabbit lung. Physiologist 33:A123, 1990.

Wiswell TE, Graziani LJ, Kornhauser MS, et al: Effects of hypocarbia on the development of cystic periventricular leukomalacia in premature infants treated with high-frequency jet ventilation. Pediatrics 98:918-924, 1996.

Wiswell TE, Graziani LJ, Kornhauser MS, et al: High-frequency jet ventilation in the early management of respiratory distress syndrome is associated with a greater risk for adverse outcomes. Pediatrics 98:1035-1043, 1996.

35

High-Frequency Oscillatory Ventilation

Reese H. Clark and Dale R. Gerstmann

I. Introduction
   A. Definition: High-frequency oscillatory ventilation (HFOV) is rapid-rate, low–tidal volume (V_T) form of mechanical ventilation.
   B. Reasons for use of HFOV
      1. To improve gas exchange in patients with severe respiratory failure
      2. To reduce ventilator-associated lung injury
         a. Prevention of volutrauma: HFOV dramatically reduces the V_T needed to maintain ventilation (normocarbia). During HFOV, the lung can be held close to mean lung volume. There is minimal change in lung volume with each delivered breath. Visually this translates to chest wall vibration that is barely perceptible. In contrast, during conventional ventilation (CV), the lung is cycled from low to high volume with each breath, such that chest rise and fall is easily visible.
         b. Reduced exposure to inspired oxygen: HFOV improves the uniformity of lung inflation, reduces intrapulmonary shunt, and improves oxygenation. The need for supplemental oxygen is reduced and exposure to oxygen free radicals is decreased.
      3. To decrease pulmonary morbidity in patients who require assisted ventilation
      4. To provide a method of assisted ventilation that allows severe pulmonary air leaks to heal
II. Comparison of Basic Parameters of HFOV and CV

Parameter	HFOV	CV
Rate (breaths/min)	0-60	180-1200
V_T (mL/kg)	4-20	0.1-5
Alveolar pressure (cm H_2O)	5-50	0.1-20
End-expiratory lung volume	Low	High
Minute ventilation (MV)	$Rate^{(0.5-1)} \times V_T^{(1.5-2)}$	$Rate \times V_T$

A. The calculation of MV determines how much carbon dioxide is removed from the lung. The MV equation shown for HFOV predicts that factors effecting V_T delivery have a larger impact on ventilation during HFOV than during CV. Changes in endotracheal tube (ETT) size, lung compliance, airway resistance, and chest wall rigidity all impact delivery of "tidal volume."

B. It is important to remember that the impedance of the respiratory system increases with frequency. During HFOV, as frequency is increased, V_T delivery and MV may decrease.

C. Some devices, such as the SensorMedics 3100A, have lower V_T output at higher frequencies. This can be compensated for by increasing the power setting.

III. Advantages of HFOV

A. Improves ventilation at lower pressure and volume swings in the lung.

B. Safer way of using "super" PEEP (positive end-expiratory pressure). The lung can be inflated to higher mean volumes without having to use high peak airway pressures to maintain ventilation (carbon dioxide removal).

C. Produces more uniform lung inflation.

D. Reduces air leak.

IV. Disadvantages of HFOV

A. As with CV, there is potential for gas trapping and the development of inadvertent PEEP. The time for exhalation during HFOV is very short. Gas delivered to the lung during the inspiratory cycle may become trapped in the lung. This "trapped" gas can cause over-inflation of the lung and lung injury (stretch injury or air leak). The propensity for gas trapping is dependent on the high-frequency device being used. Devices that facilitate exhalation are less likely to cause gas trapping than devices that depend on the passive recoil of the chest and lung.

B. Defining optimal mean lung volume is difficult, yet crucial to the safe use of HFOV.

1. Increasing lung volume results in decreasing venous return, which can be severe enough to compromise cardiac output. Overinflation of the lungs can also cause acute lung injury, especially if cardiac output is compromised.

2. Underinflation of the lungs is equally dangerous. Collapsed lungs are difficult to recruit and recruitment of collapsed lungs can be associated with significant lung injury. Atelectasis is associated with increased pulmonary vascular resistance, increased intra- and extrapulmonary shunts, and life-threatening hypoxemia.

V. Types of HFOV

A. Diaphragm HFOV with variable fractional inspiratory time (T_I): The SensorMedics 3100A oscillatory ventilator is the only HFOV device approved for use in newborns in the U.S. It is an electronically controlled diaphragm that produces pressure oscillation in the patient circuit. Adjusting the power, frequency, or fractional T_I to the diaphragm driver controls the airway pressure amplitude.

The mean airway pressure (P̄aw) is set independently from the pressure oscillations. Adjusting the bias flow or the outlet resistance in the patient circuit controls the P̄aw.

   B. Piston HFOV with a fixed fractional T_I: These types of HFOV have used a 1:1 inspiratory-to-expiratory (I:E) ratio. In healthy adult rabbits, the use of a 1:1 I:E ratio has been shown to be associated with gas trapping and inadvertent PEEP. Newer devices allow for 1:2 and 1:1 I:E ratios. The Hummingbird is the best example of this type of HFOV. This ventilator is used widely in Japan.

   C. Hybrid devices employ a Venturi to generate negative pressure during the expiratory cycle of ventilation.

 VI. Theories of Improved Ventilation during HFOV
   A. Enhanced molecular diffusion
   B. Enhanced convection (Pendelluft effect)
   C. Taylor dispersion
   D. Reduced dependence on bulk convection

 VII. Mechanisms of Oxygenation
   A. Directly related to the degree of lung inflation (lung surface area)
   B. Dependent on FiO_2
   C. Lung overinflation can lead to decreased venous return and compromised cardiac output.

 VIII. Physiologically Targeted Strategies of HFOV
   A. Poor lung inflation: The most dramatic effects of HFOV are seen in infants and children whose primary pathophysiology is decreased lung inflation. When used with continuous distending pressure (CDP) directed at recruiting lung volume, followed by careful weaning of the CDP once lung inflation is improved and FiO_2 is decreased, HFOV reduces lung injury and promotes healthy survival. This approach exploits the concept of pressure-volume hysteresis, assuming that the lung is not injured too severely and still has some recruitable volume. By using a CDP that is higher than the lung opening pressure and usually greater than that generally accepted during CV, HFOV recruits collapsed lung units. Once open, these lung units usually can be maintained open at a P̄aw lower than that used for lung recruitment.

   B. Pulmonary hypertension: HFOV can be effective in patients with pulmonary hypertension, if the process leading to the hypertension is poor lung inflation and regional hypoxia and hypercarbia. Improving lung inflation improves ventilation-perfusion matching and gas exchange, thereby relaxing the pulmonary vascular bed and decreasing pulmonary arterial pressure. HFOV is not as effective in patients with airway obstruction or in patients with poor cardiac output, especially from myocardial dysfunction. Airway obstruction attenuates the pressure signal as it is propagated across the airways to the alveoli. This attenuation decreases the alveolar ventilation and reduces ventilator efficiency. In patients with poor cardiac output, the constant high end-expiratory pressure decreases venous return and further impairs cardiac output.

IX. Reported Indications and Contraindications for HFOV: Numerous clinical reports of uncontrolled trials of the use of HFOV as a rescue technique have been published. The absolute indications and contraindications remain to be established by carefully controlled clinical trials.

A. Reported indications

1. Persistent air leak (e.g., bronchopleural fistula, pulmonary interstitial emphysema)
2. Persistent neonatal respiratory failure associated with:
   a. Respiratory distress syndrome (RDS)
   b. Pneumonia
   c. Acute respiratory distress syndrome (ARDS)
   d. Meconium aspiration syndrome (MAS)
   e. Lung hypoplasia syndromes
   f. Congenital diaphragmatic hernia (CDH)
   g. Hydrops fetalis
   h. Pulmonary hypoplasia
3. Tracheoesophageal fistula in patients who are not surgical candidates (e.g., premature infants)
4. Primary pulmonary hypertension, which is responsive to reversal of atelectasis and controlled alkalosis. HFOV may be able to produce alkalosis with less barotrauma than CV.

B. Reported contraindications

1. Airway disease associated with gas trapping: Most authors agree that HFOV is not effective in patients with airway obstruction. The use of HFOV in patients with airway disease can accentuate problems with gas trapping.
2. Shock. Appropriate use of HFOV increases mean lung volume. As lung volume increases, right atrial volume will decrease. These changes impede venous return. Reduced venous return may amplify problems with hypotension unless preload is increased through aggressive treatment of shock and its causes. These problems are identical to the problems seen with increasing levels of PEEP in CV.

X. Specific Reports and Summary of Results of Clinical Trials

A. The largest prospective study involving HFOV was reported by the HIFI Study Group (1989). Of 673 preterm infants weighing between 750 and 2000 g, 346 were assigned to receive CV and 327 to receive HFOV. No infant received surfactant. The incidence of chronic lung disease (CLD) was nearly identical in the two groups. HFOV did not reduce mortality or the level of ventilatory support during the first 28 days. HFOV was associated with an increased incidence of pneumoperitoneum of pulmonary origin, grades 3 and 4 intracranial hemorrhage, and periventricular leukomalacia (PVL). These results suggested that fixed-ratio HFOV, as used in this trial, did not offer any advantage over CV, and that it might be associated with undesirable side effects.

B. In a much smaller study (n = 98), also of non–surfactant-treated infants, Clark et al (1996) showed that HFOV could be used to reduce the incidence of CLD in premature infants with RDS without increasing the incidence of intraventricular hemorrhage (IVH). The HFOV strategy used in this study was designed to recruit lung volume. The average CDP used during HFOV was 2 to 3 cm H_2O higher than the P̄aw used during CV.

C. In a multicenter trial (n = 176), the HIFO Study Group (1996) showed that rescue HFOV could be used to reduce the incidence of air leak syndromes in infants with established severe lung disease. There was a slight increase in incidence of grades 3 and 4 IVH in those infants treated with HFOV.

D. Gerstmann et al (1996) did the first study of HFOV in which all infants received surfactant. The purpose of this study was to compare the hospital course and clinical outcome of preterm infants (35 weeks' gestation) with RDS treated with surfactant and managed with HFOV or CV as the primary mode of ventilator support. A total of 125 infants with an arterial/alveolar ratio <0.5 were studied. HFOV was used in a strategy to promote lung recruitment and maintain lung volume. Patients randomized to HFOV demonstrated the following significant findings compared with CV-treated patients: less vasopressor support; less surfactant redosing; improved oxygenation, sustained during the first 7 days; less prolonged supplemental oxygen or ventilator support; reduced treatment failures; more survivors without CLD at 30 days; less need for continuous supplemental oxygen at discharge; lower frequency of necrotizing enterocolitis; fewer abnormal hearing tests; and decreased hospital costs. In pulmonary follow-up at 6 years of age, infants randomized to HFOV had normal lung volume measurements, whereas those randomized to CV had larger than normal residual volume and decreased vital capacity.

E. Using the Infant Star HFOV and a volume recruitment strategy, Thome et al (1999) were unable to reproduce the results reported by Gerstmann et al (1996) (HFOV) or Keszler (HFJV).

F. Two recent studies show conflicting results.

1. Courtney et al (2002) studied 500 infants. Those randomly assigned to HFOV were successfully extubated earlier than infants assigned to synchronized intermittent mandatory ventilation (SIMV). Of infants assigned to HFOV, 56% were alive without need for supplemental oxygen at 36 weeks of postmenstrual age, compared to 47% of those receiving SIMV. There was no difference between the groups in the risk of IVH, cystic PVL, or other complications.

2. Johnson et al (2002) studied 400 infants who were assigned to HFOV and 397 who were assigned to CV. The composite primary outcome (death or CLD diagnosed at 36 weeks of postmenstrual age) occurred in 66% of the infants assigned to receive HFOV and 68% of those in the CV group. There were also no significant differences between the groups in a range of other secondary outcome measures, including serious brain injury and air leak.

G. Current status
   1. Animal studies show that HFOV reduces lung injury, promotes more uniform lung inflation, improves gas exchange, and prolongs the effectiveness of exogenous surfactant in experimental models of acute lung injury.
   2. Clinical studies show that the results are strategy specific. When used with a strategy designed to optimize and maintain lung inflation, HFOV can be used safely to reduce the occurrence of CLD. However, technology is ever-changing and the debate over the best surfactant and the gentlest mode of ventilation continues.
H. Air leak syndromes
   1. Pulmonary interstitial emphysema (PIE)
      a. Clark et al (1986) showed that HFOV improved gas exchange in premature infants with severe respiratory failure and PIE. Compared to previously reported data involving CV, HFOV also appeared to improve survival.
      b. Current status: PIE remains a serious complication of assisted ventilation. The introduction of surfactant has reduced the incidence of PIE but has not eliminated the disease process. HFOV improves gas exchange and appears to improve the outcome of patients with PIE. However, affected infants are at high risk for long-term pulmonary and neurologic morbidity.
   2. Pneumothoraces
      a. Blum-Hoffman et al (1988) showed that HFOV was effective in improving oxygenation and ventilation in patients with air leak syndromes. Carter et al reported similar results.
      b. Current status: Both HFJV and HFOV appear to improve gas exchange and allow for more rapid resolution of pneumothoraces.
   3. Extracorporeal membrane oxygenation (ECMO) candidates
      a. Paranka et al (1995) demonstrated that 50% of ECMO-eligible patients could be rescued with HFOV alone. The outcome of patients rescued with HFOV was as good as for those who went on to require ECMO. Patients with CDH (30%) and MAS (50%) were not as likely to respond to HFOV as were patients with pneumonia (85%) and/or RDS (90%).
      b. Vaucher et al (1996), using a different type of HFOV and a different clinical strategy, did not demonstrate results as encouraging. Patients who met criteria and were treated with ECMO had less CLD than infants who were "rescued" with alternate therapies. Walsh-Sukys presented similar findings. Both these studies show that prolonged use of HFOV or CV to avoid ECMO may increase the risk for development of CLD.
      c. Kinsella et al (1997) reported that treatment with HFOV and inhaled nitric oxide was more effective than either therapy alone in the management of babies with lung disease and persistent pulmonary hypertension of the newborn (PPHN). This finding was particularly true for infants with RDS or MAS.

    d. Current status: Results achieved with HFOV are likely to be device and strategy specific. The relative roles that surfactant, inhaled nitric oxide, liquid ventilation, HFOV, and ECMO play in the management of term infants with severe respiratory failure have not yet been determined.

I. Reported complications of HFOV

   1. Adverse cardiopulmonary interactions: It is essential to maintain the balance between adequate lung volume and cardiac preload. During HFOV, lung volume is nearly constant. Failure to maintain adequate preload and/or optimal lung volume can result in progressive hypotension and hypoxemia.

   2. Mucostasis

     a. The HFOV I:E setting affects mucus clearance from the lung. Mucus can build up in the airways during HFOV. When weaned from HFOV and returned to CV, some patients will rapidly mobilize these secretions. Airways can become occluded, and frequent suctioning may be required during the 24- to 48-hour period following HFOV. Airway trauma associated with suctioning should be avoided by passing the suction catheter only 1 cm below the endotracheal tube. Although mucostasis is an uncommon complication of HFOV, it can be life-threatening.

     b. Gerstmann et al (2001) found that premature patients with RDS who were treated with HFOV actually required less suctioning.

     c. Management of airway secretions must be individualized. Try to avoid suctioning unless clinically indicated (increasing $PaCO_2$, visible airway secretions, or decreasing oxygen saturation).

   3. Gas trapping—See preceding discussion.

   4. IVH and PVL: Recent meta-analyses suggest that the association between HFOV and poor neurologic outcome is related more to how HFOV is used than to whether it is used. HFOV can cause rapid reduction in $PaCO_2$, which can cause sudden changes in cerebral blood flow. To use HFOV safely, acute changes in ventilation, especially overventilation (i.e., hypocarbia and alkalosis), must be avoided.

XI. General and Disease-Specific Recommendations

  A. Atelectasis with diffuse radiopacification of the lung (RDS or pneumonia)

   1. The CDP required to optimize lung inflation is higher than that which is usually achieved on CV. Paw can be increased in increments of 1 to 2 cm H_2O until PaO_2 improves or the chest radiograph shows normal inflation. Evidence of overinflation or signs of cardiac compromise should be avoided. Radiographic signs of overinflation include "extra clear" lung fields, a small heart, flattened diaphragms, and more than nine posterior ribs of lung inflation. Signs of cardiac compromise include increased heart rate, decreased blood pressure, poor peripheral perfusion, and metabolic acidosis.

2. Pāw levels used in the management of uncomplicated RDS in premature infants are generally lower than those used to treat term newborns. The severity of the lung disease, the age at start of HFOV, the use of surfactant, and the presence of infection all influence the amount of pressure that is required. CDPs commonly reported are:
   a. For infants weighing <1 kg, 5 to 18 cm H_2O
   b. For infants weighing 1 to 2 kg, 6 to 20 cm H_2O
   c. For infants weighing >2 kg, 10 to 25 cm H_2O
3. Frequency is generally held constant at 10 to 15 Hz. Most clinical data report the use of 10 Hz. In infants who weigh <1 kg, extreme caution must be taken to avoid hyperventilation and alkalosis. If $PaCO_2$ is low and the pressure amplitude is <20 cm H_2O, the frequency may need to be increased in order to decrease MV and allow the $PaCO_2$ to rise to a normal range. Also, if small changes in power settings result in large changes in $PaCO_2$, ventilation control will be improved by increasing the frequency from 10 to 15 Hz.

B. MAS
   1. Some patients with MAS present with diffuse lung injury with limited pulmonary hypertension and minimal airway obstruction. These patients respond as described previously.
   2. In contrast, some newborns with MAS have severe airway obstruction and persistent pulmonary hypertension. These infants are not as responsive to HFOV.
   3. During the initiation of HFOV in patients with MAS, a chest radiograph should be obtained to assess lung inflation and to rule out evidence of gas trapping. Lowering the frequency and increasing CDP may reduce gas trapping from narrowed airways.
   4. Patients who have poor lung inflation, minimal improvement in gas exchange during HFOV, and clinical evidence of pulmonary hypertension are more likely to respond to a combination of HFOV and inhaled nitric oxide than to either therapy alone.

C. Lung hypoplasia syndromes
   1. Similar to patients with MAS, the patients most likely to respond to HFOV are those in whom the primary pathophysiologic process is poor lung inflation.
   2. Patients whose lung volumes have been optimized on HFOV, as evidenced by clear lung fields, but who still have severe pulmonary hypertension are less likely to respond to HFOV alone.
   3. Patients with both poor lung inflation and pulmonary hypertension may be best treated with a combination of HFOV and inhaled nitric oxide.

D. Air leak syndrome
   1. Patients who have severe persistent air leak (e.g., PIE or recurrent pneumothoraces) require a different approach. The goal of assisted ventilatory support must be to allow the air leak to resolve. If the air leak is unilateral, placing the involved lung in

the dependent position will increase the resistance to gas flow to this lung and promote atelectasis. Both lung collapse and decreased ventilation of the dependent lung will promote air leak resolution.

2. In addition to dependent positioning, using a strategy of HFOV that emphasizes decreasing mean airway pressure over decreasing FiO_2 will help to allow air leak resolution.

E. Idiopathic PPHN with normal lung inflation. These patients are easy to ventilate on low levels of conventional support. HFOV is not as effective in these patients and can be associated with the development of life-threatening hypoxemia if the balance between preload and lung volume is not carefully addressed.

Suggested Reading

Blum-Hoffmann E, Kopotic RJ, Mannino FL: High-frequency oscillatory ventilation combined with intermittent mandatory ventilation in critically ill neonates: 3 years of experience. Eur J Pediatr 147:392-398, 1988.

Carter JM, Gerstmann DR, Clark RH, et al: High-frequency oscillatory ventilation and extracorporeal membrane oxygenation for the treatment of acute neonatal respiratory failure. Pediatrics 85:159-164, 1990.

Clark RH: High-frequency ventilation. J Pediatr 124:661-670, 1994.

Clark RH, Dykes FD, Bachman TE, et al: Intraventricular hemorrhage and high-frequency ventilation: A meta-analysis of prospective clinical trials. Pediatrics 98:1058-1061, 1996.

Clark RH, Gerstmann DR, Null DM, et al: Pulmonary interstitial emphysema treated by high-frequency oscillatory ventilation. Crit Care Med 14:926-930, 1986.

Clark RH, Gerstmann DR, Null DM, et al: Prospective randomized comparison of high-frequency oscillatory and conventional ventilation in respiratory distress syndrome. Pediatrics 89:5-12. 1992.

Clark RH, Yoder BA, Sell MS: Prospective, randomized comparison of high-frequency oscillation and conventional ventilation in candidates for extracorporeal membrane oxygenation. J Pediatr 124:447-454, 1994.

Courtney SE, Durand DJ, Asselin JM, et al: High-frequency oscillatory ventilation versus conventional mechanical ventilation for very-low-birth-weight infants. N Engl J Med 347: 643-652, 2002.

Fredberg JJ, Allen J, Tsuda A, et al: Mechanics of the respiratory system during high-frequency ventilation. Acta Anaesthesiol Scand 90:39-45, 1989.

Gerstmann DR, deLemos RA, Clark RH: High-frequency ventilation: Issues of strategy. Clin Perinatol 18:563-580, 1991.

Gerstmann DR, Minton SD, Stoddard RA, et al: The Provo multicenter early high-frequency oscillatory ventilation trial: Improved pulmonary and clinical outcome in respiratory distress syndrome. Pediatrics 98:1044-1057, 1996.

Gerstmann, DR, Wood K, Miller A, et al. Childhood outcome following early high-frequency oscillatory ventilation for neonatal respiratory distress syndrome. Pediatrics 107:1-7, 2001.

HIFI Study Group: High-frequency oscillatory ventilation compared with conventional mechanical ventilation in the treatment of respiratory failure in preterm infants. The HIFI Study Group. N Engl J Med 320:88-93, 1989.

HIFO Study Group: Randomized study of high-frequency oscillatory ventilation in infants with severe respiratory distress syndrome. HiFO Study Group. J Pediatr 122:609-619, 1996.

Johnson AH, Peacock JL, Greenough A, et al. High-frequency oscillatory ventilation for the prevention of chronic lung disease of prematurity. N Engl J Med 347:633-642, 2002.

Keszler M, Donn S, Bucciarelli R, et al: Multi-center controlled trial of high-frequency jet ventilation and conventional ventilation in newborn infants with pulmonary interstitial emphysema. J Pediatr 119:85-93, 1991.

Kinsella JP, Truog WE, Walsh WF, et al: Randomized, multicenter trial of inhaled nitric oxide and high-frequency oscillatory ventilation in severe, persistent pulmonary hypertension of the newborn. J Pediatr 1997;131:55-62, 1997.

Paranka MS, Clark RH, Yoder BA, et al: Predictors of failure of high-frequency oscillatory ventilation in term infants with severe respiratory failure. Pediatrics 95:400-404, 1995.

Thome U, Kossel H, Lipowsky G, et al. Randomized comparison of high-frequency ventilation with high-rate intermittent positive pressure ventilation in preterm infants with respiratory failure. J Pediatr 135:39-46, 1999.

Vaucher YE, Dudell GG, Bejar R, et al: Predictors of early childhood outcome in candidates for extracorporeal membrane oxygenation. J Pediatr 128:109-117, 1996.

Walsh-Sukys MC, Tyson JE, Wright LL, et al: Persistent pulmonary hypertension of the newborn in the era before nitric oxide: Practice variation and outcomes. Pediatrics 105;14-20, 2000.

Wiswell TE, Clark RH, Null DM, et al: Tracheal and bronchial injury in high-frequency oscillatory ventilation and high-frequency flow interruption compared with conventional positive-pressure ventilation. J Pediatr 112:249-256, 1988.

Commonly Used Neonatal Ventilators

Bird VIP Gold Ventilator

36

Michael A. Becker and Steven M. Donn

I. Introduction: The Bird VIP Gold ventilator (Viasys Healthcare, Palms Springs, CA) provides both neonatal and pediatric ventilation. The ventilator breaths are synchronized in all modes. Continuous tidal volume, graphic monitoring of waveforms and mechanics are also available.

II. Monitoring
  A. Internal
    1. AC power
    2. External DC power
    3. Patient effort
    4. Demand flow (pressure-limited modality only)
    5. Peak inspiratory pressure (PIP)
    6. Mean airway pressure (Pāw)
    7. Positive end-expiratory pressure (PEEP)
    8. Rate (total breath rate)
    9. Inspiratory time (T_I) and expiratory time (T_E)
    10. I:E (inspiratory:expiratory) ratio
    11. Tidal volume (V_T) (V_{TI} = inspiratory tidal volume; V_{TE} = expiratory tidal volume)
    12. Expiratory minute volume (MV)
    13. Airway pressure monometer (aneroid gauge)
  B. Bird graphic monitor
    1. Waveforms (two of the three displayed at the same time)
      a. Flow
      b. Volume
      c. Pressure
    2. Mechanics
      a. Pressure-volume loop
      b. Flow-volume loop
    3. Trends (24-hour trend monitoring)
    4. Pulmonary mechanics calculations
      a. Compliance and C_{20}/C ratio
      b. Resistance

III. Alarms/Limits
  A. Blender input gas alarm
  B. High breath rate alarm
  C. High pressure alarm
  D. High/prolonged pressure alarm

E. High V_T

F. Low inlet gas pressure alarm

G. Low minute volume alarm

H. Low PEEP/CPAP (continuous positive airway pressure) alarm

I. Low peak pressure alarm

J. Pressure support/volume-assured pressure support (VAPS) time limit

IV. Nomenclature

A. Pressure versus volume ventilation

1. Pressure ventilation

a. The pressure is controlled.

b. The volume delivery varies with changes in compliance.

c. There are three pressure modalities on the VIP Gold ventilator: time-cycled pressure-limited (TCPL), pressure control (PC), and pressure support (PS).

2. Volume ventilation

a. The volume delivery is controlled.

b. The pressure varies with changes in compliance.

B. Assist/control (A/C) versus synchronized intermittent mandatory ventilation/pressure support (SIMV/PS)

1. A/C

a. A preset number of control breaths are delivered.

b. If the patient triggers the ventilator with a spontaneous effort, another breath of the same type is delivered.

2. SIMV/PS

a. A preset number of control breaths are delivered.

b. If the patient's spontaneous effort triggers the ventilator above the preset control rate, the additional breaths will be supported by a pressure-limited breath (PS).

C. Flow-cycling (Fig. 36-1)

1. Use of "termination sensitivity" (or expiratory trigger) enables the patient to end mechanical inspiration nearly synchronously by spontaneous breathing.

2. Inspiration ends at a percentage (almost always 5%) of the peak inspiratory flow rate rather than the preset T_I, and if properly set, this occurs before the preset T_I.

3. Flow-cycling prevents inversion of the I:E ratio during rapid breathing and greatly reduces gas trapping, which could occur in A/C at fixed T_I, because T_E is shortened the faster the patient breathes.

4. In rare instances, the patient may "choose" a T_I that is too short to provide an adequate V_T. (Switch to TCPL or PC.)

V. Modalities of Ventilation

A. TCPL

1. Continuous flow is present.

2. Mechanical breaths are pressure-limited and synchronized to the patient's own respiratory effort by flow changes that are detected by a proximal flow sensor (pneumotachograph).

3. The pressure is controlled and the volume varies with lung compliance.

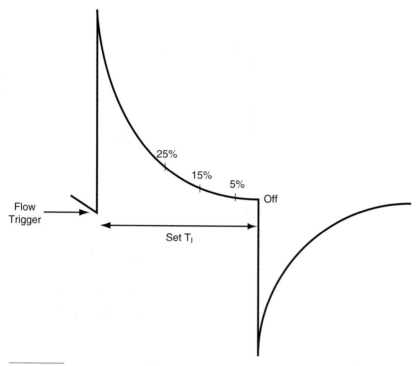

FIGURE **36-1.** Termination sensitivity or expiratory trigger. Inspiration is initiated by a change of flow at the airway. When the lungs have inflated, flow decreases at the proximal airway, which results in termination of the breath. The point of termination is clinician-adjustable, and represents a percentage of peak inspiratory flow. Thus, a 5% termination sensitivity setting means that the breath will be terminated when airway flow has decreased to 5% of peak flow (i.e., there has been a 95% decay of the curve). T_I = inspiratory time.

    B. PC
         1. A pressure-limited breath is delivered at a variable flow rate.
         2. It accelerates to peak flow and then decelerates.
         3. The endotracheal tube (ETT) resistance and patient compliance determine the flow rate, which can also be adjusted with "rise time." (See below.)
    C. PS
         1. A pressure-limited breath is patient-triggered. The patient has primary control of the inspiratory time and flow.
         2. The inspiratory flow may be adjusted with rise time, an adjustment that affects the waveform. A setting of 1 is the steepest rise. The breath will be given quickly. A setting of 7 will give the breath more slowly and may be very helpful in the management of infants with high resistance disease or small ETTs.

D. Volume-controlled (targeted)
  1. A preset volume is delivered with each breath.
    a. The volume is constant and pressure varies, depending on the patient's lung compliance.
    b. The breaths are triggered by a flow change at the flow sensor, indicating that the patient is making a respiratory effort.
    c. The minimum V_T leaving the ventilator is 10 mL.
  2. Because cuffed ETTs are not used in newborns, there is usually some leakage of delivered volume. It is more appropriate to refer to this as volume-controlled or volume-limited ventilation, rather than as volume-cycled ventilation.
E. VAPS (Fig. 36-2)
  1. VAPS begins as a variable flow, decelerating waveform, pressure-limited breath (PS type breath).

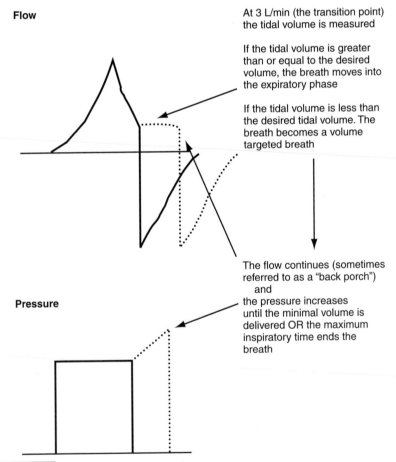

Flow

At 3 L/min (the transition point) the tidal volume is measured

If the tidal volume is greater than or equal to the desired volume, the breath moves into the expiratory phase

If the tidal volume is less than the desired tidal volume. The breath becomes a volume targeted breath

The flow continues (sometimes referred to as a "back porch") and the pressure increases until the minimal volume is delivered OR the maximum inspiratory time ends the breath

Pressure

FIGURE 36-2. Suggested algorithm for setting up volume-assured pressure support (VAPS). L/min, liters per minute.

2. A minimal volume target is set.
3. At a selected transition point, generally set at 3 L/min (the lowest setting, it gives the PS support breath the maximum time to deliver the minimal V_T), the V_T is measured.
4. If the volume target is met, the breath will flow cycle and move into the expiratory phase.
5. If the volume is not met, the breath converts from a PS breath to a volume-targeted breath. The flow continues, the inspiratory time is extended, and the pressure increases slightly until the minimal target volume is achieved or the maximum T_I limit ends the breath. This mode will deliver either patient-triggered breaths or a control rate if the patient has no effort.

F. CPAP
1. Continuous gas flow through the circuit with expiratory resistance to provide the desired PEEP.
2. May be oxygen enriched.
3. No additional volume or pressure boost is provided.

VI. Ventilation Management: The newer generations of ventilators give the clinician the opportunity to use a number of different strategies.
A. Ventilation ($PaCO_2$): Carbon dioxide removal is related to the minute ventilation (MV).

$$MV = V_T \times \text{respiratory rate}$$

Measured V_{TI} should be 4 to 8 mL/kg to avoid overinflation.

$$\text{Normal MV} = 240 - 360 \text{ mL/kg/min}$$

1. Pressure-targeted
   a. V_T is adjusted by the change in pressure or
      $\Delta P = (PIP - PEEP)$.
   b. Compliance and resistance will affect the delivered tidal volume.
2. Volume-targeted
   a. The V_{TI} delivered to the patient is determined by the set V_T minus the volume that is compressed in the ventilator circuit (and any leak).
   b. The compressed volume varies with the pressure that is generated within the circuit and patient compliance.
   c. Always monitor the measured nspiratory and expiratory volumes to determine the leak volume.
B. Oxygenation (PaO_2) is correlated directly with Paw and fraction of inspired oxygen (FiO_2).
1. Increases in PIP, T_I, PEEP, and respiratory rate all contribute to higher Paw and increased oxygenation.
2. FiO_2

VII. Weaning and Extubation (see Chapter 58)
A. Weaning from the ventilator: Weaning strategies should encourage the patient to breathe above the set respiratory rate. This is done by

decreasing the rate to the point at which the patient breathes spontaneously.

1. Pressure modes
   a. Weaning in A/C mode
      (1) It is possible to wean in either the A/C or SIMV/PS mode.
      (2) As compliance improves, the patient requires less pressure to deliver the appropriate desired V_{TI}.
   b. Weaning in SIMV/PS mode
      (1) Set the mandatory (SIMV) breath as $\Delta P = (PIP - PEEP)$ to deliver a V_{TI} of 4 to 8 mL/kg.
      (2) The PS level should be set at the same PS_{max} or slightly lower pressure, delivering a V_{TI} of 4 to 8 mL/kg.
      (3) Decrease the rate of the control breaths until all the breaths are PS breaths. (A low SIMV rate of 6/min to 10/min may be used as a safeguard.)
      (4) Extubate from a rate of zero and a $PS_{min} = 4$ mL/kg V_T.
2. Volume modes
   a. Weaning in A/C mode
      (1) Weaning in volume A/C is difficult.
      (2) Decrease the rate until the patient begins spontaneous respirations.
      (3) At rates = 40, change to SIMV/PS to continue weaning.
   b. Weaning in SIMV/PS mode
      (1) Set the volume parameter to approximately 10 to 12 mL/kg to deliver a measured V_{TI} of 5 to 6 mL/kg (will depend upon tubing compliance).
      (2) The PS should be set at the same PS_{max} (or slightly lower pressure) that is being generated by the volume breath, delivering an V_{TI} of approximately 4 to 6 mL/kg.
      (3) Decrease the rate of the control breaths until all the breaths are PS breaths. (A low SIMV rate of 6/min to 10/min may be used as a safeguard.)
      (4) Extubate from a rate of zero and a PS_{min} of 4 mL/kg V_T.
3. VAPS mode
   a. Weaning in A/C mode
      (1) VAPS A/C is generally not considered a weaning mode.
      (2) As compliance improves, the PIP may be decreased. Review waveforms for the occurrence of transitional breaths (a switch to volume-targeted breaths).
   b. Weaning in SIMV/PS mode
      (1) Decrease the rate of the control breaths until all the breaths are PS breaths.
      (2) Extubate from a rate of zero and a minimal PS level.

B. Extubation: When to extubate has always been a subjective decision. We have attempted to make it more objective with the initiation of a trial of MV.
   1. Record the MV measured by the proximal flow sensor. Do not change the respiratory support.

2. Change the ventilator mode to SIMV (CPAP), rate of zero, and no pressure support. Use of the TCPL mode is important, because in this mode the patient can breathe spontaneously from the continuous flow provided by the ventilator.
3. After 10 minutes, record the spontaneously generated MV.
4. If the spontaneous MV is 50% of the mechanically delivered MV, extubate the patient.

Suggested Reading

Donn SM (ed): Neonatal and Pediatric Pulmonary Graphics: Principles and Clinical Applications. Armonk, NY, Futura Publishing, 1998.

Donn SM, Nicks JJ, Becker MA: Flow-synchronized ventilation of preterm infants with respiratory distress syndrome. J Perinatol 14:90-94, 1994.

Donn SM, Sinha SK: Controversies in patient-triggered ventilation. Clin Perinatol 25:49-61, 1998.

Donn SM, Sinha SK: Neonatal ventilation—aspects of weaning and extubation: Physiological considerations. Perinatology 1: 317-324, 1999.

Donn SM, Sinha SK: Newer modes of mechanical ventilation for the neonate. Curr Opin Pediatr 13:99-103, 2001.

Gillespie LM, White SD, Sinha SK, Donn SM: Usefulness of the minute ventilation test in predicting successful extubation in newborn infants: A randomized controlled trial. J Perinatol 23:205-207, 2003.

Goldsmith JP, Karotkin EH (eds.): Assisted Ventilation of the Neonate, 4th ed. Philadelphia, WB Saunders, 2003.

Nicks JJ, Becker MA, Donn SM: Bronchopulmonary dysplasia: Response to pressure support ventilation. J Perinatol 14:495-497, 1994.

Sinha SK, Donn SM: Advances in neonatal conventional ventilation. Arch Dis Child 75: F135-F140, 1996.

Sinha SK, Donn SM: Neonatal ventilation—aspects of weaning and extubation: Clinical aspects. Perinatology 2:1-10, 2000.

Sinha SK, Donn SM: Weaning infants from mechanical ventilation: Art or science? Arch Dis Child 83:F64-F70, 2000.

Sinha SK, Donn SM: Newer modes of neonatal ventilation. Int J Intens Care 7:109-115, 2000.

Sinha SK, Donn SM (eds): Manual of Neonatal Respiratory Care. Armonk, NY, Futura Publishing, 2000.

Sinha SK, Donn SM: Volume controlled ventilatory modes for the newborn: Variations on a theme. Clin Perinatol 8:547-560, 2001.

Sinha SK, Donn SM, Gavey J, McCarty M: Randomised trial of volume controlled versus time cycled, pressure limited ventilation in preterm infants with respiratory distress syndrome. Arch Dis Child 77:F202-F205, 1997.

Sinha SK, Nicks JJ, Donn SM: Graphic analysis of pulmonary mechanics in neonates receiving assisted ventilation. Arch Dis Child 75:F213-F218, 1996.

Wilson BJ Jr, Becker MA, Linton ME, Donn SM: Spontaneous minute ventilation predicts readiness for extubation in mechanically ventilated preterm infants. J Perinatol 18:436-439, 1998.

Wiswell TE, Donn SM (eds): Update on mechanical ventilation and exogenous surfactant. Clin Perinatol 28:487, 2001.

37

Bear Cub 750psv Infant Ventilator

Joanne J. Nicks

I. Description
   A. The Bear Cub 750psv Infant ventilator (Viasys Health Care, Yorba Linda, CA) is pneumatically powered with 30 to 80 psig (pounds per square inch, gauge) of air and oxygen and is electronically controlled.
   B. It is designed to ventilate newborn infants and pediatric patients weighing between 500 g and 30 kg.
   C. This ventilator provides a range of modes, controls, monitors, and alarms appropriate for the targeted patient population.
   D. An optional flow sensor may be placed at the proximal airway to provide synchronized mandatory breaths and volume monitoring.
II. Breath Types and Modes of Ventilation
   A. Breath types
      1. The changeover from expiration to inspiration may be time-triggered, based on the rate setting, or flow-triggered, based on the Assist Sensitivity setting. Flow-triggering requires that the flow sensor be properly installed.
      2. Mandatory breaths are pressure-limited; however, the peak P_I may be less than the P_I setting if the Volume Limit function is activated.
      3. The changeover from inspiration to expiration may be time-cycled based on the inspiratory time (T_I) setting or flow-cycled based on a fixed termination at 10% of peak inspiratory flow. If the Volume Limit function is activated, mandatory breaths may be volume-cycled. When a breath is flow-cycled or volume-limited, the actual T_I may be less than the set T_I.
   B. Modes
      1. Assist/control (A/C): The patient may trigger mandatory breaths in excess of the preset rate, provided that the Assist Sensitivity threshold is met (flow sensor must be installed). As a result, the mandatory breaths are synchronized with the patient's breathing pattern.
      2. Flow-cycled A/C: A pressure-limited breath is delivered at a preset P_I based on the mandatory set rate, or with each patient effort that meets the Assist Sensitivity threshold. Delivered breaths may be flow-cycled when the inspiratory flow falls to 10% of the peak flow rate, or time-cycled at the preset T_I, whichever occurs first.
      3. SIMV (synchronized intermittent mandatory ventilation): In this mode, a combination of mandatory breaths and spontaneous breaths

is possible. Based on "assist windows," mandatory breaths are delivered in synchrony with the patient's breathing pattern at the preset rate (flow sensor required). In between mandatory breaths, the patient may breathe spontaneously from the preset flow base, but receives only positive end-expiratory pressure (PEEP).

4. IMV (intermittent mandatory ventilation): Mandatory breaths are delivered at preset intervals based on the rate setting without regard to the patient's breathing pattern. The patient may breath spontaneously in between mandatory breaths as in SIMV.

5. Flow-cycled SIMV: A pressure-limited breath is delivered at a preset P_I based on the mandatory set rate, in synchrony with the patient's spontaneous effort. These breaths may be flow-cycled when the inspiratory flow falls to 10% of the peak flow rate or may be time-cycled at the preset T_I limit, whichever occurs first. In between mandatory breaths, the patient may breathe spontaneously.

6. PSV (pressure support ventilation): All spontaneous efforts that reach the assist sensitivity threshold will be supported by the preset P_I and may be flow-cycled when the inspiratory flow falls to 10% of the peak flow rate, or time-cycled at the preset T_I limit, whichever occurs first. There is no mandatory rate. If the patient is apneic for the duration of the apnea alarm setting, the ventilator will deliver a backup mandatory breath at the preset pressure and T_I limit. If no patient-initiated breaths are taken during a time-out period based on the set ventilator rate or in 10 seconds, which ever is less, another backup breath will be delivered. This sequence will continue until a breath is recognized. An apnea alarm will be activated throughout this sequence.

7. SIMV/PSV: A mandatory pressure-limited breath is delivered to the patient at a preset P_I and time-cycled at the preset T_I limit, synchronized to patient effort. Any spontaneous efforts recognized by the ventilator (i.e., exceeding the assist sensitivity threshold) between mandatory breaths will be supported at the preset P_I and may be flow-cycled when the inspiratory flow falls to 10% of the peak flow rate, or time-cycled at the preset T_I limit, whichever occurs first.

8. CPAP (continuous positive airway pressure). The patient breathes spontaneously at a constant airway pressure determined by the PEEP setting. When a flow sensor is installed, spontaneous breaths are monitored by the ventilator. If the patient is apneic for the duration of the apnea alarm setting, the ventilator will deliver a backup mandatory breath at the preset pressure and T_I. If no patient-initiated breaths are taken during a time-out period based on the set ventilator rate or in 10 seconds, whichever is less, another backup breath will be delivered. This sequence will continue until a breath is recognized. An apnea alarm will be activated throughout this sequence.

III. Controls

A. Ventilation

1. PEEP/CPAP: 0 to 30 cm H_2O—Sets the level of baseline pressure.

    2. P_I: 0 to 72 cm H_2O—This is the primary determinant of delivered tidal volume (V_T).

    3. Respiratory rate: 1 to 150 breaths/min—Sets the number of mandatory breaths in SIMV and IMV and the minimum number of mandatory breaths in A/C.

    4. T_I: 0.1 to 3.0 seconds—Determines the maximum length of the inspiratory phase of mandatory breaths.

    5. Inspiratory flow: 1 to 30 L/min—Sets the flow delivered by the ventilator during the inspiratory phase of a mandatory breath.

    6. Base flow: 1 to 30 L/min—Sets the flow available to the patient for spontaneous breathing.

    7. Volume limit: 5 to 300 mL—This patented feature is unique to the Bear Cub 750psv ventilator. The preset P_I generally determines the delivered volume. A dramatic improvement in patient compliance may result in excessive V_T volume delivery unless the P_I is adjusted accordingly. The Volume Limit function allows the clinician to set a maximum V_T to be delivered. If the preset V_{TI} should be reached before achieving the preset P_I, the ventilator will terminate inspiration and cycle into the expiratory phase.

B. Oxygenation (FiO_2): 0.21 to 1.0

C. Other

    1. Assist sensitivity: 0.2 to 5.0 L/min—Sets the amount of flow which the patient must generate at the proximal airway flow sensor to trigger a mandatory breath in A/C and SIMV or a PS breath. It also sets the threshold for monitoring the patient's total breath rate in CPAP.

    2. Overpressure relief valve: 15 to 75 cm H_2O—This is a mechanical valve that provides secondary protection against excessive airway pressure. Recommended setting is 15 cm H_2O above the P_I setting.

    3. Manual breath: Push button control that delivers one mandatory breath according to the preset control settings.

IV. Monitors

A. Timing

    1. Breath rate: Reflects the total breath rate in A/C, SIMV, PS, and CPAP (flow sensor required), and the mandatory rate in IMV.

    2. Patient-initiated: Indicates that the patient has exceeded the assist sensitivity requirement for breath delivery, triggering a mechanical or spontaneous breath.

    3. Inspiratory time: Displays T_I of both mandatory and spontaneous breaths.

    4. Expiratory time: Displays T_E of mandatory breath only (i.e., time elapsed from the end of one mandatory breath to the beginning of the next).

    5. I:E ratio: Reflects the calculated relationship between the duration of inspiration to the duration of expiration for mandatory breaths only.

B. Pressure

    1. Peak P_I: Displays the maximum pressure reached during each pressure breath.

2. Mean airway pressure (Pāw): Reflects the average pressure applied to the proximal airway over time.
3. PEEP: Indicates the PEEP/CPAP measured at the proximal airway.
C. Volume (requires properly installed flow sensor)
1. Minute volume: Displays the measured exhaled MV from all breath types (i.e., mandatory and spontaneous).
2. Inspiratory tidal volume: Displays the V_{TI} measured at the proximal airway for both mandatory and spontaneous breaths.
3. Exhaled tidal volume: Displays the V_{TE} measured at the proximal airway for both mandatory and spontaneous breaths.
4. % Leak—Reflects the calculated difference between V_{TI} and V_{TE}. Helpful in assessing the need for reintubation with a larger endotracheal tube.
V. Alerts and Alarms
A. Low PEEP/CPAP: Will be activated if the measured proximal pressure falls below the set value for a minimum of 250 msec. Low PEEP/CPAP must be set within 10 cm H_2O of the PEEP setting or a Prolonged P_I alarm will be activated.
B. High breath rate: Will be activated whenever the monitored value for breath rate exceeds the alarm setting.
C. Low minute volume: Will be activated when the monitored MV falls below the set threshold (flow sensor must be attached).
D. High pressure limit: Will be activated when the proximal pressure exceeds the set threshold. Breath will be immediately terminated.
E. Low P_I: Automatically set by the ventilator based on the following algorithm:

0.25 (high pressure limit − low PEEP/CPAP) + low PEEP/CPAP

F. Apnea: Indicates that no breath has been initiated/detected in the preset time interval (e.g., 5, 10, 20, or 30 seconds).
VI. Optional Features
A. Graphics monitor: Pressure, flow, and volume waveforms
B. Computer connection: RS-232
C. Analog connection: Pressure, flow, and breath phase

Suggested Reading

Instruction Manual for BEAR CUB 750psv Infant Ventilator. Palm Springs, CA, Bear Medical Systems, 1998.

38 Newport Wave Ventilator

Robert L. Chatburn

I. Classification
  A. The Wave ventilator (Newport Medical Instruments, Newport Beach, CA) is a pressure or flow controller that may be pressure-, time-, or manually triggered; pressure- or flow-limited; and pressure-, flow-, or time-cycled.
  B. It has an optional compressor, an internal air-oxygen blender, and a gas outlet port that will power a nebulizer during inspiration.
II. Input
  A. The Wave ventilator uses 100 to 110 volts AC at 60 Hz to power the control circuitry.
  B. The pneumatic circuit operates on external compressed gas sources (i.e., air and oxygen) at 40 to 70 psig (pounds per square inch, gauge).
  C. The operator may input the mode of ventilation; pressure-triggering, pressure-limiting, and pressure-cycling thresholds (for high pressure alarm); positive end-expiratory pressure/continuous positive airway pressure (PEEP/CPAP); peak inspiratory flow rate; inspiratory time (T_I); ventilatory frequency; bias flow; and fraction of inspired oxygen (FiO_2).
III. Control Scheme
  A. Control variables
    1. The Wave ventilator controls inspiratory pressure (P_I) for all spontaneous breaths and for mandatory breaths whenever the peak pressure is limited using the Pressure Control knob.
    2. For all other breaths, the Wave ventilator controls inspiratory flow.
  B. Phase variables
    1. Trigger variables
      a. Inspiration is pressure-triggered when pressure in the patient circuit drops below the sensitivity setting. The threshold for triggering a mandatory breath is adjustable from 0.1 to 5 cm H_2O below the baseline pressure.
      b. The Wave ventilator may also be manually triggered.
    2. Limit variables
      a. Inspiration is pressure-limited during assist/control (A/C) and synchronized intermittent mandatory ventilation (SIMV) modes whenever the pressure control setting (0 to 80 cm H_2O) is lower than the natural peak inspiratory pressure (PIP) that would result from the flow and T_I settings along with the patient's lung impedance. P_I also may be limited by a mechanical

pressure relief valve, adjustable from 0 to 120 H_2O, although the primary purpose of this valve is as a safety pop-off.
  b. If the pressure control setting is high enough so that there is no pressure limit (or if it is set to off), inspiration is flow-limited. Inspiratory flow rate may be set from 1 to 100 L/min.
  c. The Wave ventilator can be volume-limited by setting inspiratory pause at 0%, 10%, 20%, or 30% of the ventilatory period, using a switch on the back of the machine.
3. Cycle variables
  a. Inspiration may be pressure-cycled when the high inspiratory pressure alarm threshold is violated. It may be set over a range of 5 to 120 cm H_2O.
  b. Inspiration cannot be volume-cycled because the Wave ventilator main flow control system does not measure instantaneous volume. Using the T_I and flow controls, the Wave is capable of delivering a tidal volume (V_T) of 5 to 2000 mL.
  c. Spontaneous breaths are flow-cycled when using pressure support. Actually, a complex mathematical control equation is used for flow cycling in this mode, relating peak flow, delivered flow, and elapsed inspiratory time. Cycling flows range from <5% to 100% of peak flow. Secondary pressure and time-cycling thresholds are automatically set as backups to the primary flow-cycling threshold.
  d. Inspiration is normally time cycled according to the T_I setting (adjustable from 0.1 to 3.0 second).
4. Baseline variables
  a. Baseline pressure may be adjusted from 0 to 45 cm H_2O using the PEEP/CPAP dial.
  b. Baseline continuous flow, or "bias flow," may be set from 0 to 30 L/min. It is controlled through feedback from the proximal airway pressure. Flow is delivered at the set rate in between breaths when proximal pressure is very close to the set baseline pressure. It is reduced or turned off at pressures above baseline.
C. Modes
1. A/C mode: During continuous mechanical ventilation, inspiration is pressure-triggered (depending on the presence of spontaneous breathing efforts and the sensitivity setting) or time-triggered (according to the the respiratory rate setting), may be pressure- or flow-limited, and is time-cycled.
2. SIMV mode
  a. In SIMV, mandatory breaths are pressure-triggered (depending on the presence of spontaneous breathing efforts and the sensitivity setting) or time-triggered (according to the frequency setting), may be pressure- or flow-limited, and are time-cycled. A mandatory breath is pressure-triggered the first time a spontaneous breathing effort is made in each ventilatory period (the ventilatory period is equal to the reciprocal of the respiratory rate). If a breathing effort is not detected during a given ventilatory period, a mandatory breath will be delivered at

the beginning of the next period. The ventilator will continue to deliver mandatory breaths according to the Respiratory Rate setting until a spontaneous breath is detected, and the sequence of events repeats itself.

    b. Spontaneous inspirations between mandatory breaths are controlled for baseline pressure (i.e., PEEP/CPAP) and are assisted to the pressure support setting (measured relative to baseline pressure). If pressure support is set at zero, breaths are supported to the baseline pressure level.

  3. Spontaneous mode: Inspiration is pressure-controlled in the spontaneous mode at the set PEEP/CPAP level. A pressure support level may also be set. The slope or rise time of pressure during pressure support is automatically controlled using "predictive learning logic" software to maintain optimal patient synchronization.

D. Control subsystems

  1. Control circuit

    a. The Wave ventilator uses pneumatic and electronic control components.

    b. Triggering and cycling signals arise from the T_I time and ventilatory frequency settings as well as from the airway pressure transducer and flow sensors.

    c. Output control signals from two pressure transducers (one monitors airway pressure and the other monitors pressure in the exhalation valve) and two redundant flow transducers (monitoring the output of the master flow control valve) are used to control flow.

    d. The exhalation manifold is controlled pneumatically.

  2. Drive mechanism

    a. The Wave ventilator uses either external compressed gas (for air and oxygen) or an electric motor and compressor (for air) in conjunction with a pressure regulator. Gas from supply lines is fed to an internal air-oxygen blender.

    b. Mixed gas leaves the blender at 28 psig and enters a rigid-walled vessel (the "accumulator"). The flow control system is driven by the pressure from the accumulator, reducing the instantaneous flow demand required for the blending system. This action allows a wide range of peak flow settings, significantly increase the peak spontaneous flow capability above the mandatory flow limit, reduces the flow required for the compressed gas supply, and improves response time. The accumulator also acts as a mixing chamber, which helps to stablize the delivered oxygen concentration within a given breath. An optional flush valve assembly allows instantaneous dumping of the accumulator to enable immediate FiO_2 changes when necessary.

  3. Output control valves

    a. All gas flow to the patient is regulated by the main flow control valve, which is a proportional solenoid valve.

  b. An electromagnetic poppet valve switches between two sources of a pneumatic signal to the exhalation valve. One source comes from the output of the master flow control valve and keeps a diaphragm-type exhalation manifold closed during assisted breaths. The other source is a pressure regulator that generates an adjustable pressure signal to control baseline pressure (i.e., PEEP/CPAP).

  c. A microprocessor coordinates the activity of both valves such that the exhalation valve closes as the flow control valve begins to deliver flow to the patient circuit.

IV. Output

  A. Waveforms

  1. The Wave ventilator delivers a rectangular flow waveform when set for volume control—that is, if the natural PIP is below the setting of the pressure control knob or if this knob is set to "off."

  2. If PIP is limited using the pressure control knob, a variety of pressure waveforms can be achieved, ranging from rectangular to triangular depending on the respiratory system mechanics and the inspiratory flow rate.

  B. Displays

  1. In addition to the various control settings, the Wave ventilator displays include visual alarm indicators (LEDs) and a digital display of preset V_T (calculated based on flow and T_I settings); measured inspiratory V_T and minute volume (MV); ventilatory rate; peak, mean, and baseline airway pressures; and peak flow.

  2. An electronic pressure gauge provides airway pressure measurement over the range of 0 to 120 cm H_2O.

  3. The Wave ventilator is usually sold with the Compass ventilator, which incorporates a heated exhalation system and allows monitoring of expiratory V_T and MV, I:E ratio, FiO_2, and expiratory flow.

V. Alarms

  A. Input power alarms: An audible alarm is activated if the electrical power is interrupted or if the air or oxygen supply falls below 32 psig.

  B. Control circuit alarms

  1. A visual "Inspiratory Time Too Long" alarm is activated if the T_I and ventilatory rate settings result in an I:E ratio greater than the preset maximum. There are two selectable maximum ratios: 1:1 and 3:1.

  2. When the T_I is set such that the preset maximum I:E ratio is violated, the ventilator will override the T_I setting to restrict the I:E to the preset value.

  3. Audible and visual "Ventilator Inoperative" alarms are activated when malfunction of the integrated circuit or ventilator occurs.

  4. There are two pressure sensors and two flow sensors in the Wave ventilator. They are automatically re-zeroed at regular intervals during use. If the drift between the pressure or flow sensors is large, the visual display flashes automatically.

C. Output alarms
  1. A low-pressure alarm is adjustable from 0 to 110 cm H_2O, and a high-pressure alarm is adjustable from 5 to 120 cm H_2O.
  2. High- and low-MV alarms are adjustable from 1 to 50 and 0 to 49 L/min, respectively (or 0.1 to 5 and 0 to 4.9 L/min).
  3. The Compass ventilator offers high- and low–expiratory MV alarms as well as high- and low-FiO_2 alarms.
VI. Unique Clinical Features
  A. The Wave ventilator is among the most versatile ventilators in its price class.
  B. It can ventilate any patient from the smallest neonate to the largest adult.
  C. Its pressure support and pressure triggering capabilities have been shown to be superior to those of most other ventilators.

Suggested Reading

Chatburn RL: Principles and practice of neonatal and pediatric mechanical ventilation. Respir Care 36:569-595, 1991.

Chatburn, RL: Ventilators. In Branson RD, Hess DR, Chatburn RL (eds): Respiratory Care Equipment. Philadelphia, JB Lippincott, 1995, pp 294-392.

Chatburn RL: Computer control of mechanical ventilation. Respir Care 49:507-515, 2004.

Chatburn RL, Primiano FP Jr: A new system for understanding modes of mechanical ventilation. Respir Care 46:604-621, 2001.

Chatburn RL: Classification of mechanical ventilators. In Tobin MJ (ed): Principles and Practice of Mechanical Ventilation. New York, McGraw-Hill, 1994, pp 37-64.

Goldsmith JP, Karotkin EH (eds): Assisted Ventilation of the Neonate, 4th ed. Philadelphia, WB Saunders, 2003.

Dräger Babylog 8000 Plus Infant Care Ventilator

39

Donald M. Null, Jr.

I. Description
   A. The Babylog 8000 Plus Ventilator (Dräger, Inc., Luebeck, Germany) is a time-cycled or volume-controlled and pressure-limited, continuous flow ventilator designed for patients weighing up to 10 kg. It is dual microprocessor–controlled.
   B. Main ventilator functions and monitor systems
      1. The ventilator front panel consists of the dial panel and display/menu key panel.
         a. The lower dial panel contains buttons for main operating modes and dial knobs for oxygen concentration, inspiratory time (T_I), inspiratory flow, peak inspiratory pressure (PIP), expiratory time (T_E), and positive end-expiratory pressure/continuous positive airway pressure (PEEP/CPAP).
         b. The main components of the display/menu key panel are the screen and below this a number of menu keys with fixed or variable function assignment.
      2. An illuminated bar graph above the screen displays current airway pressure readings.
      3. The unit also includes and Alarm Silence key, Confirm key (for acknowledging alarms or settings), Manual Inspiration key, and Calibration Configuration key.
II. Technical Data: See Table 39-1.
III. Peak Flow and Volume Measurement
   A. Parameters are measured with a heated-wire anemometer, whose sensor may be integrated into the wye (Wye sensor) or into a separate sensor adapter between the wye and the endotracheal tube (ETT) connector (ISO sensor). Theses sensors are slightly different in their flow responses. Therefore, for optimal measurement results, the sensor type needs to be selected in one of the ventilator menus. Volume is displayed as expiratory volume. Leak is calculated by the difference between inspiratory and expiratory minute volumes (MVs).
   B. Trigger function
      1. Spontaneous breathing is detected using a flow measurement. Trigger sensitivity may be set from 1 to 10 to avoid autotriggering. At the highest sensitivity setting, trigger volume is 0 and

TABLE **39-1.** Technical Data for Dräger Babylog 8000 Plus Infant Ventilator

Parameter	Range	Resolution	Accuracy
Inspiratory time (T_I)	0.1-2 sec	0.1-1 sec: 0.01 sec 1-2 sec: 0.1 sec	±10 msec
Expiratory time (T_E)	0.2-30 sec	0.2-1 sec: 0.01 sec 1-10 sec: 0.1 sec 10-30 sec: 1 sec	±10 msec
O_2 concentration %	21-100%	1%	±3%
Inspiratory flow (V_{insp})	1-30 L/min	1-10 L/min: 0.1 L/min 10-30 L/min: 0.1 L/min	±10 %
Expiratory flow (V_{exp})	1-30 L/min	1-10 L/min: 0.1 L/min 10-30 L/min: 1 L/min	±10%
Inspiratory pressure (P_I)	10-80 cm H_2O	1 cm H_2O	1 cm H_2O ±3% (measuring function)
PEEP	0-25 cm H_2O	0-10 cm H_2O: 0.1 cm H_2O >10 cm H_2O: 1 cm H_2O	1 cm H_2O ±3% (measuring function)
VE alarm limits	0-15 L/min	≤1 L/min: 0.01 L/min >1-15 L/min: 0.1 L/min	±10% (measuring function)
Delay for lower alarm limit VE	0-30 sec	1 sec	±10 msec
Apnea time	5-20 sec	1 sec	±10 msec
Tachypnea	20-200 breaths/min	5 breaths/min	1 breath/min
Tidal volume (V_{Tset})	2-100 mL	2-9.9 mL: 0.1 mL 10-19.5 mL: 0.5 mL 20-100 mL: 1 mL	Up to 5 mL: ±0.5 mL >5 mL: ±10%

PEEP, positive end-expiratory pressure.

    inspiratory flow will trigger a breath when it reaches a minimum value of 0.2 L/min.

    2. Trigger response time is 40 to 60 msec.

IV. Measurement of Lung Mechanics

    A. Dynamic compliance of the respiratory system

    B. Airway and ETT resistance

    C. Coefficient of correlation

    D. Time constant of the respiratory system

    E. Lung overdistention index, C_{20}/C

    F. Parameters are measured for each respiratory cycle of mechanical breaths and can be displayed using the display/menu key panel.

V. Rate-Volume Ratio (RVR): RVR is calculated and may be used to assess the effects of weaning. The value is displayed with lung mechanics.

VI. Modes of Ventilation

  A. CPAP (0 to 25 cm H_2O available)

  B. CMV/IMV (continuous mandatory ventilation/intermittent mandatory ventilation)

    1. Rate 1 to150 breaths/min

    2. Pressure-limited with/without plateau

  C. SIMV and A/C (synchronized intermittent mandatory ventilation and assist/control)

    1. Provided by use of heated-wire anemometer.

    2. Volume measurement triggers the device.

    3. Sensitivity settings from 1 to 10 (correspond to 0.2 to 3.0 mL trigger volume).

    4. Maximum ventilator rate in assist/control is determined by the equation

$$\text{Rate} = 1/(T_I + 0.2 \text{ sec} + T_{RT})$$

    where T_{RT} represents the response time (trigger delay).

  D. Pressure support

    1. Pressure- or volume-limited

    2. Patient-triggered

    3. Patient-terminated

    4. Leak adaptation for inspiratory trigger and termination criteria ensures sensitive and exact synchronization with leaks up to 40%.

    5. Ventilation is performed as CMV if the patient fails to trigger breaths.

  E. Volume guarantee

    1. Using a preset V_T, each supported breath provides this volume irrespective of patient effort or change in compliance or resistance.

    2. Ventilator pattern with plateau is required.

    3. Target volume may not be delivered if the maximal inspiratory pressure is set too low, if the flow is too low, or if the T_I is too short to achieve a plateau.

    4. Can be used in SIMV, A/C, and PSV.

  F. Variable inspiratory and variable expiratory flow (VIVEF)

    1. Allows independently setting inspiratory and expiratory flows.

    2. Enables user to set different flow rates for spontaneous and mechanical breaths.

    3. Using VIVEF, inspiratory flow applies to mechanical breaths, and expiratory flow applies to spontaneous breathing and during CPAP.

    4. VIVEF can be used with CPAP, CMV, A/C, SIMV, and PSV.

VII. Monitoring

  A. Features both numerical and graphic displays.

  B. Screen layout is divided into three parts.

    1. Graphics shows pressure or flow waveform.

    2. Measured value window displays numeric values (e.g., PEEP, FiO_2).

C. Menu keys below the screen are used to select monitoring functions and ventilation modes.
D. Preset values are displayed numerically on one panel.
   1. T_I, T_E, I:E ratio
   2. fset (set frequency)
   3. O_2 concentration
   4. V_{TI}, V_{TE}
   5. Pressure limit (PL), PEEP
   6. Trigger
E. Measured values, mechanics, and RVR are displayed numerically on another panel.
   1. PIP, PEEP, Paw
   2. FiO_2 (built-in oxygen sensor)
   3. ftot (total frequency)
   4. V_E, V_T
   5. Spontaneous %
   6. Leak %
F. Graphic displays are available.
   1. P waveform
   2. V waveform
   3. Trends
G. There are outputs for digital or analog interfaces.
   1. Analog provides output of measured values, data reports, and communication with patient.
   2. Digital data are transmitted using the Dräger Babylink.

Sechrist Model IV-200 SAVI Ventilator

40

S. David Ferguson

I. Modes of Ventilation
- A. Synchronized assisted ventilation of infants
- B. Conventional intermittent mandatory ventilation (IMV) (continuous flow, time-cycled, pressure-limited)
- C. Continuous positive airway pressure (CPAP)

II. Synchronized Assisted Ventilation of Infants (SAVI)
- A. Provides patient-triggered assist/control (A/C) ventilation from a Sechrist Model IV-200 ventilator.
- B. Cannot provide synchronized intermittent mandatory ventilation (SIMV).
- C. Utilizes changes in transthoracic electrical impedance that occur during spontaneous respiration to generate a trigger signal.
- D. Triggers both active inspiration and active expiration, resulting in total synchrony of breathing of infant with ventilator.

III. How SAVI Works
- A. Changes in the ratio of gas to liquid in the thorax that occur during the respiratory cycle cause a corresponding change in transthoracic electrical impedance, which:
  1. Increases during inspiration and decreases during expiration.
  2. Can be detected by conventional ECG chest leads.
  3. Can be transmitted to a neonatal cardiorespiratory monitor with a real-time analog respiratory waveform output.
  4. May be affected by changes in thoracic blood volume during the cardiac cycle (cardiac artifact).
- B. Signal detection/processing
  1. Is used to obtain an optimal respiratory impedance signal.
     a. Ensure that chest electrodes are closely applied and changed daily.
     b. Place the positive and negative chest electrodes high up in the right anterior and left posterior axillary lines, respectively.
     c. Be prepared to alter placement if good impedance signal is not obtained on the bar graph display (see later), or if there is "false triggering" at the heart rate (cardiac artifact).
  2. The neonatal cardiorespiratory monitor
     a. Processes and quantifies the inspiratory-induced impedance signal.

     b. Generates a respiratory count and respiratory waveform display on the monitor screen (impedance pneumogram).

     c. Transmits the signal via an interface cable to the impedance input socket on the Sechrist SAVI ventilator.

C. Practical points

    1. Ensure that the cardiorespiratory monitor is compatible with the Sechrist SAVI system by contacting both the manufacturer and also Sechrist Laboratories.

    2. The response time (i.e., the delay between the generation of the inspirator impedance signal and the onset of a triggered breath) will be determined largely by the monitor performance.

    3. The response time should be <80 msec.

D. Within the Sechrist SAVI ventilator:

    1. A bar graph display situated immediately above the impedance input socket on the ventilator will exhibit an ascending and descending movement to show that the impedance signal is being received.

    2. An analog voltage comparator compares the voltage generated by the inspiratory impedance input signal with a trigger voltage predetermined by the setting of the ventilator sensitivity dial chosen by the operator.

    3. When the voltage of the inspiratory impedance input signal exceeds the trigger voltage, a trigger signal is generated.

    4. Through a microprocessor, the trigger signal instructs the solenoid valve of the ventilator fluidic control circuit to turn "on," unless terminated by the detection of an expiratory phase of the impedance pneumogram.

    5. At the termination of the inspiratory phase, the microprocessor will not respond to any further signals for a lockout period of 200 msec in order to prevent breath stacking and to minimize the effects of inadvertent false triggering.

E. Initiating ventilation

    1. Set the inspiratory time at 0.3 to 0.4 seconds.

    2. Adjust the sensitivity dial so that the bar graph display reaches but does not exceed the maximum.

    3. Increasing sensitivity (turning the dial clockwise) will lower the trigger voltage so that a trigger signal will be generated earlier in the upward slope of the inspiratory phase.

    4. If autocycling occurs, reduce sensitivity (turn dial counterclockwise) to increase the trigger threshold.

F. Backup conventional mandatory ventilation

    1. A trigger breath LED will illuminate green whenever a triggered breath is delivered; the trigger rate is displayed in real time on the ventilator.

    2. If no trigger signal is generated, a control breath LED will illuminate yellow.

    3. If no trigger signal is generated for a period set by the alarm "No Trigger," an LED will illuminate red accompanied by an audible

alarm, and breaths will be delivered at a preselected rate on the same settings of inspiratory time (T_I), peak inspiratory pressure (PIP), and positive end-expiratory pressure (PEEP) as on the trigger mode.

G. Clinical points

1. Set backup rate at 20 breaths/min less than the infant's spontaneous respiratory rate, but never more than 60 breaths/min.

2. If the "No Trigger" alarm persists, increase sensitivity and check impedance input signal on the bar graph display.

3. If still not triggering, check chest electrodes and then the clinical status of the infant for air entry, pneumothorax, and $PaCO_2$.

IV. Clinical Application of SAVI

A. Indication: Respiratory failure in spontaneously breathing infants with no significant airway obstruction.

B. Practical points

1. Use CMV mode for 20 minutes after administration of surfactant before commencing A/C mode in infants with surfactant deficiency.

2. Contraindications

a. Neuromuscular disease or treatment with muscle relaxants

b. Recurrent seizures

c. Septic shock or necrotizing enterocolitis

d. Tension pneumothorax

e. Pleural effusion

f. Significant airway obstruction from pulmonary hemorrhage, meconium aspiration, or pneumonia

V. Ventilation Protocol Using SAVI

A. Position chest electrodes and connect to suitable cardiorespiratory monitor as described previously.

B. Connect monitor to Sechrist SAVI ventilator using interface cable.

C. With ventilator in CMV mode, set up as follows:

1. Flow rate: 8 to 12 L/min

2. Inspiratory time: 0.3 to 0.4 second (backup rate as described previously)

3. PIP and PEEP, depending on clinical assessment of chest expansion, air entry, and arterial blood gas results

D. Switch to SAVI by turning sensitivity dial clockwise to click "on."

E. Turn SAVI toward maximum until the bar graph display reaches but does not exceed maximum.

1. If cardiac artifact occurs, reduce sensitivity until it disappears.

2. If cardiac artifact persists, check and, if necessary, reposition chest electrodes.

3. Use flow rates of 10 to 12 L/min initially to ensure adequate tidal volume delivery.

F. Maintain target arterial blood gases by adjusting PIP and PEEP.

G. It is important to maintain $PaCO_2$ above 37.5 mm Hg (5 kPa) to prevent trigger failure.

H. Weaning

1. Reduce PIP as tolerated, depending on arterial blood gases.

2. Turn sensitivity dial counterclockwise to increase trigger threshold (but not enough to cause trigger failure).
3. Decrease bias flow from 12 L/min gradually to 8 L/min to reduce tidal volume delivered.

Suggested Reading

Visveshwara N, Freeman B, Peck M, et al: Patient-triggered synchronized assisted ventilation of newborns. Report of a preliminary study of three years experience. J Perinatol 4:347-354, 1991.

41

Servo-i Ventilator

Mary K. Buschell

I. Introduction
   A. The Servo-i ventilator (Maquet Critical Care AB, Solna, Sweden) has the capability to support ventilation of patients in all age, size and weight ranges, including very low birth weight infants.
   B. Many of its features are specific for neonatal ventilation, including flow-triggering in all modes, tubing compliance compensation, and apnea support with backup ventilation.
   C. The exhalation valve on the Servo-i ventilator is an open system that is able to provide accurate levels of positive end-expiratory pressure (PEEP) and enhances comfort of spontaneously breathing patients.
   D. The new-generation exhalation valve is necessary to use the new modality BiPAP, or bilevel ventilation.

II. Modes
   A. The Servo-i ventilator offers a variety of modes and combinations of modes.
   B. The ventilator may be set to flow-trigger in all modes of ventilation.
   C. All modes are synchronized with the patient's spontaneous breathing effort.
   D. Control modes of ventilation: Spontaneous breaths have the same characteristics (flow, inspiratory time [T_I], volume, or pressure) as the set ventilator breaths.
      1. Pressure control (PC): This mode of ventilation employs a variable flow rate that is microprocessor-controlled to provide a constant inspiratory pressure.
         a. Tidal volume (V_T) is variable
         b. Peak inspiratory pressure (PIP) is constant
         c. Pressure waveform is square
         d. Decelerating flow waveform (a variable flow rate differentiates this mode from time-cycled, pressure-limited ventilation, which incorporates a constant flow)
         e. Clinician-set parameters
            (1) PIP level (above PEEP)
            (2) T_I
            (3) Ventilator rate
            (4) PEEP
            (5) FiO_2
         f. High- and low–minute ventilation (MV) alarms

   g. High-pressure alarm
   h. Trigger sensitivity level
2. Volume control (VC)
   a. Fixed V_T
   b. Variable PIP
   c. Sinusoidal flow waveform (flow is regulated based on set tidal volume and inspiratory time)
   d. Sinusoidal pressure waveform
   e. Clinician-set parameters
      (1) V_T
      (2) T_I (controls flow rate)
      (3) Pause time (added to T_I; does not affect flow rate)
      (4) Ventilator rate
      (5) PEEP
      (6) FiO_2
      (7) High- and low-MV alarms
      (8) High-pressure alarm
3. Pressure-regulated volume control (PRVC) combines a variable flow rate with the advantage of setting a targeted V_T. When PRVC is first initiated, the ventilator delivers a VC breath to establish the approximate pressure required to deliver the set V_T and then changes to a variable flow for breath delivery. This mode produces the same flow and pressure patterns as PC but targets the V_T by monitoring delivered V_T on each breath and adjusting the PIP on the subsequent breath.
   a. V_T is set
   b. PIP is variable
   c. Decelerating flow waveform (the same as PC)
   d. Square pressure waveform
   e. Clinician-set parameters
      (1) V_T
      (2) T_I
      (3) Ventilator rate
      (4) PEEP
      (5) FiO_2
      (6) High and low MV alarms
      (7) High-pressure alarm
      (8) Trigger sensitivity level
E. Modes for spontaneously breathing patients (all breaths are patient-initiated)
   1. Volume support (VS): VS mode is used for patients with an intact respiratory drive. This mode supports the patient's inspiratory effort with an assured or targeted V_T. Backup ventilation is set so that if a patient becomes apneic in this mode, the ventilator alarm will be activated and change over to PRVC with the predetermined backup settings.
      a. V_T is set
      b. PIP settings are variable (based on lung compliance and respiratory effort)

      c. Flow is decelerating
      d. Clinician-set parameters
        (1) Minimum V_T
        (2) T_I (for backup ventilation should apnea occur)
        (3) Ventilator rate (for backup ventilation should apnea occur)
        (4) PEEP
        (5) FiO_2
        (6) High- and low-MV alarms
        (7) High-pressure alarm
        (8) Trigger sensitivity level
        (9) Inspiratory cycle off
  2. Pressure support (PS): PS mode is used for patients with an intact
     respiratory drive. This mode supports the patient's inspiratory
     effort with a set inspiratory pressure. Backup ventilation is
     automatic if the patient has apnea.
      a. V_T is variable
      b. PIP is set
      c. Decelerating flow
      d. Clinician-set parameters
        (1) Inspiratory pressure
        (2) FiO_2
        (3) PEEP
        (4) High- and low-MV alarms
        (5) High-pressure alarm
        (6) Trigger sensitivity level
        (7) Inspiratory cycle off
  3. Continuous positive airway pressure (CPAP)
      a. CPAP is a mode for spontaneously breathing patients who do
        not require any assistance in overcoming the work of breathing
        imposed by lung disease or the endotracheal tube.
      b. Clinician-set parameters
        (1) FiO_2
        (2) Pressure level
        (3) High- and low-MV alarms
        (4) High-pressure alarm
F. Combination modes of ventilation: In addition, the previously listed
  modes are offered in combination. This provides the clinician with the
  ability to support ventilator-delivered breaths and spontaneously
  triggered breaths with different parameters.
  1. Synchronized intermittent mandatory ventilation (SIMV) with
     PS (volume)
  2. SIMV with PS (pressure)
  3. SIMV/PRVC with PS
G. Automode
  1. Automode is an option that enables changing from a control mode
     (VC, PC, and PRVC) to PS or VS if the patient begins
     spontaneously breathing.
  2. If the patient fails to trigger a breath, the ventilator will automatically
     change back to the former control mode of ventilation.

      a. VC changes over to VS.

      b. PRVC changes over to VS.

      c. PC changes over to PS.

H. Control panel and display

    1. The Servo-i ventilator is equipped with a user interface/control panel that is computer-based with a luminescent screen and a combination of soft touch keys and control knobs. It features a gas delivery module.

    2. The user interface/control panel includes continuous display of set and measured values; graphic monitoring of flow, pressure, and volume; and 24-hour trend monitoring. This interface provides a choice of numerous menus and functions, including the following.

      a. Patient category indicator: The ventilator has a "patient category indicator" to set different internal parameters for adult/pediatric and neonatal ventilation, including the following:

        (1) Level of continuous flow for flow-triggering:

Adult/Pediatric	Infant
2.0 L/min	.5 L/min

        (2) Maximum inspiratory peak flow:

Adult/Pediatric	Infant
200 L/min	13 L/min

        (3) Tidal volume range:

Adult/Pediatric	Infant
100-2000 mL	5-350 mL

        (4) Apnea alarm/backup ventilation activation:

Adult/Pediatric	Infant
20 sec	10 sec

        (5) Maximum flow rate:

Adult/Pediatric	Infant
200 L/min	33 L/min

      b. Mode Indicator: Lists current mode of ventilation.

      c. Automode indicator: Indicates whether automode is on or off.

      d. Nebulizer: The ventilator may be equipped with an ultrasonic nebulizer. When the nebulizer is connected, the clinician can set the time for the nebulizer to run.

      e. Admit patient: Stores and displays individual patient information, identification number, name, age, and weight. .

      f. Status: Provides internal information on the status of the following:

        (1) Oxygen fuel cell

        (2) Battery (or batteries)

        (3) Date and time of last preuse check

        (4) Hours of operation

      (5) Barometric pressure
      (6) Gas pressures
  g. Alarm Settings
      (1) High pressure
      (2) Upper and lower MV limits
      (3) Upper and lower respiratory rate
      (4) Low PEEP
  h. Graphic display: When the unit is connected to a patient, there is a continuous display
      (1) Flow-time
      (2) Pressure-time
      (3) Volume-time
      (4) Flow-volume (optional)
      (5) Pressure-volume (optional)
  i. Digital readouts of the following are also continuously displayed.
      (1) PIP
      (2) Pāw (mean airway pressure)
      (3) PEEP
      (4) FiO_2
      (5) I:E ratio (displayed during controlled breaths)
      (6) inspiratory time
      (7) Duty cycle time (T_i/T_{tot}) during spontaneous breaths
      (8) MVe (expiratory or exhaled minute ventilation)
      (9) Inspired tidal volume
     (10) Exhaled tidal volume
     (11) End inspiratory flow
     (12) Static compliance
     (13) Elastance
     (14) Inspiratory resistance
     (15) Expiratory resistance
     (16) Work of breathing (patient)
     (17) Work of breathing (ventilator)
     (18) Time constant
     (19) Shallow breathing index
  j. Trend monitoring: The user interface has comprehensive trend monitoring, with information stored for 24 hours and a time resolution of 1, 3, 6, 12, and 24 hours. Data can be downloaded.
      (1) Measured parameters (listed above)
      (2) Ventilator changes
      (3) Alarm violations
  k. Suction Support: A suction support key offers an adjustable FiO_2 for pre- and postoxygenation, silences the ventilator, and stops flow for 60 seconds. If the patient is reconnected to the ventilator in less than 60 seconds, the ventilator resumes operation.
  l. Additional features
      (1) CO_2 monitor. The Servo-i ventilator is equipped with a port to monitor end-tidal CO_2 ($ETCO_2$) using the Novametrix $ETCO_2$ sensor.

(2) Nebulizer: The Servo-i ventilator has a port to run an ultrasonic nebulizer. The nebulizer has an automatic shut-off, which may be set to run for a maximum of 30 minutes.

(3) BiVent: BiVent is a mode of ventilation for spontaneously breathing patients that provides two levels of pressure from which the patient may breathe. It is set with both a high pressure (15 to 20 cm H_2O) with a long inspiratory time and a low pressure (1 to 5 cm H_2O) with a short inspiratory time. It is a strategy used for lung protection in disease states such as acute respiratory distress syndrome (ARDS).

SLE 2000 (HFO) and SLE 5000 Ventilators

42

J. Harry Baumer

I. Decription
   A. Valveless jet ventilator
   B. Designed for use in newborns and infants weighing up to 20 kg
   C. Constant gas flow
   D. Pressure-limited
   E. Time-cycled
   F. Volume-targeted capability (SLE 5000)
II. Modes of Ventilation
   A. Intermittent mandatory ventilation (IMV)
   B. Assist/control (A/C)
   C. Synchronized intermittent mandatory ventilation (SIMV)
   D. High-frequency oscillatory ventilation (HFOV)
   E. Combined HFOV and IMV
   F. Targeted tidal volume (V_T) ventilation (SLE 5000)
   G. Pressure support ventilation (SLE 5000)
III. Background
   A. Prototype valveless jet ventilator (CW200) was first described in 1988.
   B. Use of the prototype jet ventilator resulted in acute improvement in oxygenation in 13 newborn babies with severe respiratory disease already being ventilated with conventional ventilators.
   C. The arrangement of the prototype ventilator is shown schematically in Figure 42-1. (Although the principle is the same, it should be emphasised that this design does not specifically illustrate the SLE 2000 or SLE 5000.)
   D. The SLE 2000 was introduced in 1990, produced by Scientific Laboratory Equipment, Ltd., Croydon, UK.
   E. Subsequently in 1995, SIMV and HFOV capabilities were developed (SLE 2000 [HFO]).
   F. The SLE 5000 ventilator was introduced in 2002. Additional features include the following:
      1. Pressure support ventilation (PSV)
      2. Dual hot-wire anemometer flow sensor enabling volume-targeted ventilation
      3. Color graphic monitoring of loops and waveforms in all modes of ventilation

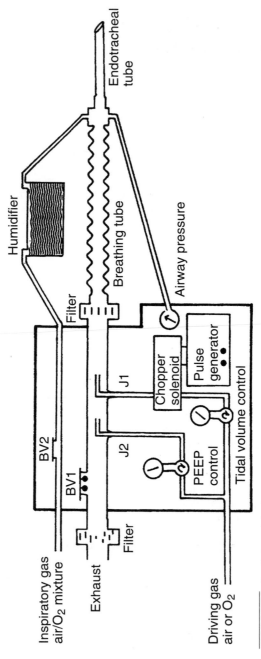

FIGURE 42-1. The design of the CW200 prototype. (Reproduced with permission of Scientific Laboratory Equipment, Ltd., Croydon, UK.)

IV. Design Details
  A. Gas supply
    1. Continuous flow of warmed, humidified gas at rate of 5 L/min.
    2. The humidified gas flow is greater than the minute volume (MV), and the space between the endotracheal tube (ETT) and the driving jet is greater than the V_T.
    3. Gas from the driving jet does not reach the infant and does not take part in gas exchange.
    4. When gas flow rate is variable, as in the conventional ventilator design, increases in gas flow may overcome the capacity of the humidifier, leading to inadequately humidified gas reaching the infant's trachea.
    5. The fixed gas flow avoids the tracheal complications that result when unhumidified gas reaches the tracheobronchial tree.
  B. Ventilator jets
    1. These jets are situated on the exhalation port of the ventilator. This consists of a removable block mounted on a manifold. The expiratory limb of the circuit attaches to the port.
    2. The jets are supplied with the same oxygen concentration as the humidified gas supply to avoid the possibility of gas dilution in the event of tubing disconnection.
    3. The pressure delivered by the jets is controlled by solenoids that are adjusted by regulators on the front panel of the ventilator. Gauges display these pressures.
    4. The driving jet delivers intermittent reverse pulses of gas to the expiratory limb. This compresses the humidified gas (5 L/min) into the ETT, providing the episodes of positive pressure for inspiration.
    5. In a conventional ventilator, the inspiratory plateau results from occlusion of the expiratory limb of the circuit by a solenoid. The compressibility of the circuit results in an attenuation of the peak inspiratory gas flow at the ETT that can be overcome by increasing the flow rate in the circuit. With a fixed resistance in the expiratory limb of the circuit, increases in flow result in rising inadvertent pressure during expiration.
    6. The driving jet replaces the solenoid used in a conventional ventilator. The driving gas from the jet acts as a pneumatic piston, with the inspiratory pressure determined by the pressure setting on the driving jet. This has two consequences.
      a. It avoids the inadvertent positive end-expiratory pressure (PEEP) that occurs when flow rates in the circuit increase.
      b. The jet produces a higher peak inspiratory flow rate, with the inspiratory plateau being reached more rapidly. This is particularly important at the higher range of respiratory frequencies used (>60 breaths/min). It results in a higher mean airway pressure, and hence improved oxygenation, at any given inspiratory time (T_I) setting.
    7. An electronic module determines the rate and duration of opening of the solenoid valve that controls the driving jet.

8. The PEEP jet (see Fig. 42-1) provides continuous gas flow throughout the respiratory cycle.

9. Oscillation is produced by rotating the jet drive by a motor situated at the rear of the exhaust block. This jet produces both an active inspiratory and expiratory flow of gas at the patient manifold. The rate of oscillation is variable up to 20 Hz.

10. Modes of oscillation
   a. Continuous oscillatory mode: This is used with the PEEP jet, which controls the mean airway pressure. The rotating oscillation jet regulator controls the pressure amplitude.
   b. Oscillation superimposed on the inspiratory pressure plateau, the expiratory phase, or both: This is achieved by the combined use of the driving and PEEP jets.

11. The benefits, or otherwise, of the combined use of oscillation and intermittent positive pressure ventilation are as yet unknown.

C. The trigger mechanism
1. Senses the rate of change of pressure at the patient manifold.
2. Detects the onset of inspiratory effort from increasing rate of reduction in pressure.
3. Has adjustable sensitivity within an uncalibrated range.
4. Adjusts backup breath rate in A/C mode. Each backup breath delivered is shown on LED with an optional audible beep.

D. Alarms
1. Power supply
2. Air supply
3. Oxygen supply
4. Microprocessor system failure
5. Inspiratory gas supply failure
6. High pressure
7. Low pressure
8. Cycle failure
9. Oscillation failure
10. Fan failure
11. Low V_T (SLE 5000 only)
12. Low minute volume (MV) (SLE 5000 only)
13. High MV (SLE 5000 only)

E. Information displayed
1. LED displays
   a. Power on
   b. Ventilator rate
   c. Inspiratory time (T_I)
   d. I:E ratio
   e. Maximum, minimum, or mean airway pressure
   f. Inspired oxygen concentration
   g. Trigger backup breath (and optional audible signal)
2. LCD display
   a. Pressure waveform
   b. High and low alarm settings
   c. Display time base (0.5 to 6 seconds)

        d. Display pressure range (up to 50 cm or ± 60 cm)
        e. Variable time base for display
        f. Display can be frozen
        g. Loops depicting flow/volume, flow/pressure, and
           volume/pressure (SLE 5000)
        h. Volume, flow waveforms (SLE 5000)
        i. Lung mechanics (SLE 5000)
  F. Other features
    1. The patient circuit has a restrictor fitted to the inspiratory side of
        the patient endotracheal manifold.
        a. The manufacturer states that this is required to ensure that
           it is possible to monitor the inspiratory limb of the circuit for
           leaks.
        b. It has also been suggested that this is required to increase the
           trigger sensitivity. The increased inspiratory resistance increases
           inspiratory effort and consequently the number of spontaneous
           breaths that will trigger the ventilator in infants <1.0 kg.
        c. The position of the restrictor is such that work of breathing
           should not be affected.
    2. A pressure waveform switch modifies the driving gas flow rate.
        This slows the rate of rise of pressure at the onset of inspiration.
    3. It is possible to deliver nitric oxide via the ventilator.
V. Performance of the SLE 2000 (HFO) ventilator
  A. Trigger sensitivity
    1. In some studies this has been defined as the proportion of infant
        breaths that trigger the ventilator. Caution is required in
        interpretation because other factors may influence the sensitivity.
        These include T_I, the use of respiratory stimulants and sedation,
        and the gestational age and neurologic state of the infant.
    2. In a comparison of four neonatal ventilators, the SLE 2000
        ventilator had a median sensitivity of 99% (range 90% to 100%)
        in a small number of babies with acute RDS, and 96.5%
        (range 59% to 100%) in infants with chronic RDS. This was at least
        as sensitive as the Sechrist IV, Infant Star, Bear Cub ventilators.
    3. A study of 22 preterm infants, which monitored interactions
        during 67,150 spontaneous respiratory cycles in 3592 15-second
        epochs, showed synchrony in only 19.5% of epochs.
    4. In a study in 12 infants, the median sensitivity was 87% (range
        19% to 100%). The sensitivity of the Infant Star ventilator using an
        abdominal capsule was significantly higher. In this study both
        ventilators had a high rate of asynchrony, with the inspiratory
        phase of the ventilator extending into the expiratory phase of the
        infant's respiration.
  B. Trigger delay
    1. Measurements of trigger delay should be interpreted with caution,
        because factors such as gestational age also will have a major
        influence.
    2. Median trigger delay was 80 msec (range 40 to 100 msec) in a
        patient-based study of 13 preterm infants with RDS.

3. Trigger delay in 40 infants with acute or chronic respiratory distress was significantly shorter than with the Bear Cub II ventilator using an airflow device, particularly in babies with chronic respiratory distress. However, the infants ventilated with the Bear Cub ventilator were more immature. The delay was not significantly different from that with the Sechrist IV and Infant Star ventilators.

4. In a further study of 12 infants with a gestational age between 24 and 27 weeks, a median delay of 112 msec (range 24 to 270 msec) was seen. A significantly shorter delay was seen in infants ventilated with the Infant Star ventilator using an abdominal surface sensor.

C. Autotriggering (Autocycling)

1. Autotriggering is a situation in which ventilator breaths occur without initiation of inspiratory efforts by the infant. This may occur spontaneously or, for example, because of water trapped in the ventilator tubing.

2. This is said to be common with the SLE 2000 ventilator at the highest sensitivity setting.

3. A different investigator found no autotriggering at the highest sensitivity setting in a study of 12 preterm infants with RDS. The importance of maintaining the ventilator circuit free of condensed water was emphasized.

4. In a study of 22 preterm infants with RDS, 19.6% of 16-second epochs was associated with autotriggering.

D. Peak inspiratory flow rate

1. The SLE 2000 ventilator was compared with the Dräger Babylog 8000 and V.I.P. Bird ventilators attached to a model lung.

2. The time to plateau was significantly shorter with the SLE 2000 ventilator than for the other ventilators when gas flow was optimized to achieve a rapid rise to plateau.

3. With the pressure wave switch set to attenuate the rise to plateau, the time to plateau seen in the SLE 2000 ventilator was similar to the minimum obtained by the the other ventilators.

4. The consequences of this difference in performance are unknown.
   a. Oxygenation at any given inspiratory time setting will be improved with a short time to plateau.
   b. It is conceivable that chronic lung damage could increase with more rapid increase in pressure.

E. Oscillation mode

1. A study of four neonatal ventilators delivering high-frequency oscillatory ventilation using a model lung showed the following:
   a. The delivered volume changed little above 10 Hz, but this effect depended upon lung compliance.
   b. ETT size had a major effect on delivered volume, emphasising the importance of using the largest size possible.
   c. The volume delivery of the SLE 2000 ventilator was comparable to that of the SensorMedics oscillator at a given setting.

    d. The reduction in delivered volume with decreasing compliance was less for the SLE 2000 ventilator than for the SensorMedics oscillator.

    e. The study concluded that optimum CO_2 elimination could be achieved with relatively low frequencies and a large ETT.

F. Studies of longer-term triggered ventilation

    1. A study of 68 infants ventilated for RDS throughout with A/C demonstrated the SLE 2000 ventilator to support infants for periods of up to 28 days. No control group was available for comparison.

    2. Retrospective analysis of nursing observations on 49 infants <28 weeks' gestation within 72 hours of birth with RDS demonstrated the following:

        a. The SLE 2000 ventilator was capable of delivering patient-triggered ventilation to infants <28 weeks' gestation.

        b. With backup rates of <40 breaths/min, the number of untriggered breaths was minimized.

        c. The triggered breath rate was 25% lower with a T_I of 0.5 second, compared to settings between 0.2 and 0.25 second.

Suggested Reading

Baumer JH, Ellis S: Patient triggered ventilation in infants under 28 weeks. Early Hum Dev 39:144-148, 1994.

Chan KN, Chakrabarti MK, Whitwam JG, et al: Assessment of a new valveless infant ventilator. Arch Dis Child 63:162-167, 1988.

Chan V, Greenough A: Neonatal patient triggered ventilators: Performance in acute and chronic lung disease. Br J Int Care 3:216-219, 1993.

deBoer RC, Jones A, Ward PS, et al: Long term trigger ventilation in neonatal respiratory distress syndrome. Arch Dis Child 68:308-311, 1993.

Laubscher B, Greenough A, Costeloe K: Performance of four neonatal high frequency oscillators. Br J Int Care 6:148-152, 1996.

43 Bunnell Life Pulse High-Frequency Jet Ventilator

Martin Keszler

I. Description
   A. The Bunnell Life Pulse is the only Food and Drug Administration (FDA)–approved neonatal high-frequency jet ventilator (HFJV) device currently available in the U.S. Other HFJV devices produced abroad have been used in Europe and elsewhere.
   B. The Life Pulse is a microprocessor-based ventilator that continuously monitors airway pressure and automatically adjusts the pressure that drives pulses of gas across the injector cannula to achieve a set peak inspiratory pressure (PIP), with a range of 8 to 50 cm H_2O.

II. Independently Set Variables
   A. Ventilator rate: 240 to 660 breaths/min = 4 to 11 Hz
   B. Inspiratory time (T_I): 0.02 to 0.034 second)
   C. Positive end-expiratory pressure (PEEP) and superimposed low rate intermittent mandatory ventilation (IMV) (when desired) are generated by a conventional ventilator used in tandem with the Life Pulse ventilator.
   D. The FiO_2 of the two ventilators can be adjusted separately (it should be maintained at the same level), or both ventilators can be supplied from a common source using a single blender.

III. Displayed Parameters
   A. PIP
   B. Mean airway pressure (Pāw)
   C. Pressure amplitude
   D. Servo pressure
   E. Alarms: Alarms are automatically set 15% above and below current levels for PIP, Pāw, and Servo pressure once the values stabilize and the ventilator reaches the "Ready" state. Subsequently, the alarm limits can be adjusted manually.
   F. An efficient low-volume humidifier is built into the device, assuring optimal heating and humidification of inspired gases.
   G. The delivery of gas is controlled by a pinch valve located in a "patient box" placed near the patient's head.
      1. The box also houses the pressure sensor.
      2. This arrangement ensures accurate pressure monitoring and efficient ventilation.

IV. Reintubation: Reintubation is not required, because a special endotracheal tube (ETT) adapter (LifePort) containing a pressure-sensing lumen and the injector port has replaced the original triple-lumen ETT tube formerly required for HFJV.

V. Suctioning: Suctioning can be done in one of two ways:

A. The jet ventilator can be placed in stand-by mode and suctioning done in the usual fashion.

B. Alternatively, suctioning can be done while the ventilator continues to operate; constant (continuous) suction is applied while the suction catheter is advanced and then withdrawn. This is necessary because unless continuous suction is applied, the jet ventilator will force gas past the suction catheter and cause overpressure.

VI. *Caution:* Clinicians should be aware that the FDA has only approved the Life Pulse jet ventilator only for the treatment of pulmonary interstitial emphysema and for rescue of infants with refractory respiratory failure complicated by air leak.

44

SensorMedics 3100A High-Frequency Oscillatory Ventilator

David J. Durand and Jeanette M. Asselin

I. Physiology of High-Frequency Oscillatory Ventilation (HFOV)
   A. Conceptual difference between conventional and high-frequency ventilation
      1. With conventional ventilation, gas is moved from the upper airway to the alveoli, primarily by *bulk flow* ("pouring gas into and out of the alveoli").
      2. With HFOV, gas movement is accomplished primarily by the *mixing* of gas in the upper airway with gas in the alveoli ("shaking gas into and out of the alveoli").
   B. Characterizing HFOV "breaths"
      1. The SensorMedics 3100A generates a pressure wave that, when analyzed at the hub of the endotracheal tube (ETT), is approximately a sine wave.
      2. This pressure wave is characterized primarily by three factors, each of which can be independently adjusted.
         a. Mean airway pressure (Pāw): The average pressure throughout the respiratory cycle
         b. Amplitude: The size of the pressure wave, or tidal volume (V_T)
         c. Frequency: The number of breaths per minute (breaths/min)
         d. The inspiratory:expiratory (I:E) ratio can also be adjusted but is kept at 1:2 for essentially all neonatal patients.
   C. Oxygenation and ventilation
      1. Oxygenation is proportional to Pāw.
         a. The higher the Pāw, the more alveoli are open throughout the respiratory cycle. This decreases atelectasis and improves ventilation-perfusion matching.
         b. Increasing Pāw increases average lung volume and is reflected by increased lung volume on chest radiography.
      2. Ventilation (or CO_2 removal) is approximately proportional to frequency × amplitude^2.
         a. This means that changes in amplitude have a greater impact on CO_2 exchange than do changes in frequency.
         b. For most patients, a frequency is chosen and left constant, whereas CO_2 exchange is affected by changing the amplitude.

3. Effect of frequency on amplitude
   a. The ETT and upper airway act as a *low-pass filter*. This means that low-frequency pressure waves are passed from the ventilator to the alveoli without being attenuated, whereas high-frequency pressure waves are attenuated. The higher the frequency, the greater the attenuation.
   b. A simplified example of the attenuation of pressure amplitude at high frequencies is outlined here. Imagine a ventilator that is set to deliver an amplitude of 20 cm H_2O (e.g., peak inspiratory pressure [PIP] 25 cm H_2O, positive end-expiratory pressure [PEEP] 5 cm H_2O).
      (1) At a low frequency (e.g., 30 breaths/min), the pressure amplitude of 20 cm H_2O is completely transmitted to the alveoli. The alveolar pressure changes from 5 to 25 cm H_2O as the ventilator cycles.
      (2) At an intermediate frequency (e.g., 120 breaths/min), the pressure amplitude will be slightly attenuated as it travels from the hub of the ETT to the alveoli, because neither the inspiratory time (T_I) nor the expiratory time (T_E) is adequate for the pressure to equalize between the upper airway and the alveoli. At the alveolar level, the breath will have a PIP of 22 and a PEEP of 8. Thus the amplitude of the breath will have been attenuated from 20 cm H_2O to 14 cm H_2O. This is the phenomenon that causes air trapping (sometimes called inadvertent PEEP) at inappropriately high rates on conventional ventilation.
      (3) At an even higher frequency (e.g., 600 breaths/min), the attenuation is far more significant. A breath with an amplitude of 20 cm H_2O at the hub of the ETT may be attenuated to less than 5 cm H_2O at the alveoli.
   c. Thus, if everything else is constant, *decreasing frequency will increase alveolar amplitude,* because at a lower frequency more of the pressure wave will be transmitted to the alveoli. Because amplitude has a greater impact on CO_2 exchange than does frequency, *decreasing frequency will increase CO_2 exchange.*
   d. This complex relationship between frequency and CO_2 exchange is one of the reasons why frequency is not the primary parameter to be adjusted when optimizing ventilation.
II. Theoretical Advantages of HFOV
   A. With HFOV, the alveolus never deflates to the degree that it does with conventional ventilation. Thus surface forces are less likely to cause atelectasis. In any patient with a tendency to develop atelectasis (e.g., patients with respiratory distress syndrome [RDS]), this should be a significant advantage because preventing atelectasis is a key element in avoiding lung injury.
   B. With HFOV, the lung is not distended as much as it is with a typical V_T; therefore, there is less chance of causing alveolar or airway overdistention, a primary cause of both acute and chronic lung injury.

Distal airway overdistention is the primary mechanism of pulmonary interstitial emphysema (PIE).

III. When to Use the SensorMedics 3100A

A. HFOV theoretically is superior to conventional ventilation for infants with any lung disease characterized by severe, homogeneous decrease in compliance and no airway involvement. The ideal HFOV patient is one with the "white-out" of severe RDS.

B. HFOV is probably better than conventional ventilation for infants with severe PIE or bronchopleural fistula. However, HFOV is probably not as effective as high-frequency jet ventilation (HFJV) in treating these patients.

C. HFOV may be better than conventional ventilation for term or near-term infants with severe nonhomogeneous disease, such as pneumonia or meconium aspiration syndrome, if atelectasis is a prominent component of the disease.

D. HFOV is probably superior to conventional ventilation for most (or all) premature infants with significant lung disease that would predispose them to development of bronchopulmonary dysplasia. Although clinical trials of high-frequency ventilation have yielded conflicting results, the most impressive data supporting the use of HFOV in this population come from a large controlled trial in which infants treated with HFOV were extubated significantly earlier and were significantly less likely to develop chronic lung disease (CLD) than infants treated with conventional ventilation in a synchronized intermittent mandatory ventilation (SIMV) mode.

IV. Mechanics of the SensorMedics 3100A: Only six parameters can be adjusted.

A. Pāw

1. Pāw is set by adjusting the pressure adjust knob.
2. Increasing Pāw recruits alveoli, leading to improved ventilation-perfusion matching, and improved oxygenation.
3. Increasing Pāw also leads to increased lung inflation, as seen on chest radiography.
4. When placing a patient on HFOV, start with a Pāw that is approximately 20% above the Pāw on conventional ventilation.
5. Follow chest radiographs closely to determine the degree of lung inflation.
   a. In most patients, the lungs should be inflated so that the top of the right hemidiaphragm is between 8 and 10 ribs.
   b. Patients on HFOV should have chest radiographs obtained frequently enough that both over- and underdistention can be avoided. A typical schedule usually includes obtaining a radiograph:
      (1) 30 to 60 minutes after starting HFOV.
      (2) 2 to 6 hours after starting HFOV.
      (3) 12 hours after starting HFOV.
      (4) 12 to 24 hours until off HFOV.
      (5) After any large (>20%) change in Pāw.
      (6) After any large (>20%) change in FiO_2.

6. Changes in Pāw.
   a. Increase Pāw if the lungs are underinflated and/or if the patient is not oxygenating adequately.
   b. Decrease Pāw if the lungs are overinflated and/or if the patient's oxygenation is improving.
   c. To cause a small change in lung inflation and/or oxygenation, change the Pāw by 10% to 20%.
   d. To cause a larger change in lung inflation and/or oxygenation, change the Pāw by 20% to 40%.

B. Amplitude is set by adjusting power (in arbitrary units) and is measured as delta pressure (cm H_2O).
   1. Increasing the power leads to an increase in the excursion of the ventilator diaphragm. This increases the amplitude of the pressure wave and is reflected in an increase in the delta pressure, which is measured at the hub of the ETT. Remember that the delta pressure is markedly attenuated by the time it reaches the alveoli.
   2. Increasing the amplitude leads to an increase in chest movement ("chest wiggle") and a decrease in $PaCO_2$.
   3. Relatively small changes (10% to 20%) in amplitude result in significant changes in $PaCO_2$.
   4. When placing a patient on HFOV, adjust the amplitude so that the patient is comfortable without much spontaneous respiratory effort, and so that the chest wiggle looks appropriate (there is no way to learn this other than through experience). Follow the $PaCO_2$ closely and consider using a transcutaneous CO_2 monitor to help with initial adjustments in amplitude.

C. Frequency, measured in Hz (1 Hz = 1 breath/sec or 60 breaths/min). For neonatal patients, frequency is usually 6 to 12 Hz (360 to 720 breaths/min).
   1. Use higher frequencies for small babies with dense lung disease and lower frequencies for large babies, babies with mild disease, and babies with nonuniform disease.
   2. In general, use a lower frequency for patients with nonhomogeneous lung disease, airway disease, or air-trapping. If a patient has an unacceptable degree of air trapping that does not respond to decreasing Pāw, consider decreasing the frequency by at least 1 to 2 Hz.
   3. Typical frequencies
      a. Preterm infant with severe RDS: 10 to 12 Hz, sometimes higher
      b. Preterm infant with mild RDS or early chronic lung disease: 8 to 10 Hz
      c. Preterm infant with significant CLD: 6 to 8 Hz
      d. Term infant with severe pneumonia or meconium aspiration: 6 Hz

D. % T_I is almost always 33%, or an I:E ratio of 1:2.

E. Flow, measured in liters per minute
   1. As with other types of ventilators, more flow is needed for large patients than for small patients.
   2. Although the ventilator is always calibrated and set up with a flow of 20 L/min, this should be decreased for premature infants. Typical flow settings are the following:

    a. Premature infant < 1000 g: Flow 6 to 8 L/min

    b. Premature infant 1500 to 2500 g: Flow 10 to 12 L/min

    c. Term infant with severe meconium aspiration: Flow 15 to 20 L/min

F. FiO_2: Adjustments in FiO_2 have the same impact on oxygenation for a patient on HFOV as they do for a patient on other forms of ventilation.

V. Optimizing Settings

  A. In general, the approach to HFOV includes avoiding the extremes of over- and underinflation, minimizing oxygen exposure, and weaning as aggressively as tolerated.

    1. Optimizing lung volume can be done only in conjunction with chest radiography. The Pāw should be adjusted so that lung volume is optimal, usually with the top of the right hemidiaphragm at approximately the level between the 8th and the 10th posterior rib.

    2. Minimizing oxygen exposure is done by increasing Pāw, as long as it does not cause overinflation, in patients with an F_iO_2 >0.35 to 0.4. Often, small increases in Pāw will allow significant reduction in FiO_2 without causing overinflation.

    3. Weaning the Pāw is done by judiciously decreasing pressure (usually in 1 cm H_2O decrements) for patients who have an F_iO_2 <0.35 to 0.4. However, if a decrease in Pāw results in a significant increase in FiO_2 or in clinical lability, the Pāw may have been weaned too much.

    4. Weaning the amplitude is done by judiciously decreasing delta pressure (usually by 10%) for patients who have a $PaCO_2$ in their "target range." However, if a decrease in amplitude results in a significant increase in PCO_2, work of breathing, or clinical lability, the amplitude has probably been weaned too far.

  B. Optimizing frequency is an imprecise process. In most cases, the frequency range listed previously is adequate. However, if the patient appears to have air trapping, manifested by an overinflated chest radiograph and poor oxygenation or ventilation, consider decreasing the frequency by 1 to 2 Hz. Remember that decreasing frequency will decrease the pressure attenuation, increasing the delivered pressure amplitude at the alveolar level, and decreasing $PaCO_2$.

VI. Weaning and Extubating from HFOV

  A. Many patients can be extubated directly from HFOV, without changing back to another mode of ventilation. In a study that showed that HFOV significantly reduced CLD, patients were placed on HFOV within the first few hours of life, and were kept on HFOV until they were extubated.

    1. Decrease both Pāw and amplitude as the patient improves.

    2. As the patient improves, and as amplitude decreases, the patient will do more spontaneous breathing. If the amplitude decreases sufficiently, the patient will essentially be on "oscillatory continuous positive airway pressure (CPAP)" rather than oscillatory ventilation.

3. When the patient is achieving most of the CO_2 elimination by spontaneous breathing, and the Pāw has been decreased sufficiently, the patient can be extubated.
4. General guidelines for extubation
    a. Patient <1000 g: Pāw = 7 to 8 cm H_2O and FiO_2 = 0.3 to 0.4
    b. Patient >1000 g: Pāw = 8 to 9 cm H_2O and FiO_2 = 0.3 to 0.4
B. Some clinicians prefer to wean patients from HFOV to another mode of ventilation before extubating. This is particularly useful in an institution that does not have many high-frequency ventilators available. In general, patients should not be weaned from HFOV until they have improved significantly.
C. General guidelines for weaning from HFOV to another form of ventilation
    1. FiO_2 <0.4
    2. Able to be ventilated at a PIP <25 cm H_2O
D. In some patients with CLD, HFOV may not be as effective as other forms of ventilation. If a patient with obvious CLD is still on HFOV at 2 to 4 weeks of age, it may be reasonable to give that patient a trial of conventional ventilation do determine which mode is more effective.

Suggested Reading

Chang H: Mechanisms of gas transport during ventilation by high-frequency oscillation. J Appl Physiol 56:553-563, 1984.

Courtney SE, Durand DJ, Asselin JM, et al: High frequency oscillatory ventilation vs conventional mechanical ventilation for very-low-birth-weight infants. N Engl J Med 347:643-652, 2002.

Durand DJ, Asselin JM, Hudak ML, et al: Early HFOV vs SIMV in VLBW infants: A pilot study of two ventilation protocols. J Perinatol 21:221-229, 2001.

Keszler M, Durand DJ: Neonatal high-frequency ventilation: Past, present, and future. Clin Perinatol 28:579-607, 2001.

Management of Common Neonatal Respiratory Diseases

Mechanisms of Respiratory Failure

45

Anne Greenough and Anthony D. Milner

I. Respiratory failure is present when there is a major abnormality of gas exchange.
   A. In an adult, the limits of normality are a PaO_2 >60 mm Hg (8 kPa).
   B. In the newborn, the oxygen tension needed to maintain the arterial saturation above 90% varies between 40 and 60 mm Hg (5.3 to 8 kPa), depending on the proportion of hemoglobin that is fetal and the arterial pH (a drop in pH of 0.2 eliminates the left shift produced by 70% of the hemoglobin being fetal). Thus, in the newborn period, respiratory failure is best defined in terms of oxygen saturation. There are, however, no agreed criteria (see later).
   C. Hypoxia may be associated with hypercarbia ($PaCO_2$ >55 mm Hg [6.7 kPa])

$$PaCO_2 \approx \frac{CO_2 \text{ production}}{\text{Alveolar ventilation}}$$

Alveolar ventilation = tidal volume − dead space × frequency

II. Respiratory failure associated with hypercarbia will occur, therefore, in situations associated with reduction in tidal volume (T_1) and/or frequency.
   A. Respiratory failure in the neonatal period may be defined as PaO_2 <50 mm Hg (6.7 kPa) in an inspired oxygen of at least 50% with/without $PaCO_2$ >50 mm Hg (6.7 kPa).
   B. Hypoxemia in the neonatal period can result from multiple causes.
      1. Ventilation-perfusion (V/Q) mismatch
         a. Distinguished by a good response to supplementary oxygen (intrapulmonary shunting)
         b. Increased physiologic dead space
         c. Found in the following conditions:
            (1) Respiratory distress syndrome (RDS)
            (2) Pneumonia
            (3) Meconium aspiration syndrome (MAS)
            (4) Bronchopulmonary dysplasia (chronic lung disease [CLD])

2. Extrapulmonary (right-to-left) shunts are distinguished by relatively little improvement with supplementary oxygen and are found in:
   (a) Pulmonary hypertension
   (b) Cyanotic congenital heart disease*
3. Methemoglobinemia*
4. Inadequate inspired oxygen *
5. Hypoventilation (reduced alveolar ventilation, reduction in tidal volume and/or frequency)
   a. Distinguished by a high $PaCO_2$ in association with hypoxemia
      (1) Reduced respiratory compliance
      (2) Found in:
         (a) RDS
         (b) Pneumonia
   b. Reduced lung volume, found in:
      (1) RDS
      (2) Pulmonary hypoplasia
   c. Compressed lung, found in:
      (1) Pneumothorax
      (2) Pleural effusion
      (3) Lobar emphysema
      (4) Cystic adenomatoid malformation
      (5) Asphyxiating thoracic dystrophy
   d. Ventilatory pump failure
      (1) Reduced central drive, found in:
         (a) Maternal opiate treatment (high levels of sedation)
         (b) Cerebral ischemia
         (c) Intracerebral hemorrhage
         (d) Apnea of prematurity
         (e) Central alveolar hypoventilation syndrome
      (2) Impaired ventilatory muscle function
      (3) Miscellaneous conditions
         (a) Drugs (corticosteroids, paralytics—synergism with aminoglycosides)
         (b) Disuse atrophy (first signs occur after 1 to 2 days of mechanical ventilation)
         (c) Protein calorie malnutrition
         (d) Disadvantageous tension-length relationship (e.g., hyperinflation—diaphragm must contract with a much higher than normal tension. When completely flat, contraction of the diaphragm draws in the lower rib cage, producing an expiratory rather than inspiratory action.)

---

*Note: although these situations produce cyanosis, it is not from respiratory failure. Cyanosis appears when the reduced hemoglobin concentration of the blood in the capillaries is more than 5 g/dL. Cyanosis, therefore, does not occur in severe anemic hypoxia (hypoxia is oxygen deficiency at the tissue level).

(e) Neuromuscular disorders (Werdnig-Hoffman disease, myotonic dystrophy)
(f) Diaphragmatic problems (hernia, eventration)
(g) Phrenic nerve palsy (birth trauma, with Erb palsy)
(4) Increased respiratory muscle workload, found in:
(a) "Obesity," chest wall edema (hydrops)
(b) Upper airway obstruction/endotracheal tube with insufficient compensatory ventilatory support
(c) Pulmonary edema, pneumonia
(d) Intrinsic (inadvertent) positive end-expiratory pressure (PEEP)
e. Disorders affecting the alveolar-capillary interface, distinguished, if incomplete, by a good response to increased supplementary oxygen
(1) Diffusion abnormalities (interstitial lung disease), such as pulmonary lymphangiectasia (Noonan syndrome)
(2) Anemia
(3) Alveolar-capillary dysplasia

Suggested Reading

Aldrich TK, Prezant DJ: Indications for mechanical ventilation. In Tobin MJ (ed): Principles and Practice of Mechanical Ventilation. New York, McGraw-Hill, 1994, pp 155-189.

Bazzy-Asaad A: Respiratory muscle function: Implications for ventilatory failure. In Haddad GG, Abman SH, Chernick V (eds): Basic Mechanisms of Pediatric Respiratory Disease, 2nd ed. Hamilton, Ontario, Canada, BC Decker, 2002, pp 250-271.

Marini JJ, Slutsky AS: Physiological basis of ventilatory support. In Lenfant C (ed): Lung Biology in Health and Disease, Vol 188. New York, Marcel Dekker, 1988.

Roussos C, Macklem PT: The respiratory muscles. N Engl J Med 307:786-797, 1982.

46 Tissue Hypoxia

Anne Greenough and Anthony D. Miller

I. Definition
   A. Tissue hypoxia occurs when oxygen transport is reduced below a critical level (i.e., below the metabolic demand), at which point either metabolism must be maintained anaerobically or tissue metabolic rate must be reduced.
   B. Under experimental conditions, if demands are kept constant, there is a biphasic response in oxygen consumption as oxygen transport is progressively reduced.
      1. Initially, oxygen consumption is independent of oxygen transport.
      2. Subsequently, oxygen consumption becomes dependent on oxygen transport and declines in proportion (physiologic supply dependency).
II. Evaluating Tissue Oxygenation
   A. There is no very good method.
   B. Mixed venous saturation identifies global tissue hypoxia, but tissue hypoxia can exist with a normal mixed venous saturation.
   C. Blood lactate levels: Elevation can be present in the absence of tissue hypoxia, particularly in patients with sepsis.
   D. Fractional oxygen extraction (FOE) increases as oxygen transport is progressively compromised. FOE can be measured by near infrared spectroscopy. Whether FOE is a reliable measure of tissue hypoxia requires further testing.
III. Oxygen Transport
   A. Determinants
      1. Cardiac output
      2. Hemoglobin concentration
      3. To a lesser extent, hemoglobin saturation
   B. Oxygen-hemoglobin dissociation curve
      1. The quaternary structure of hemoglobin determines its affinity for oxygen. By shifting the relationship of its four-component polypeptide chains, and hence a change in the position of the heme moieties, it can assume:
         a. A relaxed (R) state—favors O_2 binding
         b. A tense (T) state—decreases O_2 binding
      2. When hemoglobin takes up a small amount of the oxygen, the R state is favored and additional O_2 uptake is facilitated.
      3. The oxygen-hemoglobin dissociation curve (which relates percentage of oxygen saturation of hemoglobin to PaO_2) has a sigmoid shape.

C. Factors affecting the affinity of hemoglobin for oxygen:
1. Temperature
2. pH
3. 2,3-Diphosphoglycerate (2,3-DPG)
    a. A rise in temperature, a fall in pH (Bohr effect, elevated $PaCO_2$), or an increase in 2,3-DPG all shift the curve to the right, liberating more oxygen.
    b. The P_{50} is the PaO_2 at which the hemoglobin is half-saturated with O_2; the higher the P_{50}, the lower the affinity of hemoglobin for oxygen.
    c. A right shift of the curve means a higher P_{50} (i.e., a higher PaO_2 is required for hemoglobin to bind a given amount of O_2).
D. 2,3-DPG
1. It is formed from 3-phosphoglyceride, a product of glycolysis.
2. It is a highly charged anion that binds to the β chains of deoxygenated hemoglobin, but not to those of oxyhemoglobin.
3. 2,3-DPG concentration
    a. Increased by:
        (1) Thyroid hormones
        (2) Growth hormones
        (3) Androgens
        (4) Exercise
        (5) Ascent to high altitude (secondary to alkalosis)
    b. Decreased by:
        (1) Acidosis (which inhibits red blood cell glycolysis)
        (2) Fetal hemoglobin (HbF) has a greater affinity for O_2 than adult hemoglobin (HbA); this is caused by the poor binding of 2,3-DPG to the δ chains of HbF. Increasing concentrations of 2,3-DPG have much less effect on altering the P_{50} if HbF rather than HbA is present.
IV. Response to Reduced Oxygen Transport
A. From low cardiac output (if chronic, 2,3-DPG increases unless there is systemic academia)
B. From anemia
1. Cardiac output and oxygen extraction increase.
2. If chronic, the HbO_2 dissociation curve shifts to the right.
C. From alveolar hypoxemia
1. Increased cardiac output and oxygen extraction
2. Increased hemoglobin
V. Oxygen Extraction Increases Progressively: Oxygen transport is reduced if oxygen consumption remains constant.
A. Alterations in vascular resistance with adjustments to the microcirculation—opening of previously closed capillaries. This has three positive effects:
1. The increase in capillary density decreases the distance for diffusion between the blood and site of oxygen utilization.
2. It increases the lateral surface area for diffusion.
3. The increase in cross-sectional area of the capillaries reduces the blood linear velocity and increases the transit time for diffusion.

B. Changes in hemoglobin oxygen affinity
   1. Increase in hydrogen (H^+) concentration results in a right shift of the dissociation curve.
   2. Changes occur in the 2,3-DPG concentration.
   3. The concentration of 2,3-DPG is regulated by red blood cell H^+ concentration (because the rate-limiting enzyme is pH sensitive): A high pH stimulates 2,3-DPG synthesis.
   4. Deoxyhemoglobin provides better buffering than oxyhemoglobin and thereby raises red blood cell pH; thus, low venous oxygen promotes DPG synthesis.*

VI. Consequences of Tissue Hypoxia
   A. Reduced oxidative phosphorylation
   B. Electron transport chain slowed
   C. Reduced phosphorylation of adenosine-5'-diphosphate (ADP) to adenosine-5'-triphosphate (ATP)
   D. Increased adenosine-5'-monophosphate (AMP), which is rapidly catabolized to inosine and hypoxanthine during hypoxia.
   E. Creatinine phosphate acts as a "supplementary" energy reservoir if creatinine kinase is available but becomes rapidly depleted.
   F. ADP can be phosphorylated anaerobically, but this is much less efficient than aerobic metabolism. During aerobic glycolysis, production of ATP is 19 times greater than it is under anerobic conditions (i.e, production of 38 mmol versus 2 mmol of ATP). Lactic acid accumulates.
   G. Adverse effect on immune function and inflammation
      1. Increased neutrophil sequestration
      2. Increased vascular permeability
      3. Decreased cellular immune function

Suggested Reading

Lister G: Oxygen transport and consumption. In Gluckman PD, Heymann MA (eds): Pediatrics and Perinatology—The Scientific Basis, 2nd ed. London, Edward Arnold, 1996, pp 778-790.
Lister G, Farhey J: Oxygen transport. In Haddad GG, Abman SH, Cherick V (eds): Basic Mechanisms of Pediatric Respiratory Disease, 2nd ed. Hamiton, Ontario, Canada, BC Decker, 2002, pp 184-199.
Wardle SP, Weindling AM: Peripheral fractional oxygen extraction and other measures of tissue oxygenation to guide blood transfusions in preterm infants. Semin Perinatol 25:60-64, 2001.

---

*Note: This adaptive mechanism is less prominent in young infants with high levels of HgF because HbF binds 2,3-DPG poorly and its synthesis is inhibited by unbound DPG.

Indications for Mechanical Ventilation

47

Anne Greenough and Anthony D. Milner

I. Absolute Indications
   A. In the delivery room
      1. Failure to establish adequate spontaneous respiration immediately after delivery despite adequate face mask ventilation.
      2. Persistent bradycardia unresponsive to face mask ventilation.
      3. A large diaphragmatic hernia: Affected infants should be intubated, ventilated, and paralyzed from birth to stop them from swallowing, which increases the dimensions of the bowel and worsens respiratory failure.
   B. In the neonatal intensive care unit (NICU)
      1. Sudden collapse with apnea and bradycardia and failure to establish satisfactory ventilation after a short period of face mask ventilation.
      2. Massive pulmonary hemorrhage: Such infants should be intubated, preferably paralyzed, and ventilated with high levels of positive end-expiratory pressure (PEEP).
II. Relative Indications
   A. In the delivery room
      1. Infants <28 weeks of gestational age may be electively intubated unless vigorous at birth.
      2. Infants <32 weeks of gestational age may be electively intubated to receive prophylactic surfactant therapy. (Note: In some centers, continuous positive airway pressure is used as an alternative to elective intubation and mechanical ventilation.)
   B. In the NICU
      1. Worsening respiratory failure: The criteria will depend upon the gestational age of the infant.
         a. 28 weeks of gestational age: Arterial carbon dioxide tension ($PaCO_2$) >50 to 55 mm Hg (6.7 to 7.3 kPa), the lower limit being used if associated with a pH <7.25 and/or arterial oxygen tension (PaO_2) <50 to 60 mm Hg (6.7 to 8 kPa) in a fractional inspired oxygen (FiO_2) >0.40, although if the infant only has poor oxygenation, nasal continuous positive airway pressure (CPAP) may be tried first.
         b. 28 to 34 weeks of gestational age: $PaCO_2$ >50 to 55 mm Hg (6.7 to 7.0 kPa), the lower limit being used if the pH is <7.25 and/or PaO_2 <50 to 60 mm Hg (6.7 to 8 kPa) in an FiO_2 >0.6, if nasal CPAP has failed to improve blood gas tensions.

    c. >35 weeks of gestational age: If the $PaCO_2$ exceeds 60 mm Hg (8 kPa) with a pH <7.25 and/or PaO_2 <45 mm Hg (6 kPa) in an FiO_2 of >0.80. CPAP is usually less well tolerated in mature infants. (Note: In centers that prefer to use CPAP rather than intubation and mechanical ventilation, more severe blood gas abnormalities are used as criteria for intubation.)

2. Stabilization of infants at risk for sudden collapse
    a. Small preterm infants with recurrent apnea unresponsive to nasal CPAP and administration of methylxanthines
    b. Severe sepsis
    c. Need to maintain airway patency
3. To maintain control of carbon dioxide tension:
    a. Persistent pulmonary hypertension
    b. Following severe asphyxia

Suggested Reading

Greenough A, Milner AD (eds): Neonatal Respiratory Disorders, 2nd ed. London, Edward Arnold, 2004.

Respiratory Distress Syndrome

48

Steven M. Donn and Sunil K. Sinha

I. Description
   A. Respiratory distress syndrome (RDS) is a primary pulmonary disorder
      that accompanies prematurity, specifically immaturity of the lungs,
      and to a lesser extent the airways. It is a disease of progressive
      atelectasis, which in its most severe form can lead to severe respiratory
      failure and death.
   B. The incidence and severity of RDS is generally inversely related to
      gestational age. Approximate incidence:
      1. 24 weeks: >80 %
      2. 28 weeks: 70%
      3. 32 weeks: 25%
      4. 36 weeks: 5%
II. Pathophysiology
   A. Biochemical abnormalities
      1. The major hallmark of RDS is a deficiency of surfactant, which
         leads to higher surface tension at the alveolar surface and interferes
         with the normal exchange of respiratory gases.
      2. The higher surface tension requires greater distending pressure to
         inflate the alveoli, according to the LaPlace law:

$$P = 2T/r$$

where P = pressure, T = surface tension, and r = radius.
      3. As the radius of the alveolus decreases (atelectasis) and as surface
         tension increases, the amount of pressure required to overcome
         these forces increases.
   B. Morphologic/anatomic abnormalities
      1. The number of functional alveoli (and thus the surface area available
         for gas exchange) decreases with decreasing gestational age.
      2. With extreme prematurity (23 to 25 weeks), the distance from the
         alveolus or terminal bronchiole to the nearest adjacent capillary
         increases, thus increasing the diffusion barrier and interfering with
         oxygen transport from lung to blood.
      3. The airways of the preterm infant are incompletely formed and lack
         sufficient cartilage to remain patent. This can lead to collapse and
         increased airway resistance.

    4. The chest wall of the preterm newborn is more compliant than the lungs, tending to collapse when the infant attempts to increase negative intrathoracic pressure.

  C. Functional abnormalities

    1. Decreased compliance

    2. Increased resistance

    3. Ventilation-perfusion abnormalities

    4. Impaired gas exchange

    5. Increased work of breathing

  D. Histopathologic abnormalities

    1. RDS was originally referred to as hyaline membrane disease (HMD) as a result of the typical postmortem findings in nonsurvivors.

    2. Macroscopic findings

      a. Decreased aeration

      b. Firm, rubbery, "liver-like" lungs

    3. Microscopic findings

      a. Airspaces filled with an eosinophilic-staining exudate composed of a proteinaceous material, with and without inflammatory cells.

      b. Edema in the airspaces

      c. Alveolar collapse

      d. Squamous metaplasia of respiratory epithelium

      e. Distended lymphatics

      f. Thickening of pulmonary arterioles

III. Clinical Manifestations of RDS

  A. Tachypnea: The affected infant breathes rapidly, attempting to compensate for small tidal volume (V_T) by increasing respiratory frequency.

  B. Flaring of the ala nasi: This increases the cross-sectional area of the nasal passages and decreases upper airway resistance.

  C. Grunting: This is an attempt by the infant to produce positive end-expiratory pressure (PEEP) by exhaling against a closed glottis. Its purpose is to maintain some degree of alveolar volume (distention) so that the radius of the alveolus is larger and the amount of work needed to expand it further is less than if the radius were smaller.

  D. Retractions: The infant utilizes the accessory muscles of respiration, such as the intercostals, to help overcome the increased pressure required to inflate the lungs.

  E. Cyanosis: This is a reflection of impaired oxygenation, in which there is more than 5 g/dL of deoxygenated hemoglobin.

IV. Radiographic Findings

  A. The classic description is a "ground glass" or "reticulogranular" pattern with air bronchograms (see Chapter 20).

  B. Severe cases with near-total atelectasis may show complete opacification of the lung fields ("white-out").

  C. Extremely preterm infants with a minimal number of alveoli may actually have clear lung fields.

  D. Most infants cases will have diminished lung volumes (unless positive pressure is being applied).

V. Laboratory Abnormalities

  A. Arterial oxygen tension is usually decreased.

B. Arterial carbon dioxide tension initially may be normal if the infant is able to compensate (tachypnea), but it is usually increased.

C. Blood pH may reflect respiratory acidosis (from hypercarbia), metabolic acidosis (from tissue hypoxia), or mixed acidosis.

VI. Diagnosis

A. Clinical evidence of respiratory distress

B. Radiographic findings

C. Laboratory abnormalities from impaired gas exchange

VII. Differential Diagnoses

A. Sepsis/pneumonia, especially group B streptococcal infection, which can produce a nearly identical radiographic picture

B. Transient tachypnea of the newborn

C. Pulmonary malformations (e.g., cystic adenomatoid malformation, congenital lobar emphysema, diaphragmatic hernia)

D. Extrapulmonary abnormalities (e.g., vascular ring, ascites, abdominal mass)

VIII. Treatment

A. Establish adequate gas exchange.

1. If the infant is only mildly affected and has reasonable respiratory effort and effective ventilation, only an increase in the FiO_2 may be necessary. This can be provided by an oxygen hood or nasal cannula.

2. If the infant is exhibiting evidence of alveolar hypoventilation ($PaCO_2$ >50 mm Hg [6.7 kPa]), or hypoxemia (PaO_2 <50 mm Hg [6.7 kPa] in FiO_2 = 0.5), some form of positive pressure ventilation is indicated.

   a. Consider the use of continuous positive airway pressure (CPAP) if the infant has reasonable spontaneous respiratory effort and has only minimal hypercarbia (see Chapter 24). A level of 4 to 6 cm H_2O should be used.

   b. Consider endotracheal intubation and mechanical ventilation the following conditions exist:

      (1) Hypercarbia ($PaCO_2$ >60 mm Hg [8 kPa])

      (2) Hypoxemia (PaO_2 <50 mm Hg [6.7 kPa])

      (3) Decreased respiratory drive or apnea

      (4) Need to maintain airway patency

      (5) Plan to administer surfactant replacement therapy

   c. Mechanical ventilation

      (1) The goal is to achieve adequate pulmonary gas exchange while decreasing the patient's work of breathing.

      (2) Either conventional mechanical ventilation or high-frequency ventilation can be used.

      (3) RDS is a disorder of low lung volume; therefore the approach should be one that delivers an appropriate V_T while minimizing the risks of complications (see later).

B. Surfactant replacement therapy (see Chapter 60)

1. The development and use of surfactant replacement therapy has revolutionized the treatment of RDS.

2. Numerous preparations (natural, synthetic, and semisynthetic) are now available.

3. Types of intervention
   a. Prophylaxis: Infant is immediately intubated and given surfactant as close to the first breath as possible.
   b. Rescue: Infant is not treated until the diagnosis is established.
4. Dose and interval are different for each preparation.
5. Although there is little doubt as to efficacy, the treatment is very expensive.

C. Adjunctive measures
   1. Maintain adequate blood pressure (and hence pulmonary blood flow) with judicious use of blood volume expanders and pressors.
   2. Maintain adequate oxygen-carrying capacity in infants with a high oxygen (FiO_2 >0.4) requirement.
   3. Maintain physiologic pH but do not give sodium bicarbonate if hypercarbia is present.
   4. Maintain adequate sedation/analgesia (see Chapter 62).
   5. Provide adequate nutrition but avoid excessive non-nitrogen calories, which can increase CO_2 production and exacerbate hypercarbia.
   6. Observe closely for signs of complications, especially infection.

IX. Complications
   A. Respiratory
      1. Air leaks
         a. Pneumomediastinum
         b. Pulmonary interstitial emphysema
         c. Pneumothorax
         d. Pneumopericardium
         e. Pneumoperitoneum (transdiaphragmatic)
         f. Subcutaneous emphysema
      2. Airway injury
      3. Pulmonary hemorrhage (see Chapter 68)
      4. Chronic lung disease (bronchopulmonary dysplasia) (See Chapters 55 to 57.)
   B. Cardiac
      1. Patent ductus arteriosus (see Chapter 67)
      2. Congestive heart failure
      3. Pulmonary hypertension
      4. Cor pulmonale
   C. Neurologic (see Chapter 70)
      1. Relationship to intraventricular hemorrhage
      2. Relationship to periventricular leukomalacia
      3. Neurodevelopmental impact
   D. Infectious
      1. Nosocomial and acquired pneumonia
      2. Sepsis

X. Prenatal Treatments and Conditions That Impact RDS
   A. Antenatal treatment of the mother with corticosteroids has been demonstrated to reduce the incidence and severity of RDS, particularly if given between 28 and 32 weeks of gestation.
      1. Betamethasone
      2. Dexamethasone

B. Other agents have been explored but results are thus far unconvincing.
  1. Thyroid hormone
  2. Thyrotropin
C. Accelerated pulmonary (i.e., surfactant system) maturation is seen in the following:
  1. Intrauterine growth retardation
  2. Infants of substance-abusing mothers
  3. Prolonged rupture of the membranes
D. Delayed pulmonary maturation is seen in the following:
  1. Infants of diabetic mothers
  2. Rh-sensitized fetuses
  3. Infants of hypothyroid mothers
  4. Infants who are hypothyroid

Suggested Reading

Cotton RB: Pathophysiology of hyaline membrane disease (excluding surfactant). In Polin RA, Fox WW (eds): Fetal and Neonatal Physiology, 2nd ed. Philadelphia, WB Saunders, 1998, pp 1165-1174.

Kattwinkel J: Surfactant: Evolving issues. Clin Perinatol 25:17-32, 1998.

Martin GI, Sindel BD: Neonatal management of the very low birth weight infant: The use of surfactant. Clin Perinatol 19:461-468, 1992.

Nelson M, Becker MA, Donn SM: Basic neonatal respiratory disorders. In Donn SM (ed): Neonatal and Pediatric Pulmonary Graphics: Principles and Clinical Applications. Armonk, NY, Futura Publishing, 1998, pp 253-278.

Robertson B, Halliday HL: Principles of surfactant replacement. Biochim Biophys Acta 1408:346-361, 1998.

Walsh MC, Carlo WA, Miller MJ: Respiratory diseases of the newborn. In Carlo WA, Chatburn RL (eds): Neonatal Respiratory Care, 2nd ed. Chicago, Year Book Medical Publishers, 1988, pp 260-288.

49

Pneumonia in the Newborn Infant

Elvira Parravicini and Richard A. Polin

I. Background
   A. An estimated 800,000 deaths occur worldwide from respiratory infections in newborn infants.
   B. Four varieties of pneumonia occur in newborn infants (differ in pathogens and routes of acquisition).
      1. Congenital pneumonia: Acquired by transplacental transmission of TORCH* agents
      2. Intrauterine pneumonia: Associated with intrauterine bacterial infection (chorioamnionitis/choriodeciduitis)
      3. Pneumonia acquired during birth: Caused by organisms colonizing the genital tract
      4. Pneumonia acquired after birth: Onset of symptoms in the first month of life, acquired in the nursery (nosocomial infection) or at home
   C. Lung host defenses
      1. Local and systemic host defenses are diminished in newborn infants.
         a. Lack of secretory IgA in the nasopharynx and upper airway
         b. Absence of protective antibody for common bacterial pathogens (e.g., group B streptococcus [GBS])
         c. Lower complement levels
         d. Diminished phagocyte function (chemotaxis, phagocytosis, and killing)
         e. Slower development of inflammatory responses
      2. Endotracheal tubes promote colonization of the trachea and injure the mucosa (portal for entry); oxygen interferes with ciliary function and mucosal integrity.
II. Congenital Pneumonia
   A. Toxoplasmosis
      1. Pathology
         a. Widened and edematous alveolar septa are infiltrated with mononuclear cells.
         b. Walls of small blood vessels are infiltrated with lymphocytes and mononuclear cells.

---

*Acronym meaning *t*oxoplasmosis, *o*ther agents, *r*ubella, *c*ytomegalovirus, and *h*erpes simplex.

       c. Parasites may be found in endothelial cells and the epithelium lining small airways.
  2. Manifestations
       a. Infected infants may be asymptomatic (75%), present with neurologic findings (chorioretinitis, hydrocephalus, and calcification), or exhibit a generalized systemic illness (e.g., intrauterine growth retardation [IUGR], hepatosplenomegaly, pneumonia).
       b. Pneumonia is observed in 20% to 40% of infants with generalized disease. Infants exhibit signs of respiratory distress/sepsis along with other manifestations of systemic disease (e.g., hepatosplenomegaly).
       c. Respiratory distress may result from superinfection with other pathogens.
  3. Diagnosis
       a. Demonstration of tachyzoites in tissue is definitive.
       b. Demonstration of IgM antibodies to *Toxoplasma gondii* in cord or neonatal sera is diagnostic.
       c. There is a high incidence of false-negative results with the IgM indirect immunofluorescent antibody (IFA) test.
       d. The double-sandwich IgM-capture ELISA and the IgM immunosorbent agglutination assay (ISAGA) have a lower incidence of false-positive results.
       e. All infants with positive tests at birth should have repeat tests at 10 days of age to confirm infection.
  4. Treatment and prognosis
       a. Pyrimethamine and sulfidiazene (plus folinic acid).
       b. Most infants survive with good supportive care; however, up to 30% of treated infants with ophthalmologic or neurologic manifestations at birth exhibit neurologic sequelae.
B. Cytomegalovirus (CMV)
  1. Pathology
       a. Inclusion bodies in alveolar cells
       b. Minimal inflammatory reaction
  2. Manifestations
       a. CMV is the most common congenital infection (~1% of all newborns).
       b. Only 10% to 15% of congenitally infected newborns have clinically apparent disease.
       c. A diffuse interstitial pneumonitis occurs in <1% of congenitally infected, symptomatic infants.
       d. Common signs of congenital infection include IUGR, hepatosplenomegaly, microcephaly, jaundice, and petechiae.
  3. Diagnosis
       a. Viral isolation from urine or other infected fluids is best.
       b. Anti-CMV IgM is diagnostic.
  4. Treatment and prognosis: Ganciclovir is being investigated as a therapeutic agent, but its use should be limited to controlled trials.

C. Herpes simplex virus
1. Pathology: Diffuse interstitial pneumonitis that progresses to a hemorrhagic pneumonitis
2. Manifestations
   a. Most HSV infections in the neonate are symptomatic, but 20% of infants never develop vesicles.
   b. Three varieties: Localized disease (skin, eye, or mouth), encephalitis with or without localized disease, and disseminated infection.
   c. Half the infants are born prematurely. Respiratory distress syndrome (RDS) must always be a consideration.
   d. Infants with disseminated infection usually present with signs of bacterial sepsis or shock, liver dysfunction (hepatitis), and respiratory distress at 9 to 11 days of life.
3. Diagnosis
   a. Viral cultures (oropharyngeal and respiratory secretions) and a rectal swab
   b. Lumbar puncture with viral culture and polymerase chain reaction (PCR) (75% of affected infants have meningoencephalitis)
   c. Direct immunofluorescence of skin lesion specimens
4. Treatment and prognosis
   a. Intravenous acyclovir and supportive care.
   b. Mortality exceeds 80% and many survivors are neurologically impaired.
D. *Treponema pallidum*
1. Pathology
   a. "Pneumonia alba" is characterized grossly as heavy, firm, yellow-white enlarged lungs.
   b. There is a marked increase in connective tissue in the interalveolar septa and the interstitium and collapse of the alveolar spaces.
2. Manifestations
   a. Early congenital syphilis occurs before 2 years of age.
   b. Two thirds of infected infants are asymptomatic.
   c. Early congenital syphilis should be suspected in any infant with unexplained prematurity, hydrops, or an enlarged placenta.
   d. Pneumonia is an uncommon manifestation.
   e. Common manifestations of early congenital syphilis include hepatosplenomegaly, anemia, leukopenia or leukocytosis, generalized lymphadenopathy, rhinitis, nephrotic syndrome, maculopapular rash, bony abnormalities, and leptomeningitis.
3. Diagnosis
   a. Confirmation of *T. pallidum* by dark-field microscopy.
   b. VDRL/RPR (venereal disease research laboratory/rapid plasma reagin) antibody titers in infant that are fourfold greater than maternal titers.
   c. IgM by FTA-ABS (fluorescent treponemal antibody absorption) testing has a 20% to 39% incidence of false-negative results and a 10% incidence of false-positive results.

      4. Treatment and prognosis
        a. All symptomatic newborn infants with a positive RPR should be treated as if they have congenital infection.
        b. Penicillin is the drug of choice.
        c. The earlier treatment is initiated, the greater the likelihood of a good outcome (prevention of stigmata).
III. Pneumonia Acquired before, during, or after Birth
    A. Background: Time of presentation varies.
      1. The onset of respiratory distress immediately after birth suggests aspiration of infected amniotic fluid while in utero.
      2. The "delayed" presentation (1 to 3 days) results from colonization of mucoepithelial surfaces and seeding of the bloodstream from that site.
    B. Pathology
      1. Dense cellular exudate, congestion, hemorrhage, and necrosis.
      2. *Staphylococcus aureus* and *Klebsiella* may cause microabscesses and pneumatoceles.
      3. Hyaline membranes are common (especially in preterm infants), and bacteria may be seen with the hyaline membranes
    C. Pathophysiology of lung injury
      1. Direct invasion of lung tissue by bacteria: Bacterial pathogens secrete microbial enzymes and toxins that disrupt cell membranes, disturb metabolism, and interfere with the supply of nutrients.
      2. Indirect injury secondary to the host inflammatory response, mediated by phagocytes and inflammatory cascades (cytokines, complement, and coagulation).
      3. Airway obstruction caused by inflammatory debris.
      4. Alteration in surfactant composition and function (secondary to leak of proteinaceous material or presence of meconium).
    D. Disturbances in lung function
      1. Increased airway resistance from inflammatory debris and airway smooth muscle
      2. Decreased lung compliance (atelectasis and parenchymal inflammation)
      3. Ventilation-perfusion abnormalities (intrapulmonary shunts)
      4. Pulmonary hypertension secondary to release of vasoactive mediators
      5. Alveolar diffusion barriers
    E. Epidemiology
      1. Identical to that of early-onset bacterial sepsis
      2. Risk factors
        a. Prematurity
        b. Male gender
        c. Colonization with a known pathogen, such as (GBS)
        d. Recurrent maternal urinary tract infection (UTI)
        e. Prolonged rupture of membranes >18 hours
        f. Signs of chorioamnionitis (maternal fever >100.4° F [38° C]), abdominal tenderness, foul-smelling or cloudy amniotic fluid)
          (1) Chorioamnionitis can be subclinical or clinical.

      (2) Subclinical chorioamnionitis may be a risk factor for chronic lung disease (CLD) (see "Atypical Pneumonia: *Ureaplasma urealyticum*" later).

F. Pathogenesis

    1. Infection begins with colonization of the maternal genital tract.

    2. Organisms that colonize the cervix, vagina, or rectum spread upward into the amniotic cavity through intact or ruptured membranes (causing amnionitis).

    3. The fetus either inhales infected amniotic fluid (and exhibits immediate onset of respiratory distress) or is colonized and becomes symptomatic after an asymptomatic interval.

G. Bacterial pathogens

    1. *Streptococcus agalactiae* (GBS)

       a. Most common bacterial pathogen

       b. From 15% to 40% of women are colonized with GBS.

       c. In the absence of intrapartum antibiotics, the vertical transmission rate is ~50%, and the risk of infection (sepsis and pneumonia) in colonized infants is 1% to 2%.

    2. *Escherichia coli*

       a. Fifty percent of women are colonized with K1 *E. coli* at the time of delivery, and vertical transmission occurs 70% of the time.

       b. Forty percent of the strains causing early-onset sepsis/pneumonia are K1-containing *E. coli.*

       c. Risk of disease in colonized infants is 1% to 2%.

    3. *Listeria monocytogenes*

       a. Almost all cases originate from ingestion of contaminated food.

       b. Fecal carriage rate ranges from 1% to 5%.

       c. *L. monocytogenes* can be transmitted to the fetus transplacentally or via an ascending infection.

       d. Infection commonly results in preterm delivery.

       e. Maternal influenza-like infection precedes delivery in 50% of cases.

    4. Other pathogens: *Enterobacter* sp., *Enterococcus, Haemophilus* sp., *Klebsiella, S. aureus,* coagulase-negative *Staphylococcus, Streptococcus viridans,* and group A streptococcus

H. Clinical history (suggestive of sepsis/pneumonia)

    1. Prolonged rupture of membranes >18 hours

    2. Signs and symptoms of chorioamnionitis

    3. Colonization with GBS (Adequate intrapartum therapy lowers the risk of infection by 85% to 90%.)

    4. Maternal UTI

    5. Preterm premature rupture of membranes

    6. Preterm labor

    7. Unexplained fetal tachycardia

    8. Meconium (decreases the antibacterial properties of amniotic fluid)

I. Clinical manifestations

    1. Signs of sepsis/pneumonia can be subtle (tachypnea) or overt (grunting, flaring, retracting).

    2. Pulmonary findings

       a. Tachypnea (respiratory rate >60/min)

   b. Grunting
   c. Flaring
   d. Retractions
   e. Rales or rhonchi
   f. Cyanosis
   g. Change in the quality of secretions (serosanguineous or purulent)
3. Systemic findings (nonpulmonary)
   a. Apnea
   b. Lethargy
   c. Irritability
   d. Hypothermia, hyperthermia, or temperature instability
   e. Poor perfusion or hypotension (manifested as oliguria or metabolic acidosis)
   f. Pulmonary hypertension
   g. Abdominal distention
J. Diagnosis
   1. General concepts
      a. Laboratory testing (in general) is not useful for identifying infants who are likely to have bacterial sepsis/pneumonia (i.e., most laboratory tests have a low positive predictive value).
      b. Testing is helpful in deciding which infants are *not* likely to be infected and who do *not* require antibiotics (high negative predictive value).
      c. In infants with proven sepsis/pneumonia, laboratory tests (e.g., white blood cell count, neutrophil indices, acute phase reactants) obtained at birth frequently are normal. Tests obtained 8 to 12 hours following birth have a higher likelihood of being abnormal.
      d. The only absolutely sure way to make the diagnosis of bacterial sepsis/pneumonia is to recover an organism from a normally sterile site (blood, urine, cerebrospinal fluid, pleural fluid). The presence of bacteria in a tracheal aspirate obtained *immediately after intubation* is presumptive evidence of infection.
      e. Infants with sepsis/pneumonia can be asymptomatic at the time of birth.
      f. All symptomatic infants should be tested and treated. Some infants exhibit transient signs and symptoms that resolve quickly (within a few hours of birth), and these infants may not require treatment.
   2. Cultures
      a. A positive blood culture is the "gold standard" for detection of bacteremia in the newborn. Therefore, a blood culture is required in every infant with suspected sepsis.
      b. Urine cultures are rarely positive in infants with early-onset bacterial sepsis and should not be routinely obtained.
      c. A lumbar puncture should be performed in all infants with a positive blood culture and in symptomatic infants with a high probability of infection based on adjunct laboratory studies.

Lumbar puncture should be deferred in any infant who is clinically unstable or who has an uncorrected bleeding diathesis.

3. Adjunct laboratory tests

    a. Neutrophil indices (absolute neutrophil count, absolute band count, and immature-to-total neutrophil [I/T] ratio) are more useful than total leukocyte counts.

    b. Neutrophil indices suggestive of infection are an absolute neutrophil count <1750/mm³, an absolute band count >2000/mm³, and an I/T ratio ≥ 0.2.

    c. C-reactive protein (CRP) (an acute phase reactant) is a useful adjunct test.

       (1) Values rise slowly in infected infants. Therefore, a CRP obtained at birth is not as useful.

       (2) A CRP ≥1 mg/dL is considered positive.

    d. Sepsis screens: Suggested algorithms for the management of asymptomatic infants (<35 weeks or ≥35 weeks) and symptomatic infants are shown in Figure 49-1. These algorithms use a combination of laboratory tests (neutrophil indices [I/T ratio, absolute neutrophil count, and absolute band count] and CRP) to help with decisions about antibiotics.

       (1) Sepsis screens are most useful for identifying infants with a low probability of infection (i.e., who do not require antibiotics or who no longer require antibiotics).

       (2) Sepsis screens are not very useful for identifying infected infants (the positive predictive value is <40%).

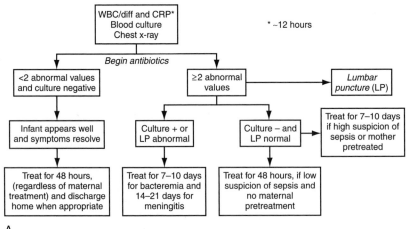

FIGURE **49-1.** Evaluation of (**A**) symptomatic infants and (**B** and **C**) asymptomatic infants at <35 weeks' (**B**) and ≥35 weeks' (**C**) gestation with >1 risk factor for neonatal sepsis. CRP, C-reactive protein; Diff, differentials; Px, physical.

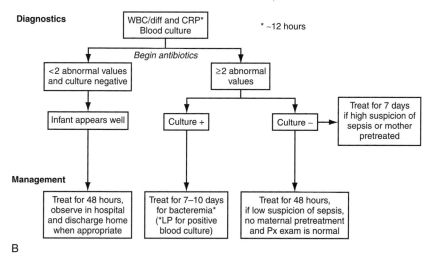

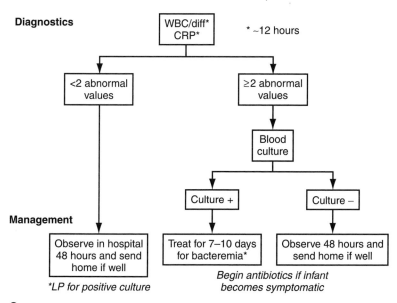

Figure 49-1. Continued.

(3) Antibiotics are not required for asymptomatic infants ≥35 weeks' gestation, unless the sepsis screen is positive or the infant becomes symptomatic.

(4) Antibiotics should be started at birth if the infant is:
  (a) <35 weeks' gestation with risk factors for sepsis (listed previously).
  (b) Symptomatic (regardless of gestational age).

(5) In applying these algorithms, major risk factors for sepsis are:
  (a) Prolonged rupture of membranes >18 hours.
  (b) Signs and symptoms of chorioamnionitis (fever ≥100.4° F [≥38° C]), uterine tenderness, foul-smelling or cloudy amniotic fluid).
  (c) Colonization with GBS.

(6) A positive sepsis screen is defined as two abnormal values obtained concurrently (see Figure 49-1).

4. Chest radiographs
  a. In preterm infants, the radiographic appearance of pneumonia may be indistinguishable from that of (i.e., ground-glass appearance and air bronchograms).
  b. In term infants, pneumonia more commonly causes hyperinflation with increased central peribronchial infiltrates and scattered subsegmental atelectasis.
  c. Other findings include effusions/empyema, hyperinflation, and pneumatoceles (suggestive of *S. aureus*).

K. Management
  1. Broad-spectrum antibiotics
    a. Choice depends on the predominant pathogen causing sepsis and the antibiotic sensitivity patterns for the microorganisms causing early-onset sepsis in a given region.
    b. Empiric therapy must cover both gram-positive and gram-negative organisms.
    c. The most commonly used combination is ampicillin and an aminoglycoside (frequently gentamicin). Ampicillin and cefotaxime are an effective alternative, but this combination has been associated with the development of resistance.
    d. After an organism has been identified, the antibiotic therapy should be tailored according to the sensitivities.
      (1) *L. monocytogenes* infection is treated with a combination of ampicillin and an aminoglycoside antibiotic.
      (2) Enterococcus infection is treated either with ampicillin and an aminoglycoside antibiotic or vancomycin, depending on sensitivities.
      (3) *S. agalactiae* infection is treated with penicillin or ampicillin.
      (4) *S. aureus* infection is treated with penicillinase-resistant penicillins (e.g., methicillin) or cephalosporins. Infection with methicillin-resistant organisms is treated with vancomycin.
      (5) *Pseudomonas aeruginosa* infections are commonly treated with ticarcillin or carbenicillin and an aminoglycoside, but most organisms are also sensitive to ceftazidime.

       (6) Most other gram-negative infections can be treated with aminoglycoside antibiotics or cefotaxime.

    e. Duration of therapy usually is 7 to 10 days (3 weeks or longer for *S. aureus* infections).

  2. Supportive care

    a. Hemodynamic support (volume and pressors) to assure adequate systemic perfusion.

    b. Nutritional support: Parenteral nutrition for any infant who will not be able to tolerate enteral feedings.

    c. Respiratory support

       (1) Oxygen to maintain saturation of 88% to 92%. A higher range (92% to 95%) is preferred for term and near-term infants with pulmonary hypertension.

       (2) Use the least invasive form of respiratory support to achieve adequate oxygenation and ventilation.

       (3) Chest physiotherapy (vibration and percussion) once the infant is clinically stable.

       (4) Judicious use of suctioning

       (5) Drainage of pleural effusions if lung function is compromised.

    d. Nitric oxide for term and near-term infants with persistent hypoxemia despite maximal ventilatory support.

    e. Extracorporeal membrane oxygenation for term and near-term infants unresponsive to the preceding measures if criteria are met.

    f. Benefit from the use of surfactant is unproved, but anecdotal reports suggest efficacy. Inflammation may inactivate surfactant.

 L. Prevention

  1. The incidence of early-onset sepsis/pneumonia caused by GBS can be diminished by intrapartum administration of antibiotics. The following "high-risk" women should be treated.

    a. Previous infant with invasive disease

    b. GBS bacteriuria during pregnancy

    c. Positive GBS screening culture during pregnancy (unless a planned cesarean delivery, in the absence of labor or amniotic membrane rupture, is performed)

    d. Unknown GBS status (culture not done, incomplete, or results unknown) and any of the following:

       (1) Delivery at <37 weeks' gestation

       (2) Amniotic membrane rupture ≥18 hours

       (3) Intrapartum temperature ≥100.4° F (≥38° C)

  2. The incidence of early-onset sepsis/pneumonia can be reduced in women with preterm premature rupture of membranes by administering ampicillin and erythromycin for 7 to 10 days.

IV. Atypical Pneumonia: *Ureaplasma urealyticum*

 A. Transmission

  1. Although *U. Urealyticum* is a frequently found in the lower genital tract of asymptomatic women, isolation of *U. urealyticum* from the chorion or amnion has been associated with premature labor and chorioamnionitis.

2. The vertical transmission rate ranges from 25% to 60% and is highest in preterm infants.
3. Transmission occurs in utero by ascending infection or at delivery through an infected vaginal canal.

B. Pathology
1. Patchy exudate of polymorphonuclear cells and swollen vacuolated macrophages in bronchioles and alveoli.
2. Prominent interstitial fibrosis of lung tissue (possible association with CLD).

C. Manifestations
1. *U. Urealyticum* infection of the newborn is associated with pneumonia, meningitis, and osteomyelitis.
2. Pneumonia resembling RDS usually develops in premature infants, accompanied by leukopenia and thrombocytopenia.
3. Radiographs: Radiating streakiness, coarse patchy infiltrates, subtle haziness, and diffuse granularity indistinguishable from RDS and precocious dysplastic changes (possible association with CLD).

D. Diagnosis
1. Cultures (blood, urine, nasopharyngeal secretions, endotracheal aspirates) require special media and long incubation times.
2. PCR has a better sensitivity than culture, and results are available in less than 24 hours.
3. Serologic tests (*U. Urealyticum* IgG and IgM) have limited value.

E. Treatment and prognosis
1. Prophylactic treatment of *U. Urealyticum*–colonized women in preterm labor failed to decrease mortality and morbidity, and it is not recommended.
2. Erythromycin is the drug of choice for infections that do not involve the CNS. (A risk of hypertrophic pyloric stenosis has been reported with use of erythromycin.)
3. Long-term morbidities include increased stay in the NICU and possible association with CLD.

V. *Chlamydia trachomatis*
A. Transmission
1. In women colonized with *C. trachomatis*, 50% to 75% of offspring become colonized at the time of delivery, of whom 30% develop conjunctivitis and 20% develop pneumonia.
2. Systematic screening and treatment of chlamydial infection during pregnancy markedly decreases perinatally acquired infections.

B. Pathology
1. Intra-alveolar inflammation with a mild degree of interstitial reaction.
2. Alveolar lining cells contain intracytoplasmic inclusions.

C. Manifestations
1. At 4 to 2 weeks of age, newborns infected with *C. trachomatis* present with purulent conjunctivitis and/or respiratory distress.
2. Clinical findings include tachypnea, rales, and, rarely, wheezing. Significant laboratory findings include eosinophilia and elevated serum immunoglobulins. Chest radiography shows hyperinflation and bilateral diffuse, nonspecific infiltrates.

   D. Diagnosis
      1. Definitive diagnosis is made by culture (conjunctiva, nasopharynx, vagina or rectum) and by nucleic acid amplification. Because *Chlamydia* is an obligate intracellular organism, culture specimens must contain epithelial cells.
      2. In infants with pneumonia, the detection of a specific IgM ($\geq$1:32) is diagnostic.
   E. Treatment and prognosis: Erythromycin is the treatment of choice (risk of hypertrophic pyloric stenosis).
VI. Nosocomial Infections and Ventilator-Associated Pneumonia (VAP)
   A. General concepts
      1. In the absence of mechanical ventilation, pneumonia is an uncommon presentation in infants with hospital-acquired infections.
      2. Pneumonia in the hospitalized newborn infant results either from dissemination of microorganisms from colonized mucosal sites or aspiration of food or gastric contents.
         a. Endotracheal tubes and suctioning can disrupt mucosal integrity and promote dissemination.
         b. On rare occasions, microorganisms may be transmitted from contaminated equipment.
      3. VAP has a reported incidence of 6.5 per 1000 ventilator days.
      4. The diagnosis of VAP requires the presence of new and persistent focal radiographic infiltrates in a ventilated infant occurring >48 hours after NICU admission.
   B. Risk factors for nosocomial sepsis/pneumonia
      1. Prematurity (most important)
      2. Parenteral nutrition
      3. Mechanical ventilation
      4. Central venous catheters
      5. Steroids for CLD
      6. H-2 blockers (to decrease gastric acidity)
      7. Low serum IgG levels
      8. Overcrowding and understaffing
   C. Bacterial and fungal pathogens
      1. *Candida* sp.
      2. *S. aureus*
      3. Enteric organisms (*E. coli, Serratia marcescens, Klebsiella* sp., *Enterobacter cloacae, Citrobacter diversus,* and *P. aeruginosa*)
   D. Diagnosis
      1. Pneumonia should be suspected in any hospitalized newborn infant who exhibits a deterioration in respiratory status unexplained by other events or conditions.
      2. A change in the characteristics of the secretions may be an early clinical sign.
      3. Sepsis may be suspected because of increased apnea, hypothermia, hyperthermia, feeding intolerance, or abdominal distention.
      4. Blood cultures may or may not be positive in infants with VAP.

5. Tracheal aspirates for culture are not helpful because they merely identify which microorganisms are colonizing the airway (not necessarily those causing disease).

6. Chest radiographs may indicate new or focal infiltrates, but in infants with CLD, the distinction from atelectasis is difficult.

7. Adjunct laboratory studies are not as helpful as with early-onset sepsis; however, infants with serious bacterial or fungal infections commonly exhibit an increase in total white blood cell count, an increased percentage of immature forms, and thrombocytopenia.

E. Management

1. Broad-spectrum antibiotics to treat common pathogens (usually a combination of vancomycin and an aminoglycoside antibiotic)

2. When there is an outbreak of pneumonia from a resistant microorganism, empiric therapy should target those pathogens. (Note: Any cluster of infections or an infection due to an unusual pathogen [e.g., *Citrobacter*] should be investigated by the hospital's infection control service.)

3. Amphotericin or fluconazole for fungal infections

4. Hemodynamic and respiratory support as noted previously

VII. Respiratory Syncytial Virus (RSV)

A. Background

1. Although RSV infections are rare in the first weeks of life, epidemics in newborns have been described.

2. RSV pneumonia and bronchiolitis constitute the leading cause of infant hospitalization and are the most common viral causes of death in children in the first year of life.

3. RSV is spread by contact with infected nasal secretions. The virus can live up to 7 hours on countertops, gloves, and cloths, and up to 30 minutes on skin.

4. Risk factors for severe RSV infection in infants include prematurity, CLD, and congenital heart disease (CHD).

B. Pathology: Necrosis of the bronchiolar epithelium and peribronchiolar infiltrate of lymphocytes and mononuclear cells

1. Filling of alveolar spaces with fluid

2. Multinucleated giant cells circumscribed by large syncytia

C. Manifestations

1. Upper respiratory tract infection, pneumonia, bronchiolitis, and apnea in premature infants.

2. Clinical findings include respiratory distress with tachypnea, wheezing, and radiographic evidence of hyperaeration of the lungs. In most patients, symptoms and signs are resolved by 7 days.

3. RSV infection increases an infant's risk for wheezing or asthma for up to 7 years and has been associated with sudden infant death syndrome.

D. Diagnosis

1. Rapid diagnostic assays (immunofluorescence and enzyme immunoassay) using nasopharyngeal specimens are reliable.

2. Virus can be isolated in cell culture (3 to 5 days) on nasopharyngeal specimens.

3. Serologic tests can be used for confirmation.

E. Prevention

1. In absence of a safe and effective vaccine, passive immunization has been licensed in the U.S. for prevention of RSV infection. Two products are available: RSV intravenous immune globulin (IVIG), a polyclonal hyperimmune globulin, and palivizumab, a humanized monoclonal antibody that is administered intramuscularly.

2. These products are not approved for treatment of the disease.

3. Disadvantages of RSV IVIG include the need for intravenous route of administration, interference with response to vaccines, and the theoretical risk for new or existing viral infections (derived from human blood product).

4. Both products are recommended for RSV prophylaxis by the American Academy of Pediatrics (AAP) for all high-risk infants, including:

   a. Premature infants with gestational age ≤32 weeks without CLD.

   b. Infants born at <28 weeks' gestation may benefit from RSV seasonal prophylaxis whenever that occurs during the first 12 months of life.

   c. Infants born at 29 to 32 weeks' gestation up to 6 months of postnatal age.

   d. All infants with CLD requiring medical therapy.

   e. All infants with hemodynamically significant cyanotic or acyanotic CHD. The highest risk groups include infants with cyanotic CHD, infants requiring medications for congestive heart failure, and infants with pulmonary hypertension.

5. Prophylaxis should be considered for infants born with gestational age 32 to 35 weeks when supplemental risk factors are present.

6. Administration is given monthly throughout the RSV season.

F. Treatment and prognosis

1. Primary treatment is supportive (hydration, ventilatory support as needed).

2. Ribavirin has antiviral activity in vitro (use of aerosol treatment remains controversial).

Suggested Reading

AAP—Committee on Infectious Diseases and Committee on Fetus and Newborn: Policy Statement. Revised Indications for the Use of Palivizumab and Respiratory Syncytial Virus Immune Globulin Intravenous for the Prevention of Respiratory Syncytial Virus Infections. 2003.

Ablow RC, Gross I, Effman EL, et al: The radiographic features of early onset group B streptococcal neonatal sepsis. Radiology 127:771-777, 1977.

Apisarnthanarak A, Holzmann-Pazgal G, Hamvas A, et al: Disseminated fungal infections in very-low-birthweight infants: Clinical manifestations and epidemiology. Pediatrics 73:144-149, 1984.

Barker JA, McLean SD, Jordan GD, et al: Primary neonatal herpes simplex virus pneumonia. Pediatr Infec Dis J 9:285-289, 1990.

Barnett ED, Klein JO: Bacterial infections of the respiratory tract. In Remington JS, Klein JO (eds): Infectious Diseases of the Fetus and Newborn. Philadelphia, WB Saunders, 2001, pp 999-1013.

Barton L, Hodgman JE, Pavlova Z: Causes of death in the extremely low birth weight infant. Pediatrics 103:446-451, 1999.

Bortolussi R, Thompson TR, Ferrieri P: Early-onset pneumococcal sepsis in newborn infants. Pediatrics 60:352-355, 1977.

Campbell JR: Neonatal pneumonia. Semin Respir Infect 11:155-162, 1996.

Edell DS, Davidson JJ, Mulvihill DM, Majure M: A common presentation of an uncommon cause of neonatal respiratory distress: Pneumonia alba. Pediatr Pulmonol 15:376-379, 1993.

Gerberding KM, Eisenhut CC, Engle WA, Cohen MD: Congenital *Candida* pneumonia and sepsis: A case report and review of the literature. J Perinatol 9:159-161, 1989.

Glustein JZ, Kaplan M: *Enterobacter cloacae* causing pneumatocele in a neonate. Acta Paediatr 83:990-991, 1994.

Goncalves LF, Chaiworapongsa T, Romero R: Intrauterine infection and prematurity. Ment Retard Dev Disabil Res Rev 8:3-13, 2002.

Gray J, Geoerge RH, Durbin GM, et al: An outbreak of *Bacillus cereus* respiratory tract infections on a neonatal unit due to contaminated ventilator circuits. J Hosp Infect 41:19-22, 1999.

Gronek P, Schmale J, Soditt V, et al: Bronchoalveolar inflammation following airway infection in preterm infants with chronic lung disease. Pediatr Pulmonol 31:331-338, 2001.

Hammerschlag MR: *Chlamydia trachomatis* and *Chlamydia pneumoniae* infection in children and adolescents. Pediatr Rev 25:43-51, 2004.

Haney PJ, Bohlman M, Sun CC: Radiographic findings in neonatal pneumonia. AJR Am J Roentgenol 143:23-26, 1984.

Joffe S, Escobar GJ, Black SB, et al: Rehospitalization for respiratory syncytial virus among premature infants. Pediatrics 104:894-899, 1999.

Kotecha S, Hodge R, Shaber A, et al: Pulmonary *Ureaplasma urealyticum* is associated with the development of acute lung inflammation and chronic lung disease in preterm infants. Pediatr Res 55:61-68, 2004.

Lau YL, Hey E: Sensitivity and specificity of daily tracheal aspirate cultures in predicting organisms causing bacteremia in ventilated neonates. Pediatr Infect Dis J 10:290-294, 1991.

Numazaki K, Asanuma H, Niida Y: *Chlamydia trachomatis* infection in early neonatal period. BMC Infect Dis 3:2, 2003.

Rowen JL, Rench MA, Kozinetz CA, et al: Endotracheal colonization with *Candida* enhances risk of systemic candidiasis in very low birthweight neonates. J Pediatr 124:789-794, 1994.

Shamir R, Horev G, Merlob P, Nutman J: *Citrobacter diversus* lung abscess in a preterm infant. Pediatr Infect Dis J 9:221-222, 1990.

Skevaki C, Kafetzis DA: *Ureaplasma urealyticum* airway colonization and pulmonary outcome in neonates. Expert Rev Anti-infect Ther 1:183-191, 2003.

Stagno S, Cytomegalovirus. In Remington JS, Klein JO (eds): Infectious Diseases of the Fetus and Newborn. Philadephia, WB Saunders, 2001, pp 389-424.

Viscardi RM, Manimtim WM, Sun CJ, et al: Lung pathology in premature infants with *Ureaplasma urealyticum* infection. Pediatr Develop Pat 5:141-150, 2002.

Webber S, Wilkinson AR, Lindsell D, et al: Neonatal pneumonia. Arch Dis Child 65:207-211, 1990.

Meconium Aspiration Syndrome

50

Thomas E. Wiswell

I. Overview
  A. Meconium-stained amniotic fluid (MSAF).
    1. MSAF occurs in ~13% of all deliveries.
    2. Meconium passage may be a marker of antepartum or intrapartum compromise (e.g., hypoxemia or umbilical cord compression).
    3. Passage of meconium may also be a maturational event. MSAF is rarely noted in infants born before 37 weeks' gestation, but may occur in 35% or more of infants born at 42 weeks' gestation.
  B. Meconium aspiration syndrome (MAS)
    1. Definition: Respiratory distress in an infant born through MSAF whose symptoms cannot be otherwise explained.
    2. MAS occurs in 4% to 5% of newborns born through MSAF.
    3. Aspiration most commonly occurs in utero. Aspiration with the initial postnatal breaths appears to be considerably less common.
    4. The thicker the MSAF consistency, the greater the likelihood of MAS.
    5. The more depressed the baby (as reflected by the need for positive pressure ventilation or by low Apgar scores), the greater the likelihood of MAS.
    6. Of those infants born with MAS, 30% to 60% require mechanical ventilation, 10% to 25% develop pneumothoraces, and 2% to 5% die.
    7. 50% to 70% of infants with persistent pulmonary hypertension of the newborn (PPHN) have MAS as an underlying disorder.
II. Pathophysiology
  A. Complex mechanisms are involved (Fig. 50-1).
  B. At any given moment, several of these mechanisms may be influencing the degree of respiratory distress.
III. Prevention of MAS
  A. Amnioinfusion trials
    1. Initial reports from the late 1980s and early 1990s indicated that amnioinfusion for thick-consistency MSAF improved Apgar scores and prevented MAS.
    2. A recent very large, international, randomized, controlled trial indicated that this therapy does not reduce the risk of MAS.
  B. Oropharyngeal suctioning
    1. Based on anecdotal experience, this has been a widely performed procedure for the past three decades.

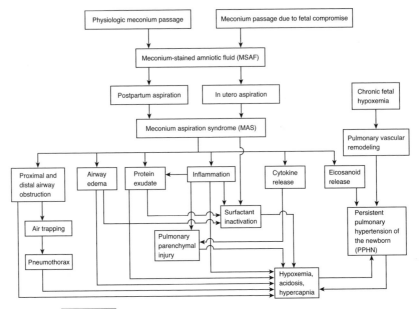

FIGURE 50-1. Pathophysiology of meconium aspiration syndrome (MAS).

2. A recent large, international, randomized, controlled trial indicates that intrapartum naso- and oropharyngeal suctioning does not reduce the incidence of MAS.

C. Potentially dangerous maneuvers of no proven benefit
  1. Cricoid pressure: Application of pressure to the infant's airway to prevent intratracheal meconium from descending into the lungs.
  2. Epiglottal blockage: Insertion of one to three fingers into the child's airway to manually "close" the epiglottis over the glottis to prevent aspiration.
  3. Thoracic compression: Encircling the infant's chest and applying pressure in an attempt to prevent deep inspiration prior to endotracheal cleansing.
  4. None of these maneuvers has been scientifically validated and all are potentially dangerous (trauma, vagal stimulation, or induction of deep inhalation with chest recoil upon removing encircling hands).

D. Endotracheal intubation and intratracheal suctioning in the delivery room
  1. A large trial indicated that endotracheal intubation is of no benefit in the apparently vigorous infant born through MSAF of any consistency (apparent vigor was defined within the first 10 to 15 seconds of life by a heart rate >100 BPM, spontaneous respirations, and reasonable tone).
  2. Endotracheal intubation and suctioning should be performed in infants born through MSAF if they are depressed, if they need

positive pressure ventilation, or if they are initially apparently vigorous, but subsequently manifest any respiratory distress within the first minutes of life.

IV. Radiographic Findings
   A. Radiographic findings among infants with MAS include:
      1. Diffuse, patchy infiltrates
      2. Consolidation
      3. Atelectasis
      4. Pleural effusions
      5. Air leaks (pneumothorax, pneumomediastinum)
      6. Hyperinflation
      7. "Wet-lung" appearance similar to findings seen with transient tachypnea of the newborn
      8. Hypovascularity
      9. Apparently clear, virtually normal appearance
   B. Correlation of radiographic findings with disease severity
      1. One early study indicated direct correlation between severity of MAS and degree of radiographic abnormalities.
      2. Other studies found no such correlation. Patients with minimal signs may have strikingly abnormal chest radiographs, whereas the sickest infant may have a virtually normal chest radiograph.

V. Conventional Management of MAS
   A. Chest physiotherapy (CPT)
      1. Objectives of CPT are to prevent accumulation of debris, improve mobilization of airway secretions, and improve oxygenation.
      2. CPT consists of postural drainage, percussion, vibration, saline lavage, and suctioning (oropharyngeal and intratracheal).
      3. Although commonly performed in both the delivery room and the NICU, CPT for MAS has never been studied in clinical trials, and its benefits are unproved.
   B. Oxygen
      1. The goal is to maintain acceptable systemic oxygenation. Generally, this consists of sustaining peripheral oxygen saturation levels between 92% and 97% or arterial partial pressure of oxygen (PaO_2) levels between 60 and 80 mm Hg (8 and 10.7 kPa).
      2. Because of the potential for air trapping and air leaks, some clinicians advocate increasing the fraction of inspired oxygen (FiO_2) to 1.0 before implementing more aggressive therapy (e.g., mechanical ventilation). Typically, however, once FiO_2 requirements exceed 0.60, more aggressive therapy (CPAP or mechanical ventilation) is instituted.
      3. Oxygen is also a pulmonary vasodilator. Because aberrant pulmonary vasoconstriction frequently accompanies MAS, clinicians often attempt to maintain higher than usual oxygenation early in the course of the disorder ([saturation 98% to 100% or PaO_2 100 to 120 mm Hg [13.3 to 16 kPa]) or even higher. However, the latter practice has not been validated in clinical trials.
      4. Supplemental oxygen is used in conjunction with more aggressive therapy.

C. Continuous positive airway pressure (CPAP)
   1. CPAP is often begun once FiO_2 requirements exceed 0.50 to 0.60 or if the patient exhibits substantial respiratory distress. Some clinicians, however, prefer to move directly to mechanical ventilation without a trial of CPAP.
   2. CPAP is provided most commonly in newborns intranasally via prongs inserted into the nostrils. CPAP may also be administered via a face mask or an endotracheal tube (ETT).
   3. Major potential complications of CPAP are air trapping and increased functional residual capacity. These factors may contribute to air leaks and to decreased venous return to the heart, further compromising the infant.
   4. There is limited published information concerning the use of CPAP in children with MAS.

D. Conventional mechanical ventilation
   1. Mechanical ventilators typically are time-cycled and pressure-limited. Some clinicians avoid volume-targeted ventilators because of an unsubstantiated fear of air leaks.
   2. Multiple strategies have been advocated.
      a. Settings (e.g., pressure, rate, I:E ratio, FiO_2) are used that will maintain arterial blood gases within normal ranges.
      b. Hyperventilation is used to achieve respiratory alkalosis in an attempt to attain pulmonary vasodilation.
      c. "Gentle" ventilation permits higher $PaCO_2$ levels and lower pH and PaO_2 levels in an attempt to prevent lung injury (from barotrauma or volutrauma) and avoid potential side effects such as hypocarbia and alkalosis.
   3. To date, there have been no prospective, randomized trials comparing any of the various mechanical ventilator strategies in the management of MAS. Therefore no single approach can be considered optimal.

E. Other conventional therapies
   1. Sedation
   2. Paralysis
   3. Systemic alkalosis from parenteral administration of sodium bicarbonate
   4. Use of pressors (dopamine, dobutamine) or fluid boluses to maintain high systemic blood pressure
   5. None of these therapies have been rigorously investigated in infants with MAS.

VI. Nonconventional Management (not the standard of care!)
   A. High-frequency (HF) ventilation
      1. Includes both HF jet ventilation and HF oscillatory ventilation.
      2. Trials in animal models of MAS have generally shown no benefit.
      3. Limited human anecdotal experience has been touted as indicating efficacy.
      4. To date, there are no published prospective human trials that have documented either form of HF ventilation to be more efficacious than conventional ventilation in the management of MAS.

B. Bolus exogenous surfactant
   1. Rationale
      a. Meconium produces a concentration-dependent direct inactivation of a newborn's endogenous surfactant.
      b. Meconium has a direct cytotoxic effect on the type II pneumocyte.
      c. Meconium causes decreased levels of surfactant proteins A and B.
   2. In the largest randomized, controlled trial assessing bolus surfactant use in term-gestation infants with respiratory failure (51% of whom had MAS), surfactant-treated infants with MAS had a decreased need for extracorporeal membrane oxygenation (ECMO). However, there were no differences in mortality, duration of mechanical ventilation or oxygen therapy, or total hospital days.
   3. An alternative approach has been the use of dilute surfactant to lavage the lungs of infants with MAS.
      a. Several different techniques have been used, as have several different surfactants.
      b. In the sole randomized, controlled trial assessing dilute, surfactant lavage, infants receiving this therapy had a more rapid and sustained improvement in oxygenation, as well as a shorter ventilator course, compared to controls.
   4. Currently no commercially available surfactant is FDA-approved for either bolus or lavage use in MAS in the U.S.
   5. Further trials are necessary to assess this therapy.
C. Inhaled nitric oxide (NO)(see Chapter 63)
   1. Results of several trials in newborns have been published (1996 to 1999). Approximately half of the babies in these trials had MAS.
   2. Among babies with MAS in the various studies with NO, there was a slight decrease in the need for ECMO. However, there were no significant differences in mortality, length of hospitalization, or duration of mechanical ventilation.
   3. Currently, inhaled NO should be considered in infants with concomitant persistent pulmonary hypertension who are not responding to conventional therapy.
D. Steroid therapy
   1. Rationale: Treatment of profound inflammation occurring within hours of aspiration.
   2. Steroids may be administered systemically or via the inhalation route.
   3. Animal data are intriguing; limited human data show some benefit.
   4. Additional clinical trials are warranted involving infants with substantial MAS who require mechanical ventilation.
F. Extracorporeal membrane oxygenation (ECMO) (see Chapter 64)
   1. ECMO is a therapy of last resort and is used when mortality is estimated to be >50% to 80%.
   2. Of more than 15,000 newborns treated with ECMO since the mid-1980s, 30% to 35% had MAS as the underlying respiratory disorder.

3. Compared to ECMO-treated infants with other disorders, those with MAS have the shortest duration of cardiopulmonary bypass and the highest survival rates.

4. Venous-arterial bypass is still the most commonly used form of ECMO in infants with MAS. In most centers, this requires sacrifice of the right carotid artery and the right jugular vein.

5. ECMO survivors have morbidity rates of 20% to 40%. It is unknown how much of this morbidity is from pre-existing conditions rather than from ECMO.

VII. Summary

A. MAS remains a common cause of respiratory distress among newborns.

B. Of the various therapies used in the management of MAS, few have been adequately investigated.

C. Further work is needed to elucidate optimal management of MAS.

Suggested Reading

Cleary GM, Wiswell TE: Meconium-stained amniotic fluid and the meconium aspiration syndrome: An update. Pediatr Clin N Am 45:511-529,1998.

Fraser W, Hofmeyr J, Lede R, et al: An international randomized controlled trial of amnioinfusion for thickly meconium-stained amniotic fluid. Am J Obstet Gynecol 191:S3, 2004.

Moses D, Holm B, Spitale P, et al: Inhibition of pulmonary surfactant function by meconium. Am J Obstet Gynecol 164:477-481, 1991.

The Neonatal Inhaled Nitric Oxide Study Group: Inhaled nitric oxide in full-term and nearly full-term infants with hypoxic respiratory failure. N Engl J Med 336:597-604,1997.

Vain N, Szyld E, Prudent L, et al: Oro- and nasopharyngeal suctioning of meconium-stained neonates before delivery of their shoulders: Results of the international, multicentre, randomised, controlled trial. Lancet 364:597-602, 2004.

Wiswell TE, Gannon M, Jacob JJ, et al: Delivery room management of the apparently vigorous meconium-stained neonate: Results of the multicenter, international collaborative trial. Pediatrics 105:1-7, 2000.

Wiswell TE: Advances in the management of the meconium aspiration syndrome. Acat Paediatr Scand 436(Suppl):28-30, 2001.

Wiswell TE: Extended use of surfactant therapy. Clin Perinatol 28:695-711, 2001.

Wiswell, TE, Knight GR, Finer NN, et al: A multicenter, randomized, controlled trial comparing Surfaxin (Lucinactant) lavage with standard care for treatment of meconium aspiration syndrome. Pediatrics 109:1081-1087, 2002.

Persistent Pulmonary Hypertension of the Newborn

51

Robert E. Schumacher and Steven M. Donn

I. Introduction
   A. Persistent pulmonary hypertension of the newborn (PPHN) is a condition in which pulmonary vascular resistance (PVR) is elevated, usually from a failure of the normal postbirth decrease in PVR. This leads to a variable degree of right-to-left shunting through persistent fetal channels, the foramen ovale and ductus arteriosus, and severe hypoxemia. A similar clinical picture can arise from decreased systemic vascular resistance (SVR) or any condition in which the PVR:SVR ratio is >1.
   B. PVR may be elevated as a result of an "appropriate" response to an underlying acute pathologic state (e.g., pneumothorax or pneumonia) or as a result of structural abnormalities of the pulmonary vascular bed.
   C. Although the disorder is also referred to as persistent fetal circulation (PFC), this is a misnomer, because the fetal organ of respiration, the placenta, has been removed, and the infant is dependent upon the lungs for gas exchange.
II. Pulmonary Vascular Development
   A. Alveolar development is primarily a postbirth event. Intra-acinar vascular development is thus also a postbirth phenomenon. As a consequence, at birth there is a decreased cross-sectional area available for pulmonary blood flow and obligate high vascular resistance.
   B. In the newborn, complete vascular smooth muscle development does not extend to the level of the acinus. Abnormally large amounts of in utero pulmonary blood flow (such as in premature closure of the ductus arteriosus) may contribute to structural/muscular changes in the pulmonary vascular system and increased PVR.
   C. Some increase in pulmonary vascular muscle mass occurs at the end of gestation; thus true structurally based PPHN is uncommon in the preterm infant.
   D. A number of nonstructural (and hence more reversible) factors may significantly impact pulmonary vascular reactivity and pressure, including arterial O_2 and CO_2 tensions and pH. Hypoxia, hypercarbia, and acidosis cause vasoconstriction and elevate pulmonary artery pressure, and their presence may lead to maladaptation from fetal to neonatal (adult-type) circulation.

III. Pathogenesis
   A. Normal pulmonary vascular morphology/myocardial dysfunction or increased vascular reactivity from vasoconstrictive stimuli
      1. Associated with asphyxia
         a. Vasoconstrictive effects of hypoxia, hypercarbia, acidosis.
         b. Myocardial dysfunction (especially left-ventricle) leading to pulmonary venous hypertension and subsequent PPHN with right-to-left shunting through the ductus arteriosus.
      2. Associated with meconium aspiration syndrome
         a. Alveolar hypoxia results in vasoconstriction.
         b. Gas trapping and lung overdistention contribute to increased PVR.
         c. Concomitant effects of severe parenchymal lung disease.
         d. Some infants will also have morphologic changes in pulmonary vasculature (see later).
      3. Sepsis/pneumonia
         a. Infection initiates an inflammatory response.
         b. Release of cytokines and other vascular mediators increases PVR.
         c. Severe parenchymal lung disease aggravates hypoxemia.
      4. Thrombus or microthrombus formation with release of vasoactive mediators
      5. Hyperviscosity syndrome, although in some newborn models using fetal hemoglobin one cannot elevate PVR:SVR ratio
   B. Morphologically abnormal pulmonary vasculature
      1. Abnormal extension of vascular smooth muscle, with thickening and increased resistance deeper into the pulmonary vascular tree (may be related to chronic intrauterine hypoxia)
         a. Some cases of meconium aspiration syndrome
         b. In utero closure of the ductus arteriosus
         c. Idiopathic PPHN
      2. Abnormally small lungs with decreased cross-sectional area of the pulmonary vascular bed and muscular thickening and distal extension
         a. Pulmonary hypoplasia (primary or secondary)
         b. Congenital diaphragmatic hernia
         c. Cystic adenomatoid malformation
   C. Structurally abnormal heart disease
      1. Left ventricular outflow tract obstruction
      2. Anomalous pulmonary venous return
      3. Ebstein anomaly
      4. Left ventricular cardiomyopathy
      5. Any structural abnormality resulting in an obligate right-to-left shunt
IV. Diagnosis
   A. Differential diagnoses of hypoxemia in the term or near-term infant
      1. Primary pulmonary disease
      2. Cyanotic congenital heart disease
      3. PPHN, with or without lung disease
   B. Initial work-up
      1. History
         a. Evidence of infection
         b. Meconium-stained amniotic fluid

     c. Intrauterine growth retardation (IUGR)/uteroplacental insufficiency (e.g., postmaturity, dysmaturity)

     d. Maternal aspirin use (premature ductal closure)

  2. Physical examination (findings nonspecific, but may help to suggest etiologic considerations)

     a. Heart murmur

     b. Abnormal breath sounds

     c. Inequality of pulses

     d. Scaphoid abdomen

     e. Potter facies

  3. Chest radiograph (nonspecific, but may suggest or exclude associated conditions)

  4. Arterial blood gas determination (attempt to correct ventilation and acid-base abnormalities before attributing hypoxemia to PPHN)

C. Hyperoxia test

  1. Expose infant to 1.0 FiO_2 for 10 to 15 minutes.

  2. Expected responses

     a. Parenchymal lung disease: PaO_2 should rise.

     b. Cyanotic congenital heart disease: No change in PaO_2.

     c. PPHN: PaO_2 may rise slightly but usually does not.

D. Simultaneous evaluation of pre- and postductal oxygenation

  1. Obtain simultaneous arterial blood gas samples from preductal (right radial artery) and postductal (umbilical or posterior tibial artery) sites.

  2. If there is a gradient (20 mm Hg [2.7 kPa] higher in the preductal PaO_2), a right-to-left ductal shunt may be inferred. Low values from both sites does not rule out PPHN; shunting may still be occurring at the level of the foramen ovale. If both values are high and essentially equal, PPHN is unlikely to be present.

  3. Double-site (e.g., right arm and either leg) transcutaneous oxygen monitoring or pulse oximetry can also be used to detect the presence of a ductal shunt.

E. Hyperoxia-hyperventilation test

  1. Hypoxemia and acidosis augment pulmonary vasoconstriction.

  2. Alkalosis and hyperoxia decrease PVR.

  3. Method

     a. Hyperventilate infant (either mechanically or manually) using 1.0 FiO_2 for 10 to 15 minutes.

     b. Attempt to decrease $PaCO_2$ (usually to 25 to 30 mm Hg [3.3 to 4.0 kPa]), and increase pH to 7.5 range.

     c. Obtain arterial blood gas measurements.

     d. Profound prolonged changes in pCO_2 may alter cerebral blood flow. Use this test with caution.

  4. Results

     a. A dramatic response (increase in PaO_2), along with marked lability, generally suggests PPHN.

     b. Must differentiate whether increase in PaO_2 came from induced alkalosis and hyperoxia or as a result of increased mean airway pressure during test.

    F. Echocardiography
        1. Will rule out congenital heart disease.
        2. Evaluates myocardial function.
        3. May enable direct visualization of shunting (Doppler blood flow).
        4. Estimates pulmonary artery pressure from regurgitant
           tricuspid jet (see Chapter 22).
 V. Treatment
    A. Prenatal
        1. Pregnancies complicated by conditions associated with PPHN
           (e.g., congenital diaphragmatic hernia, prolonged
           oligohydramnios) should be referred to a high-risk center capable
           of caring for the infant following delivery.
        2. Identification and appropriate obstetric management of other
           at-risk pregnancies (e.g., meconium-staining, chorioamnionitis,
           postdate).
    B. Postnatal
        1. Adequate resuscitation
        2. Avoidance of hypothermia, hypovolemia, and hypoglycemia
        3. Avoidance of acidosis, hypoxia, and hypercarbia
        4. Prompt treatment of suspected sepsis, hypotension, and other
           problems
    C. Establish the diagnosis.
    D. General supportive measures
        1. Use an appropriate ventilatory strategy and mode.
        2. Ensure adequate systemic blood pressure.
        3. Maintain adequate oxygen-carrying capacity (hemoglobin >15 mg/dL)
        4. Treat the underlying disorder.
            a. Surfactant replacement for RDS
            b. Antibiotics, if indicated
            c. Correction of mechanical problems (e.g., ascites, pleural
               effusions, pneumothorax)
    E. Mechanical ventilation
        1. The initial approach should be to establish adequate normal
           ventilation while correcting underlying pulmonary disease,
           if present. Both conventional mechanical ventilation and
           high-frequency ventilation have been used.
        2. There is a paucity of literature defining the optimal approach to the
           ventilatory management of PPHN. Two diametrically opposed
           approaches have been suggested, but clinical investigation
           comparing them is lacking.
            a. Conservative ventilation uses the least amount of support
               possible to achieve gas exchange and pH that are marginally
               acceptable. The aim is to decrease the level of ventilatory
               support to the lowest possible, so that lung hyperexpansion
               (which contributes to PVR) and barotrauma are avoided. PaO_2
               levels of 40 to 45 mm Hg (5.7 to 6.0 kPa), $PaCO_2$ levels of 55 to
               60 mm Hg (7.7 to 8.0 kPa), and pH levels of 7.25 are tolerated.
               In usual clinical practice, oxygen saturation values better reflect
               blood oxygen content; hence many clinicians opt to follow these
               values rather than PaO_2 values. Additionally, although PVR is

responsive to alveolar oxygen content, there is a paucity of human evidence suggesting that it is PaO_2-responsive. From this perspective, keeping $PaO_2 >$"x" seems an unhelpful approach.

b. Hyperventilation and alkalosis: This approach attempts to take advantage of the vasodilatory effects of alkalosis and hypocarbia on the pulmonary vasculature. The $PaCO_2$ is decreased to the "critical" value, below which there is a sharp rise in PaO_2. Alkalosis can be augmented by infusion of sodium bicarbonate (although recent evidence suggests that this increases morbidity). pH levels are usually kept above 7.5. However cerebral blood flow also responds to pCO_2 (decreased flow at low pCO_2) and there is epidemiologic evidence associating low values with long-term motor disability in children. Hence, this approach has fallen out of favor.

c. Many clinicians favor a "middle-of-the-road" or an "avoid acidosis and hypercarbia" approach, in which physiologically normal blood gases and pH are targeted by using ventilator support.

3. No matter which approach is chosen, remember that infants with PPHN demonstrate extreme lability. It is usually better to attempt several small ventilator/FiO_2 changes than one large one.

4. A transitional phase of PPHN occurs at 3 to 5 days of age. Vascular reactivity diminishes and support can be decreased at a faster rate.

F. Pharmacotherapy

1. Maintain adequate cardiac output and systemic blood pressure. The degree of right-to-left shunting depends upon the pulmonary-to-systemic gradient. Avoidance of systemic hypotension is critical. CVP monitoring may be of benefit.

   a. Correct hypovolemia by administering volume expanders.

   b. Administer cardiotonic agents (e.g., dopamine, dobutamine, epinephrine)

2. Correct acidosis.

   a. Sodium bicarbonate may be given as a bolus (1 to 3 mEq/kg) or as a continuous infusion (≤ 1.0 mEq/hr). Avoid hypernatremia; assure adequate ventilation.

   b. Tris-hydroxyaminomethane (THAM, 0.3 M) can be given even if $PaCO_2$ is elevated. Dose is 4 to 8 mL/kg. Observe for hypokalemia, hypoglycemia, and respiratory depression.

3. Pulmonary vasodilating agents

   a. Inhaled nitric oxide (NO) (see Chapter 63): Inhaled NO has been successful in the treatment of PPHN. Given by inhalational route. Potential toxicities include methemoglobinemia and lung injury from metabolites formed during the oxidation of NO.

   b. Other agents

      (1) Prostacyclin

      (2) Sudenafil

4. Extracorporeal membrane oxygenation (See Chapter 64.)

   a. A rescue modality is generally used when predicted mortality from PPHN is high.

   b. Overall survival exceeds 80% and is dependent upon underlying disease; there are lower rates for congenital diaphragmatic hernia and pulmonary hypoplasia.

    c. There are long-term sequelae in about 20% of infants, equivalent to those reported in infants surviving PPHN who are treated by conventional means.

Suggested Reading

Donn SM: Alternatives to ECMO. Arch Dis Child 70:F81-F84, 1994.

Kinsella JP, Shaffer E, Neish SR, et al: Low-dose inhalational nitric oxide in persistent pulmonary hypertension of the newborn. Lancet 340:818-822, 1992.

Peckham GJ, Fox WW: Physiological factors affecting pulmonary artery pressures in infants with persistent pulmonary hypertension. J Pediatr 93:1005-1110, 1978.

Roberts JD, Polaner DM, Lang P, et al: Inhaled nitric oxide in persistent pulmonary hypertension of the newborn. Lancet 340:818-821, 1992.

Walsh MC, Stork EK: Persistent pulmonary hypertension of the newborn: Rational therapy based on pathophysiology. Clin Perinatol 28:609-627, 2001.

Wung JT, James LS, Kilchevsky E, et al: Management of infants with severe respiratory failure and persistence of the fetal circulation, without hyperventilation. Pediatrics 76:488-493, 1985.

Congenital Diaphragmatic Hernia

52

David J. Field

I. Background
   A. Embryology: Congenital diaphragmatic hernia (CDH) is failure of normal development of the diaphragm during the 1st trimester. There are four types:
      1. Complete absence of the diaphragm; rare, most severe, worst prognosis.
      2. Failure of normal development of the diaphragm anteriorly; only 2% of cases.
      3. Failure of the diaphragm to close posteriorly; most common (≈1 in 5000 births)—85% left-sided, 10% right-sided, 5% bilateral.
      4. Eventration: Not a true hernia; results from a failure of muscle development in the primitive diaphragm (not considered further here).
   B. CDH can be part of a syndrome (e.g., Fryns) or associated with a chromosomal anomaly (e.g., trisomy 13 or 18); prognosis is worse in such cases.
   C. Pathophysiology
      1. Compression of both lungs during pregnancy results in hypoplasia, especially in the ipsilateral lung.
      2. In the most severe cases, cardiac function can also be compromised in utero.
      3. After delivery, gaseous distention of the gut in the chest results in further cardiorespiratory compromise.
      4. Pulmonary hypoplasia and poor oxygenation following delivery commonly result in severe persistent pulmonary hypertension of the newborn (PPHN).
      5. In mild cases, cardiopulmonary development and function may be sufficient to enable normal extrauterine adaptation with presentation at a later stage.
II. Presentation and Diagnosis
   A. Antenatal
      1. Uusally, CDH can be detected on a routine maternal sonographic scan during the second or third trimester; herniated abdominal viscera and mediastinal shift should be identifiable. However, a scan reported as "normal" does not conclusively exclude the diagnosis.

   2. Right-sided lesions are more difficult to detect because of the
      similar echogenicity of lung and liver.
   3. Polyhydramnios is commonly seen.
   4. Various other anomalies have been noted in association with CDH.
B. Postnatal (when not suspected antenatally) presentations
   1. At delivery, with failure to respond to normal resuscitative
      measures. In such cases a barrel chest and scaphoid abdomen may
      be noted.
   2. Within the first 48 hours of life with respiratory distress.
   3. In later childhood, when signs can be varied and may be respiratory
      and/or gastroenterologic in nature. Currently <5% of cases present
      in this manner.
C. Differential diagnosis: Cystic lesions of the lung (most commonly
   cystic adenomatoid malformation) and growths or effusions that
   render one hemithorax opaque can cause confusion.
D. Investigations: Antenatal ultrasound findings or clinical presentation
   alone may strongly suggest the diagnosis. Useful additional
   investigations include the following:
   1. Chest radiograph (essential)
   2. Contrast studies—used to confirm presence of stomach/gut in the
      chest—rarely necessary
   3. Ultrasound or (rarely) isotope study to document position of the liver
   4. CT scan (rarely)
III. Predicting Outcome: CDH produces a spectrum of pathology, ranging
   from very mild (causing minimal compromise) to severe (incompatible
   with life) pulmonary hypoplasia. Significant numbers fall into the latter
   category. Can they be identified in order that pointless exposure to
   surgery and intensive care can be avoided? A variety of techniques have
   been used, but none have been uniformly successful. Still commonly
   attempted, indicators of poor prognosis include:
A. Antenatal sonographic scans (polyhydramnios, reduced chest
   circumference, significant mediastinal shift, reduced fetal breathing)
B. Postnatal chest radiograph (intrathoracic stomach, estimated degree
   of pulmonary hypoplasia)
C. Postnatal lung function (lung volumes, pulmonary compliance)
D. Echocardiography (ventricular thickness)
IV. Management
A. Antenatal: Once a diagnosis is made, families should be counseled by
   the obstetrician, neonatologist, and pediatric surgeon regarding
   available options:
   1. Termination (criteria and regulations vary markedly among countries)
   2. Continuing the pregnancy and performing postnatal repair
   3. Prenatal fetal surgery—practiced in only a few centers around the
      world. Current results are poor. Repair often induces premature
      delivery.
B. At delivery in cases diagnosed antenatally
   1. Avoid distention of the GI tract by face mask ventilation.
      a. Intubate and ventilate as soon as possible (i.e., in the delivery
         room). Consider elective paralysis.

     b. Pass a nasogastric tube in the delivery room, ensure that there is free drainage, and aspirate it every 30 minutes. Alternatively, insert a Replogle tube and use continuous suction.

  2. Minimize factors that could precipitate PPHN:

     a. Use adequate sedation.

     b. Ensure adequate ventilation.

C. In the NICU, preoperatively:

  1. In infants who are not diagnosed antenatally but present soon after delivery with respiratory distress, efforts should be made to minimize PPHN and avoid gaseous distention of the bowel.

  2. Establish continuous monitoring. Invasive blood pressure/arterial access is essential. (Remember that samples obtained from sites other than the right arm will be affected by right-to-left shunting.) Central venous pressure monitoring, if available via the umbilical vein, is helpful in fluid management.

  3. Ensure adequate systemic blood pressure (maintains tissue perfusion and minimizes right-to-left shunting). Infusion of both volume and inotropes may be required. Take care not to induce fluid overload.

  4. Provide adequate ventilatory support. Local policy usually governs the first choice. Both conventional and oscillatory ventilation can be used with success. Aim to provide stability as a minimum (i.e., sufficient oxygenation to prevent metabolic acidosis, sufficient control of CO_2 elimination to prevent respiratory acidosis). If this cannot be achieved despite maximum support (including extracorporeal membrane oxygenation [ECMO]), the infant should be considered nonviable. The clinical condition of those babies who are stabilized should be optimized prior to surgery. Again, local practice often governs the timing of surgery; however, evidence to support specific criteria is weak.

  5. Introduce pulmonary vasodilators as indicated. PPHN is a common and major complication of CDH. Nitric oxide empirically would appear to be the agent of choice, but data in relation to CDH suggest that its use is unhelpful.

  6. Surfactant: No clear role for surfactant has been established, but it is commonly used.

D. Surgical repair is clearly essential but should be attempted only when the baby is stable. It may be performed through the abdomen (allows correction of associated malrotation at the same time) or chest (large defect may require use of a patch).

E. Postoperative care

  1. Essentially the same pattern of management as that used preoperatively is recommended.

  2. Failure to wean the infant from respiratory support in the days following operation may indicate pulmonary hypoplasia that is incompatible with life.

F. ECMO is clearly able to provide stability and to control PPHN; however, no evidence of benefit over other forms of care in terms of long-term outcome has been demonstrated.

V. Outcomes
   A. Short-term: Because they are hospital based, almost all published results are difficult to interpret. Inherent flaws include the following:
      1. Contain referral bias.
      2. Do not clarify the effect of antenatal counseling and selective termination.
      3. May exclude high-risk groups, such as those with associated anomalies. A survival rate of 50% to 60% beyond the neonatal period represents a good result.
   B. Medium-term: A proportion of infants who survive the neonatal period will die in the first 2 years of life as a result of pulmonary hypertension/hypoplasia.
   C. Long-term
      1. Respiratory outcome reflects the severity of the initial lesion and the amount and type of respiratory support required.
      2. Survivors are at significant risk for neurodevelopmental delay, presumably secondary to problems in the perinatal period and other medical problems (e.g., volvulus, gastroesophageal reflux, chronic lung disease).
VI. New Approaches under Development
   A. Tracheal occlusion in utero can raise intrapulmonary pressure and reduce the gut from the chest. Clinically significant improvements in lung growth have not yet been demonstrated. This procedure may also produce secondary problems (e.g., hydrops).
   B. Liquid ventilation (see Chapter 65) may be able to maintain gas exchange while encouraging increased lung volume. It has been used in association with ECMO on an investigational basis.
   C. Minimally invasive repair techniques have been developed but have not proved more beneficial than conventional approaches.

Suggested Reading

Arca MJ, Barnhart DC, Lelli L, et al: Early experience with minimally invasive repair of congenital diaphragmatic hernia: Results and lessons learned. J Pediatr Surg 38:1563-1568, 2003.

Cannon C, Dildy GA, Ward R, et al: A population-based study of congenital diaphragmatic hernia in Utah: 1988-1994. Obstet Gynecol 87:959-963, 1996.

Finer NN, Barrington KJ: Nitric oxide for respiratory failure in infants born at or near term. Cochrane Database Syst Rev CD000399, 2000.

Graf JL, Gibbs DL, Adzick NS, et al: Fetal hydrops after in utero tracheal occlusion. J Pediatr Surg 32:214-215, 1997.

Hirschl RB, Philip WF, Glick L, et al: A prospective randomized pilot trial of perfluorocarbon-induced lung growth in newborns with congenital diaphragmatic hernia. J Pediatr Surg 38:283-289, 2003.

Kinsella JP, Truog WE, Walsh WF, et al: Randomized, multicenter trial of inhaled nitric oxide and high-frequency oscillatory ventilation in severe, persistent pulmonary hypertension of the newborn. J Pediatr 131:55-62, 1997.

Nio M, Haase G, Kennaugh J, et al: A prospective randomized trial of delayed versus immediate repair of congenital diaphragmatic hernia. J Pediatr Surg 29:618-621, 1994.

Nobuhara KK, Lund DP, Mitchell J, et al: Long-term outlook for survivors of congenital diaphragmatic hernia. Clin Perinatol 23:873-887, 1996.

Pranikoff T, Gauger PG, Hirschl RB: Partial liquid ventilation in newborn patients with congenital diaphragmatic hernia. J Pediatr Surg 31:613-618, 1996.

Pulmonary Hypoplasia/ Agenesis

53

David J. Field

I. Classification
   A. Pulmonary
      1. Agenesis: Failure of one or both lung buds to develop at the very beginning of lung development. Agenesis can be isolated or part of a syndrome Bilateral agenesis is always fatal. Unilateral defect may be asymptomatic.
      2. Hypoplasia (structural)
         a. Primary: Rare defect that may be associated with other congenital anomalies
         b. Secondary: Consequence of any lesion that impairs normal development (Table 53-1)
      3. Hypoplasia (biochemical), primary: A few cases have been identified that present with features of pulmonary hypoplasia but are structurally normal lungs. Abnormalities of surfactant have been identified, in particular the absence of surfactant protein B.
   B. Vascular
      1. Macroscopic: Atresia of the main pulmonary trunk can disrupt normal pulmonary vascular development; however, pulmonary function is usually satisfactory. Presentation is with severe cyanosis, which can be remedied by improving pulmonary blood flow.
      2. Microscopic: Pulmonary vasculature can be disrupted at the alveolar level and result in severely reduced gas exchange. Dysplasia is rare, but a small number of patterns have been recognized to date (e.g., malalignment of the pulmonary veins, alveolar capillary dysplasia).
II. Pathophysiology: The exact pathophysiology varies with the underlying mechanism.
   A. Reduced lung capacity (secondary to thoracic dystrophy)

TABLE 53-1. Factors That Can Impair Lung Growth in Utero

Compression of chest (e.g., oligohydramnios—all causes)
Compression of lung (e.g., effusion, diaphragmatic hernia)
Reduction in fetal breathing (e.g., neuromuscular disorder)

    B. Structural immaturity (secondary to oligohydramnios)

    C. Diffusion deficit (secondary to malalignment of the pulmonary veins)

    D. The main functional problem that results from all the above is pulmonary insufficiency. The main clinical problem tends to be oxygen transfer.

III. Diagnosis

    A. Antenatal: Diagnosis may be suggested by the maternal antenatal ultrasound scan (e.g., severe oligohydramnios, small fetal chest cavity).

    B. Postnatal: Diagnosis may be apparent immediately after birth if hypoplasia is severe (i.e., infant cannot be resuscitated or is in severe respiratory distress from birth) or is part of recognizable syndrome (e.g., oligohydramnios sequence). When the infant presents later with apparently isolated mild to moderate respiratory distress, diagnosis may be delayed. Syndromes either primarily or secondarily associated with pulmonary hypoplasia should be considered. Similarly, conditions that can mimic these signs (e.g., infection) should be excluded. In all cases in which hypoplasia is the possible diagnosis, the following should be considered:

       1. Genetics consult

       2. Measurement of lung volumes

       3. Measurement of pulmonary compliance

       4. Examination of surfactant genotype

       5. Lung biopsy

    C. The choice of investigation will vary with severity of the infant's problem. In severe respiratory failure, lung biopsy may be performed as a terminal event to permit diagnosis and counseling about future pregnancies (see later). If respiratory problems are less severe (e.g., unexplained persistent tachypnea), assessment of pulmonary mechanics is appropriate.

IV. Management

    A. Antenatal: If a diagnosis of pulmonary hypoplasia is made in utero, the family should be counseled by the obstetrician, neonatologist, clinical geneticist, and surgeon (if appropriate). Potential options will vary according to:

       1. Diagnosis and prognosis

       2. Degree of diagnostic certainty resulting from the evaluation. Essentially parents must decide between:

          a. Termination of pregnancy (criteria and regulations vary markedly among countries).

          b. Continuing the pregnancy with postnatal intervention and "treatment."

          c. Antenatal intervention, practiced only in relation to certain conditions (e.g., bilateral pleural effusions). Results vary with both the nature and severity of underlying problem. Evidence of benefit from such interventions has not been established.

    B. At delivery, standard resuscitation should take place. When indicated by antenatal scans, special measures (e.g., draining pleural effusions) should be performed. Vigorous resuscitation of infants with small-volume lungs often results in pneumothorax. If dysmorphic features in the infant indicate a lethal syndrome, or if oxygenation proves impossible, intensive care may be withdrawn.

C. In the NICU:

1. Establish routine monitoring. Invasive blood pressure/arterial access is essential in the severest cases; central venous pressure monitoring, if available via the umbilical vein, is of great help in fluid management.

2. Ensure adequate systemic blood pressure (maintain tissue perfusion and minimize right-to-left shunting). Infusion of fluids and inotropes may be required. Take care not to induce fluid overload.

3. Provide adequate respiratory support. Infants with mild hypoplasia may not require ventilation. For those requiring invasive support, local practice usually governs the first choice; both conventional and high-frequency ventilation can be used with success. Aim to provide stability of blood gases (i.e., sufficient oxygenation to prevent metabolic acidosis). More aggressive ventilation may induce pulmonary damage and further impair lung function. If blood gas control proves impossible despite maximum support, the infant should be considered nonviable.

4. Introduce pulmonary vasodilators as indicated; pulmonary hypertension is often a complication. Doppler studies may help confirm the diagnosis. Inhaled nitric oxide appears to be the agent of choice.

5. There is no clear role for surfactant in this situation, but it is frequently used in an attempt to rescue a deteriorating baby.

6. Extracorporeal membrane oxygenation (ECMO) is clearly able to provide stability, but there is no evidence of benefit over other forms of care in pulmonary hypoplasia.

7. A role for the use of partial liquid ventilation has not been established.

8. Investigate to confirm the diagnosis. When there are no clear features to support a diagnosis of pulmonary hypoplasia, routine tests should exclude all other causes of respiratory distress.

V. Pulmonary Hypoplasia: Pulmonary hypoplasia results from a large number of different conditions. The prognosis is governed mainly by the etiology and any associated anomalies.

A. Mild cases often become asymptomatic with growth. Abnormalities of function can still be measured in later childhood.

B. Infants with moderate hypoplasia can survive with intensive care but often need long-term respiratory support. The effect of growth is uncertain, and death in later childhood can occur.

C. Severely affected babies die despite full support. No current intervention is known to help in such cases.

VI. Counseling about Future Pregnancies: Some infants will be affected by conditions that can recur in future pregnancies. A proportion of severely affected cases cannot be diagnosed without examination of lung tissue. Lung biopsy may be impossible to perform safely while the infant is alive. Postmortem studies should be made whenever possible. If permission for postmortem examination is not obtained, an open or needle biopsy of the lung obtained soon after death may a tissue diagnosis (in many areas, consent to do so is required).

Suggested Reading

Aiton NR, Fox GF, Hannam S, et al: Pulmonary hypoplasia presenting as persistent tachypnea in the first few months of life. BMJ 312:1149-1150, 1996.

DeMello D: Pulmonary pathology. Semin Neonatol 9:311-329, 2004.

DiFiore JW, Wilson JM: Lung development. Semin Pediatr Surg 3:221-232, 1994.

Kilbride HW, Yeast J, Thibeault DW: Defining limits of survival: Lethal pulmonary hypoplasia after midtrimester premature rupture of membranes. Am J Obstet Gynecol 175:675-681, 1996.

Major D, Cadenas M, Cloutier R, et al: Morphometrics of normal and hypoplastic lungs in preterm lambs with gas and partial liquid ventilation. Pediatr Surg Int 12:121-125, 1997.

McIntosh N, Harrison A: Prolonged premature rupture of membranes in the preterm infant: A 7-year study. Eur J Obstet Gynecol Reprod Biol 47:1-6, 1994.

Nogee LM, deMello DE, Dehner LP, Colten HR: Deficiency of pulmonary surfactant protein B in congenital pulmonary alveolar proteinosis. N Engl J Med 328:404-410, 1993.

Sirkin W, O'Hara BP, Cox PN, et al: Alveolar capillary dysplasia: Lung biopsy diagnosis, nitric oxide responsiveness, and bronchial generation count. Pediatr Pathol Lab Med 17:125-132, 1997.

Apnea Syndromes

54

Alan R. Spitzer

I. Terminology
   A. Apnea is the absence of respiratory airflow.
   B. There is no universally accepted definition of pathologic apnea. When discussed in this chapter, however, pathologic apnea refers to the cessation of respiratory airflow for >20 seconds, or a briefer pause associated with abrupt onset of pallor, cyanosis, bradycardia, or hypotonia. It has been demonstrated that many completely well infants occasionally have events that could be defined as pathologic apnea, and these events seem to have no serious long-term consequences.
   C. Apnea of infancy (AOI) is pathologic apnea that presents in an infant who is >37 weeks' gestational age for which no specific cause can be identified.
   D. Apnea of prematurity (AOP) is pathologic apnea or excessive periodic breathing in preterm infants (<37 weeks' gestational age).
   E. Periodic breathing (PB) is a respiratory pattern in which there are three or more consecutive central pauses of >3 seconds, separated by <20 seconds of breathing between each pause. The relationship of periodic breathing to pathologic apnea is not well understood, but it appears to reflect immaturity of respiratory control.
   F. Apparent life-threatening event (ALTE) refers to an event that is frightening to the observer and is characterized by some combination of apnea, color change, marked change in muscle tone, choking, and gagging.
   G. Sudden infant death syndrome (SIDS) is the unexpected death of an infant between 1 month and 1 year of age that remains unexplained after a review of the past medical records of the child, a postmortem examination, and a death scene investigation. To date, no etiology of SIDS has been defined, and it appears likely that SIDS represents a final common pathway for a number of unrelated clinical phenomena. For children to die of SIDS, it is also probable that the triple-risk theory of SIDS must be satisfied (Fig. 54-1).
II. Etiology of Apnea (Table 54-1)
   A. All children and adults occasionally demonstrate apnea. Apnea may be normal if it is brief, infrequent, and not associated with any underlying problems.
   B. If abnormal, apnea represents a sign rather than a specific pathologic process. Many diverse conditions can be associated with pathologic apnea.

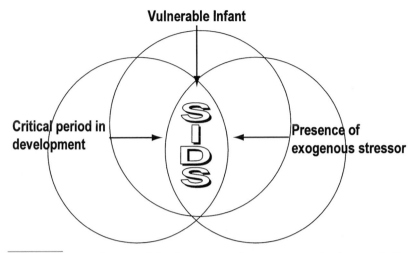

Figure 54-1. Venn diagram of the three events that must occur simultaneously for a death from SIDS to result: The infant must be vulnerable, due to genetic factors or past medical history; reach a critical period during development; and be subjected to a stressor that triggers SIDS. (Adapted from Filiano JJ, Kinney HC: A perspective on neuropathologic findings in victims of the sudden infant death syndrome: The triple-risk model. Biol Neonate 65:194-197, 1994.)

Table 54-1. Medical Conditions Associated with Pathologic Apnea

Acute Conditions	Chronic Conditions
Thermal instability	Apnea of prematurity
Infection (meningitis, bacteremia, respiratory syncytial virus infection, pertussis, infantile botulism)	Gastrointestinal reflux disease
CNS pathology (seizure, intracranial hemorrhage, including child abuse)	Airway obstruction (congenital anomaly, sleep apnea)
Metabolic disturbances (inborn errors of metabolism, hypernatremia, hyponatremia, hypoglycemia, hypocalcemia)	Cardiac disease (dysrhythmia, marked shunt including patent ductusarteriosus)
Airway obstruction (neck flexion, laryngospasm)	CNS pathology (seizure, hemorrhage, malformation including Arnold-Chiari)
Necrotizing enterocolitis	Marked anemia
Postsurgical apnea	Chronic lung disease
Drug-induced	CAHS (Ondine curse)
	Idiopathic

III. Risk Groups for Apnea
   A. Premature infants
      1. An interplay of an immature ventilatory center, impaired central and peripheral nervous system chemoreceptors, and functional obstruction of the upper airway results in AOP.
      2. Approximately 25% to 70% of premature infants have AOP during hospitalization in the NICU. The more immature an infant, the greater the likelihood of clinical apnea.
      3. Apnea in premature infants is predominantly central apnea.
   B. Term infants
      1. Approximately 2% to 3% of term infants will have apnea in the weeks shortly after birth.
      2. Term infants rarely need to be treated for their apnea.
   C. Infantile pathologic gastroesophageal reflux disease (GERD)
      1. The peak period of onset is 1 to 4 months of age.
      2. Manifestations include esophagitis, failure to thrive, recurrent pneumonia, intractable wheezing, and obstructive apnea.
      3. Groups with the greatest risk for pathologic GERD include premature infants, neurologically impaired children, infants with underlying lung disease (cystic fibrosis or chronic lung disease [CLD]), and children who require gastrostomy feedings.
      4. Although about 50% of infants will "spit up" in the first months of life, very few will have pathologic GERD that requires therapy.
   D. ALTE
      1. Occurs in 0.5% to 6% of all infants at some time in the first 6 months of life.
      2. Represents a clinical presentation rather than a specific disease process.
      3. Causes include systemic infections, upper airway obstruction, seizures, GERD, cardiac disease, idiopathic apnea, and bradycardia.
      4. There is an increased incidence of SIDS in these children, especially if vigorous resuscitation during sleep is needed.
   E. Siblings of SIDS victims
      1. Two- to fourfold increase in the incidence of SIDS in siblings of SIDS victims has been demonstrated in numerous studies.
      2. Infanticide and hereditary disorders must be considered, especially if more than one child in a family has died of SIDS.
   F. Chronic conditions, such as CLD and tracheostomy dependency
   G. Neurologic birth injury
      1. Children with perinatal hypoxic-ischemic injury following difficult deliveries often have apnea for a period of time.
      2. The duration of apnea in these children may reflect the severity of injury.
   H. Central alveolar hypoventilation syndrome (CAHS) (Ondine curse)
      1. CAHS is characterized by the inability to regulate ventilation during sleep secondary to inadequate output from brainstem centers.
      2. The diagnosis of CAHS should be considered when persistent pathologic central apnea or ventilator dependency exists in the presence of minimal pulmonary disease.
      3. CAHS is associated infrequently with Hirschsprung disease.

TABLE 54-2. Risk Factors for Sudden Infant Death Syndrome (SIDS)

Modifiable	Less Modifiable
Prone sleep position*	Prematurity
Tobacco exposure	Young mother
Inadequate health care	Poorly educated mother
Lack of breast-feeding	Poverty
Day care situations in which a child is placed prone when accustomed to supine sleep position	Low birth weight/intrauterine retardation
	Colder climate
	Previous apparent life-threatening event

*Risk for SIDS for infants in the prone sleep position is greater if there has been a recent illness, the child sleeps on soft bedding surfaces, gas-trapping objects (e.g., pillows, stuffed animals) are present in the crib, or swaddling is used.

IV. SIDS
  A. SIDS is the leading cause of postneonatal infant mortality (0.6 infant deaths per 1000 live births).
  B. Peak age of occurrence is 2 to 4 months, with the majority (95%) of deaths occurring by age 6 months.
  C. SIDS is a statistically rare event with poor predictability.
  D. There are multiple risk factors (Table 54-2).
  E. Etiology is unknown.
V. Approach to the Infant with Apnea (Table 54-3)
  A. Cardiopulmonary stabilization
  B. Detailed history and physical examination

TABLE 54-3. Diagnostic Clues for Infants with Apnea or ALTE

Clinical Features	Underlying Pathology
Choking during feeding	Pharyngeal dyscoordination, laryngospasm, GERD
Postfeeding spitting, color change, posturing (back arching)	GERD
Abnormal eye movement, muscle tone change, and postictal activity; abnormal neurologic findings, developmental delay	Seizures
Fever, activity change, recalcitrant apnea	Serious bacterial infection
Family history of SIDS or ALTE; presence of bruising	Familial disorder (inborn error of metabolism), child abuse

ALTE, apparent life-threatening event; GERD, gastroesophageal reflux disease; SIDS, sudden infant death syndrome.

TABLE **54-4.** When to Hospitalize an Infant with Suspected Apnea

Ill appearance
Frequent clinical episodes or monitor alarms
Initiation of resuscitation
Color change (i.e., cyanosis or duskiness)
Change in muscle tone
Discrepancy in medical history
Extreme parental anxiety

    C. The diagnostic evaluation is directed by the clinical presentation and the infant's associated findings.

    D. Indications for hospitalization of infants with apnea are summarized in Table 54-4.

VI. Diagnostic Considerations

    A. CBC and cultures of blood, urine, and spinal fluid are necessary if a serious bacterial infection is suspected.

    B. Continuous multichannel recording (Fig. 54-2):

        1. Measures chest wall movement, nasal/oral airflow (or change in air temperature), oxygen saturation, and heart rate trend.

        2. Categorizes apnea.

           a. Central apnea: Absence of nasal airflow and chest wall movement

           b. Obstructive apnea: Lack of airflow in the presence of chest wall movement

           c. Mixed apnea: Combination of central and obstructive apnea

        3. Sensitivity and chance of finding abnormal events are improved if multichannel recording is performed continuously for at least 18 to 24 hours.

        4. A two-channel pneumogram (which measures only chest wall excursion and heart rate trend) provides insufficient information in many cases, because it does not detect obstructive events.

    C. Intraesophageal pH recording should be used with multichannel recording if GERD is suspected (Fig. 54-3).

    D. A radiographic contrast swallow study is useful if the infant has signs of swallowing dysfunction or anatomic anomalies such as esophageal web and tracheoesophageal fistula.

    E. A gastric-emptying study and an abdominal sonogram are useful if there is a clinical picture of a generalized gastrointestinal motility disorder or pyloric stenosis.

    F. A chest radiograph and a radionuclide milk scan are helpful if the infant has persistent, yet unexplained, lower airway signs.

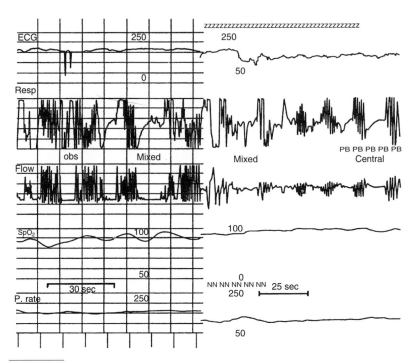

FIGURE 54-2. The three types of apnea commonly observed on a multichannel recording: obstructive, mixed, and central (with periodic breathing [PB]). The left side of the tracing was performed with an end-tidal CO_2 monitor, and the right side was performed using a nasal thermistor probe. The top channel shows averaged heart rate, the second channel shows thoracic impedance, and the third channel indicates nasal airflow. The bottom two channels are the oxygen saturation recording and the heart rate from the saturation monitor, which shows concordance with the heart rate from chest wall recording. Absence of nasal airflow indicates periods of apnea. ECG, electrocardiogram; Obs, obstructive apnea; P. rate, pulse rate; resp, respiration; SpO_2, oxygen saturation. (Courtesy of Joseph DeCristofaro, MD.)

G. Upper airway evaluation (including a lateral neck radiograph and otolaryngology evaluation with possible laryngoscopy or bronchoscopy) is useful if there is fixed or recurrent stridor, as well as unexplained pathologic obstructive apnea.

H. An EEG should be considered in infants suspected of apneic seizures or having persistent pathologic central apnea without an identifiable cause.

I. Imaging studies of the brain are necessary in the presence of developmental delay, suspicion of an intracranial hemorrhage (including child abuse), dysmorphic features, an abnormal neurologic examination, or mental status changes. In general, MRI is the study of choice.

J. Measurements of serum ammonia, as well as of urine and serum amino acids and organic acids, are useful if a metabolic

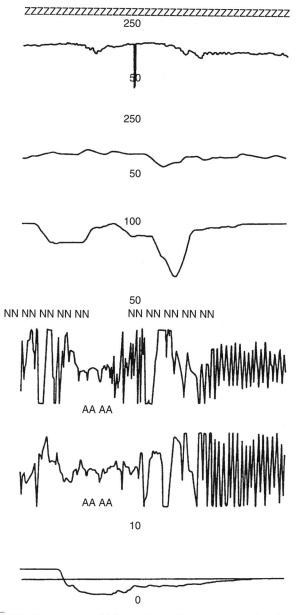

FIGURE 54-3. This figure is a multichannel recording of an episode of gastroesophageal reflux (GER) triggering an episode of apnea. The top channel is the averaged heart rate from the electrocardiogram (ECG) monitor, the next channel is heart rate from the pulse oximeter, the third channel indicates the oxygen saturation, the fourth channel is the thermistor probe indicated nasal airflow, and the fifth channel shows thoracic impedance. The bottom channel is the esophageal pH probe; the straight line indicates a pH of 4.0, below which significant esophageal acidity is denoted. AA, apnea; NN, normal. (Courtesy of Joseph DeCristofaro, MD.)

disorder is suspected. Filter-paper supplemental newborn metabolic screening also may be useful in some cases.

K. Serum electrolytes and glucose can help diagnose a recent stressful condition, a metabolic process, or chronic hypoventilation.

L. An echocardiogram and a cardiology referral are necessary if the history or physical examination suggests cardiac disease (e.g., feeding difficulties, heart murmur, and cyanosis).

M. An ECG is useful when severe unexplained tachycardia or bradycardia exists. Cardiac conduction abnormalities (e.g., prolonged QT syndrome) are rare but important causes of infant apnea.

N. A stool specimen for botulism is helpful if the apneic infant has associated constipation and hypotonia.

O. A polysomnogram is useful in older children with sleep apnea associated with features such as bizarre behaviors, abnormal body movements, and nocturnal enuresis. This multichannel recording includes an EEG, a chin muscle EMG, and an electro-oculogram.

VII. Treatment

A. The therapy of an apneic infant, as with the evaluation, must be directed at identifying and managing the underlying cause. As with many medical conditions, if the cause is not removed, the signs will usually reappear.

B. Apnea of prematurity

1. Xanthine derivatives (i.e., caffeine, theophylline)

a. Proposed mechanisms include stimulation of skeletal and diaphragmatic muscle contraction, increase in the ventilator center's sensitivity to CO_2, and stimulation of the central respiratory drive.

b. Dosage

(1) Active caffeine alkaloid: 2.5 mg/kg daily (5 mg/kg/day of caffeine citrate) 24 hours after a loading dose of 10 mg/kg of active caffeine.

(2) Theophylline: 1 to 2 mg/kg every 8 hours after a loading dose of 5 to 6 mg/kg.

c. Therapeutic serum concentrations

(1) Caffeine: 5 to 25 mg/L

(2) Theophylline: 5 to 10 mg/L (higher concentrations may be necessary in some cases).

d. Side effects include nausea, vomiting, CNS excitability, seizures, tachycardia, and cardiac arrhythmia. Serious toxic effects are rare at serum levels >20 mg/L.

e. Caution is necessary if there is an intercurrent viral illness, if certain drugs (primarily metabolized by the liver) are being administered, and if coexisting seizures (lowers seizure threshold) or coexisting GERD (lowers esophageal sphincter tone) is present.

f. The wider therapeutic range and longer half-life of caffeine compared with theophylline results in less frequent monitoring of drug concentrations and less serious toxicity.

g. Use is controversial because of concerns regarding potential neurotoxicity.
2. Continuous positive airway pressure (CPAP)
   a. Proposed mechanism
      (1) Improvement in oxygenation
      (2) Maintenance of upper airway patency
      (3) Reduction in intercostal-phrenic inhibitory reflex
      (4) Alteration of Hering-Breuer deflation reflex
   b. Indications
      (1) Poor response to xanthine derivatives
      (2) Obstructive apnea and inability to maintain airway patency
   c. Low positive pressure (2 to 5 cm H_2O by nasal prongs is suggested as a starting point; some infants may need 7 to 10 cm H_2O)
C. Pathologic GERD
   1. Nonpharmacologic therapy
      a. Small, frequent, thickened feedings (e.g., rice cereal in formula)
      b. Postprandial prone-elevated position
      c. Avoid the use of an infant car seat immediately following a feeding
   2. Pharmacologic therapy
      a. Consider for any child who does not respond to traditional therapy or who has documented GERD.
      b. Metoclopramide
         (1) Stimulates gastroesophageal motility and increases lower esophageal sphincter tone.
         (2) Side effects include restlessness, drowsiness, and extrapyramidal symptoms.
         (3) Avoid in the presence of bowel obstruction.
         (4) Dosage: 0.1 mg/kg/dose up to four times daily (30 minutes prior to meals and at bedtime).
      c. Histamine: H_2-receptor antagonists are useful for symptomatic esophagitis (e.g., back arching, irritability) or if the infant has had a protracted medical course.
      d. Omeprazole
         (1) Proton pump inhibitor
         (2) Useful if there has been a poor response to traditional pharmacologic agents
         (3) Long-term safety unknown
D. Protective strategies to prevent SIDS (Table 54-5)
   1. Good health care
   2. Supine sleep position for healthy infants
      a. Reduces SIDS rates by 40% to 50%
      b. Proposed harmful mechanisms that may enhance risk of SIDS with infant in prone position
         (1) Airway obstruction
         (2) Inadequate oxygenation and hypercarbia from rebreathing
         (3) Thermal stress

TABLE 54-5. Protective Strategies to Prevent Sudden Infant Death Syndrome (SIDS)

Good health care
Supine sleep position for healthy infants (term and premature)
Avoid prone sleep position in a child who has been sleeping in supine position (especially in day care setting)
Avoid soft bedding (e.g., sheepskin)
Avoid gas-trapping objects (e.g., pillows, stuffed animals, crib bumpers) near infant's head
Smoke-free environment
Avoidance of alcohol and drug use by cosleeper
Documented home monitor

    (4) Decreased cerebral blood flow
    (5) Efficient or deeper sleep
  c. No proven increased risk of aspiration, GERD, or ALTE
3. Consider the prone position if any of the following are present:
  a. Severe GERD
  b. Certain upper airway anomalies (e.g., Pierre Robin syndrome)
  c. Serious ongoing respiratory disease in premature infant
4. Factors that increase the risk of SIDS with the infant in the prone position
  a. Recent illness
  b. Soft bedding (e.g., sheepskin)
  c. Thermal insulation (e.g., swaddling, no central heating)
  d. Placement of gas-trapping objects (e.g., pillows, stuffed animals, crib bumpers) near the infant's head
5. A smoke-free environment is very beneficial.
6. Parents should avoid alcohol and drug use if cosleeping
7. Documented home monitors (Fig. 54-4)
  a. Measured parameters
    (1) Chest wall movement (central apnea) and heart rate trends
    (2) Monitor compliance
  b. Benefits/uses
    (1) Alerts caregivers to potentially serious central apnea or bradycardia
    (2) Eases transition of a technology-dependent child
    (3) Shortens the hospital stay of a symptomatic, premature, apneic infant
    (4) Guides pharmacologic therapy
    (5) Alleviates family anxiety
    (6) Reduces risk of SIDS (controversial)

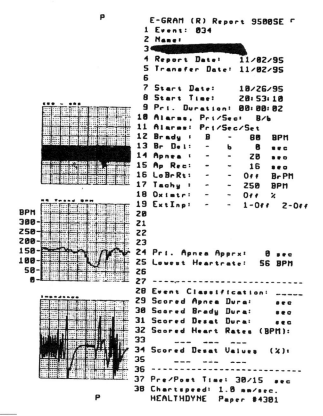

```
                  P        E-GRAM (R) Report 9500SE
                           1 Event:  034
                           2 Name:
                           3
                           4 Report Date:   11/02/95
                           5 Transfer Date:  11/02/95
                           6
                           7 Start Date:    10/26/95
                           8 Start Time:    20:53:10
                           9 Pri. Duration: 00:00:02
                          10 Alarms, Pri/Sec:  B/b
                          11 Alarms: Pri/Sec/Set
                          12 Brady :  B   -    80   BPM
                          13 Br Del:  -   b     8   sec
                          14 Apnea :  -   -    20   sec
                          15 Ap Rec:  -   -    16   sec
                          16 LoBrRt:  -   -    Off  BrPM
                          17 Tachy :  -   -    250  BPM
                          18 Oximtr:  -   -    Off  %
                          19 ExtInp:  -   -    1-Off  2-Off
  BPM                     20
  300-                    21
  250-                    22
  200-                    23
  150-                    24 Pri. Apnea Apprx:    0  sec
  100-                    25 Lowest Heartrate:   56  BPM
   50-                    26
    0-                    27 ------------------------------
                          28 Event Classification:  _____
                          29 Scored Apnea Dura:       sec
                          30 Scored Brady Dura:       sec
                          31 Scored Desat Dura:       sec
                          32 Scored Heart Rates (BPM):
                          33     ---   ---   ---
                          34 Scored Desat Values  (%):
                          35     ---   ---   ---
                          36 ------------------------------
                          37 Pre/Post Time: 30/15   sec
                          38 Chartspeed: 1.0 mm/sec.
                  P          HEALTHDYNE   Paper #4301
```

FIGURE 54-4. Documented home monitor recording of an infant with central apnea. The episode lasted for 16 seconds with a heart rate decrease to 56 BPM.

   c. Indications
     (1) Premature infant with pathologic apnea or of very young gestational age
     (2) Infant with GERD and associated apnea or bradycardia
     (3) Infant with ALTE
     (4) Sibling of infant who died of SIDS
     (5) Infant with certain underlying neurologic, cardiac, or pulmonary conditions (e.g., tracheostomy, central alveolar hypoventilation syndrome)
   d. Special consideration cases
     (1) Infant with oxygen dependency
     (2) Infant with apneic seizures
     (3) Technology-dependent child
     (4) Infant with critically ill medical course
   e. Limitations
     (1) False alarms (especially in older infants)
     (2) Misguided faith in and overdependence on monitor technology

(3) Additional family stress in some cases

(4) Poor compliance

(5) Limitation as a diagnostic tool (e.g., obstructive apnea)

(6) Dermatologic problems (skin irritation) from the monitor leads

(7) Vulnerable child syndrome

(8) Sibling jealousy

f. Criteria for discontinuation of monitoring

(1) Discontinue 4 to 6 weeks after last significant clinical or documented event.

(2) Discontinue after 4 weeks free of events if the infant has a self-limited or treated condition (e.g., GERD, respiratory syncytial virus).

(3) Discontinue at age 6 months or 1 month beyond the age of sibling's death if the infant is an asymptomatic sibling of a SIDS victim.

g. Key to safe, less stressful use of a home monitor: A comprehensive program of evaluation, treatment, and follow-up

(1) Cardiopulmonary resuscitation (CPR) and monitor training for primary caregivers

(2) 24-Hour availability of vendor repair team and qualified support staff

(3) Regular review of recordings by an experienced professional

(4) Frequent communication among the experienced monitor professional, the family, and the primary medical provider

SUGGESTED READING

American Academy of Pediatrics Task Force on Prolonged Infantile Apnea: Prolonged infantile apnea. Pediatrics 76:129-131, 1985.

American Academy of Pediatrics Task Force on Infant Positioning and SIDS: Positioning and SIDS. Pediatrics 89:1120-1126, 1992.

American Academy of Pediatrics Task Force on Infant Positioning and SIDS: Update. Pediatrics 98:1216-1218, 1996.

American Academy of Pediatrics Committee on Fetus and Newborn: Apnea, sudden infant death syndrome, home monitoring. Pediatrics 111:914-917, 2003.

DiFranza JR, Aligne CA, Weitzman M: Prenatal and postnatal environmental tobacco smoke exposure and children's health. Pediatrics 113:1007-1115, 2004.

Eichenwald EC, Blackwell M. Lloyd JS, et al: Inter-neonatal intensive care unit variation in discharge timing: Influence of apnea and feeding management. Pediatrics 108:928-933, 2001.

Getahun D, Demissie K, Lu SE, Rhods GG: Sudden infant death syndrome among twin births: United States, 1995-1998. J Perinatol 24:544-551, 2004.

Gibson E, Spinner S. Cullen JA, et al: Documented home apnea monitoring: Effect on compliance, duration of monitoring, and validation of alarm reporting. Clin Pediatr 35:505-513, 1996.

Henderson-Smart DJ, Ponsonby AL, Murphy E: Reducing the risk of sudden infant death syndrome: A review of the scientific literature. J Pediatr Child Health 34:213-219, 1998.

Horne RS, Franco P, Adamson RM, et al: Influences of maternal cigarette smoking on infant arousability. Early Hum Dev 79:49-58, 2004.

Hunt CE, Corwin MJ, Baird T, et al: Cardiorespiratory events detected by home memory monitoring during early infancy and one-year neurodevelopmental outcome. J Pediatr 145:465-471, 2004.

Krous HF, Beckwith JB, Byard RW, et al: Sudden infant death syndrome and unclassified sudden infant deaths: A definitional and diagnostic approach. Pediatrics 114:234-238, 2004.

Malloy MH: Sudden infant death syndrome among extremely premature infants: United States 1997-1999. J Perinatol 24:181-187, 2004.

National Institutes of Health Consensus Development Conference on Infantile Apnea and Home Monitoring: Sept. 29 to Oct. 1, 1980. Pediatrics 79:292-299, 1987.

Peter CS, Sprodowski N, Bohnhorst B, et al: Gastroesophageal reflux and apnea of prematurity: No temporal relationship. Pediatrics 109:8-11, 2002.

Ramanathan R, Corwin MJ, Hunt CE, et al: Cardiorespiratory events recorded on home monitors: Comparison of healthy infants with those at increased risk for SIDS. JAMA 285:2199-207, 2001.

Spitzer AR: Apnea and home cardiorespiratory monitoring. In McConnel MS (ed): Guidelines for Pediatric Home Health Care. Elk Grove Village, Ill. American Academy of Pediatrics Publications, 2002, pp 357-387.

Sridhar R, Thach BT, Kelly DH, Henslee JA: Characterization of successful and failed autoresuscitation of human infants, including those dying of SIDS. Pediatr Pulmonol 36:113-122, 2003.

Weese-Mayer DE, Corwin MJ, Peucker MR, et al: Comparison of apnea identified by respiratory inductance plethysmography with that detected by end-tidal CO_2 of thermistor. Am J Resp Crit Care Med. 162:471-480, 2000.

Weese-Mayer DE, Berry-Kravis EM, Zhou L, et al: Sudden infant death syndrome: Case-control frequency differences at genes pertinent to early autonomic nervous system embryological development. Pediatr Res 56:391-395, 2004.

Willinger M, Hoffman HJ, Hartford RB: Infant sleep position and risk for sudden infant death syndrome: report of meeting held January 13 and 14, 1994, National Institutes of Health, Bethesda, Maryland. Pediatrics 93:814-819, 1994.

55 Chronic Lung Disease: Etiology and Pathogenesis

Linda Genen and Jonathan M. Davis

I. Introduction
  A. Bronchopulmonary dysplasia (BPD), also known as CLD, is a condition that develops in newborns treated with oxygen and mechanical ventilation for a primary lung disorder.
  B. Approximately 10,000 new cases occur yearly in the U.S., and 10% to 15% of these infants subsequently die in the first year of life. BPD has become the most common form of CLD in infants.
II. Definition
  A. BPD is generally defined as the presence of chronic respiratory signs, a persistent oxygen requirement, and an abnormal chest radiograph at 1 month of age or at 36 weeks corrected age. Unfortunately, this definition lacks specificity and fails to account for important clinical distinctions related to extremes of prematurity and wide variability in criteria for the use of prolonged oxygen therapy.
  B. A consensus conference of the National Institutes of Health suggested a new definition of BPD/CLD (Table 55-1) that incorporates many elements of previous definitions and attempts to categorize the severity of CLD.
  C. Recently, a physiologic assessment of the need for oxygen at 36 weeks corrected age has been proposed in order to better standardize the definition of CLD.
III. Incidence: Incidence depends on the definition used and the gestational age of the population studied. Although surfactant treatment has improved overall survival of premature infants, the incidence of CLD remains approximately 30% to 40% (inversely proportional to gestational age at birth). With the use of standardized oxygen saturation monitoring involved in the physiologic definition, the incidence may be further decreased by as much as 10%.
IV. Pathogenesis (Fig. 55-1)
  A. Barotrauma: Initial injury is the result of the primary disease process (e.g., respiratory distress syndrome [RDS]). Superimposed mechanical ventilation adds to the lung injury. Inflammatory cascade is then activated, leading to greater injury and CLD.
  B. Oxygen/antioxidants
    1. A balance exists between antioxidant defenses and the production of reactive oxygen species (ROS) (Table 55-2), which are molecules

TABLE 55-1. National Institutes of Health Consensus Conference: Diagnostic Criteria for Establishing BPD

Criteria	Gestational Age	
	<32 weeks	*>32 weeks*
Time point of postnatal age	36 weeks PMA or discharge to home, whichever comes first	>28 days but <56 days or discharge to home, whichever comes first
Assessment	Treatment with oxygen	>21% for at least 28 days
Mild BPD	Breathing room air at 36 weeks of age or discharge, whichever comes first	Breathing room air at 56 days PMA or discharge, whichever comes first
Moderate BPD	Need for <30% O_2 at 36 weeks PMA or discharge, whichever comes first	Need for <30% O_2 at 56 days postnatally or discharge, whichever comes first
Severe BPD	Need for > 30% $O_2 \pm$ PPV or CPAP at 36 weeks PMA or discharge, whichever comes first	Need for >30% $O_2 \pm$ PPV or CPAP at 56 days postnatal age or discharge, whichever comes first

BPD, bronchopulmonary dysplasia; CPAP, continuous positive airway pressure; PMA, postmenstrual age; PPV, positive pressure ventilation.

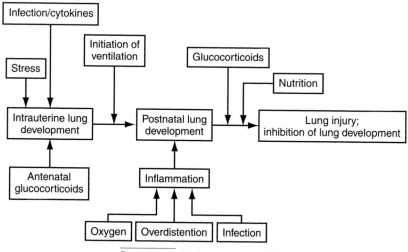

FIGURE 55-1. Pathogenesis of BPD.

TABLE 55-2. Reactive Oxygen Species and Relevant Antioxidants

Radical	Symbol	Antioxidant
Superoxide anion	O_2^-	Superoxide dismutase, uric acid, vitamin E
Singlet oxygen	$^1O_2$	β-Carotene, uric acid, vitamin E
Hydrogen peroxide	H_2O_2	Catalase, glutathione peroxidase, glutathione
Hydroxyl radical	$OH^·$	Vitamins C, E
Peroxide radical	LOO^o (L = lipid)	Vitamins C, E
Hydroperoxyl radical	LOOH (L = lipid)	Glutathione transferase, glutathione peroxidase
Peroxynitrite	$ONOO^-$	Superoxide dismutase

with extra electrons in their outer ring that are toxic to tissues, causing direct damage to growth factors, antiproteases, cell membranes and nucleic acids (Table 55-2).

2. The balance may be disturbed by increased ROS production under conditions of hyperoxia, ischemia/reperfusion, or inflammation.
3. The premature newborn may be more susceptible to free radical damage because antioxidant defenses (which develop at a rate similar to pulmonary surfactant) may be relatively deficient at birth.

C. Inflammation
  1. Inflammation plays an important role in the pathogenesis of CLD and permits a unifying hypothesis.
  2. Early elevations (by 12 hours of age) of cytokines (IL-6, IL-8) are followed by neutrophil/mononuclear cell influx, leading to increased elastase activity and protease/antiprotease imbalance.
  3. This leads to decreased epithelial/endothelial cell integrity, pulmonary edema, and exudate.
  4. Antenatal infection and inflammation (chorioamnionitis, funisitis) may "prime the lung," predisposing to the development of CLD.

D. Infection
  1. Group B streptococcus, gram-negative bacteria (increasing with the use of broad-spectrum antibiotics during labor to eradicate group B streptococcus)
  2. *Ureaplasma urealyticum*

E. Nutrition
  1. Inadequate calories
  2. Deficiency in essential nutrients (vital components for immunologic and antioxidant defenses)
  3. Vitamin deficiencies (vitamin A)
  4. Decreased polyunsaturated fatty acids (PUFAs).

F. Fluids and patent ductus arteriosus (PDA): PDA and CLD have been associated with increased fluid administration. Early closure of the

PDA (indomethacin or surgical ligation) has not substantially affected the incidence of CLD.

G. Genetics: Family history of atopy and asthma. Low levels of TNF-α associated with the adenine allele of TNF-a-238 may reduce the risk and severity of CLD.

V. Pathophysiologic Changes

   A. Clinical assessment: Toce et al (1984) suggested a clinical scoring system.

   B. Radiographic aspects: The abnormalities first described by Northway et al (1967) are no longer usually seen. New radiographic classifications have been developed.

   C. Cardiovascular changes include abnormal pulmonary circulation (endothelial cell degeneration and proliferation, medial muscle hypertrophy, peripheral extension of smooth muscle, and vascular obliteration), increased pulmonary vascular resistance, and cor pulmonale.

   D. Pulmonary mechanics

      1. Initially, pulmonary resistance and airway reactivity are increased. Later, expiratory flow limitation may become more significant.

      2. Increased resistance causes increased work of breathing and V/Q mismatch.

      3. Functional residual capacity may be reduced initially because of atelectasis but can increase in later stages from air trapping and hyperinflation.

      4. Reduction of lung compliance

   E. Pathologic changes

      1. Large upper airways (trachea, main bronchi)

         a. Earliest histologic changes are patchy loss of cilia from columnar epithelial cells. Mucosal edema and/or necrosis (focal or diffuse) may lead to ulceration and granulation tissue formation.

         b. Inflammatory cells and granulation tissue (area of the endotracheal tube tip) are infiltrated.

         c. Mucosal cells regenerate or are replaced by stratified squamous or metaplastic epithelium.

      2. Terminal bronchioles and alveolar ducts: Necrotizing bronchiolitis and fibroblast proliferation and activation may lead to peribronchial fibrosis and obliterative fibroproliferative bronchiolitis.

      3. Alveoli

         a. Earliest findings involve interstitial and/or alveolar edema.

         b. Later, areas of atelectasis, inflammation, exudate, and fibroblast proliferation are seen.

         c. Finally, areas of atelectasis alternating with areas of marked hyperinflation develop.

         d. More recent findings in extremely premature infants reveal alveolar simplification and failure of secondary alveolar crests to form normal alveoli (epithelial and endothelial cell growth abnormalities).

VI. Outcome (See Chapter 57)

   A. Most infants with CLD ultimately achieve normal lung function and thrive. They are at higher risk for death in the first year of life and for long-term complications.

B. In childhood, there is an increased risk for chronic respiratory problems such as reactive airway disease.

C. Cardiac function: Cor pulmonale may develop.

D. Infection: Increased susceptibility to viral infections (respiratory syncytial virus [RSV], influenza). Prophylactic treatment with Synagis (MedImmune, Gaithersberg, MD) is recommended during the RSV season (<2 years of age).

E. Growth failure and neurodevelopmental abnormalities are increased. In contrast, severity of CLD is not a major predictor of neurologic outcome.

VII. Prevention

A. Antenatal steroids for mothers delivering prematurely may reduce the severity and incidence of BPD/CLD.

B. Early use of nasal continuous positive airway pressure (CPAP) (with or without transient intubation and surfactant administration) in infants with RDS may eliminate the need for mechanical ventilation and facilitate earlier extubation.

C. Synchronized nasal intermittent positive-pressure ventilation (SNIPPV) is an effective method of augmenting the beneficial effects of nasal CPAP in preterm infants in the postextubation period.

D. Exogenous surfactant reduces mortality and the severity of CLD, although the total number of survivors with CLD will increase.

E. Treatment of symptomatic PDA (fluid restriction, diuretics, indomethacin, and/or surgery).

F. Ventilator pressures and FiO_2 should be reduced as low and as soon as possible.

G. Nutritional support: vitamins (A, C, E) and minerals (selenium, copper, zinc, manganese).

H. Prophylactic treatment with recombinant human superoxide dismutase (rhSOD)

1. Cell culture studies demonstrate prevention of cell damage from hyperoxia with the addition of rhSOD.

2. Various studies of animal models have shown reduction in acute hyperoxic lung injury with administration of rhSOD. Studies in newborn piglets showed that intratracheal administration of rhSOD prevented inflammatory changes and acute lung injury from hyperoxia and mechanical ventilation. The rhSOD was rapidly incorporated into a variety of cell types in the lung and remained active for 48 to 72 hours. Genetically engineered mice overexpressing SOD had improved survival, whereas mice with disrupted SOD genes died sooner when exposed to prolonged hyperoxia compared to diploid controls.

3. Multicenter collaborative trials using prophylactic, intratracheal rhSOD in premature infants at high risk for developing BPD have recently been completed. Premature infants (birth weight 600 to 1200 g) receiving intratracheal instillation of rhSOD at birth had significantly fewer episodes (44%) of respiratory illness (wheezing,

asthma, pulmonary infections) severe enough to require treatment with bronchodilators or corticosteroids at 1 year corrected age compared to placebo controls. There were also significant reductions in hospital readmissions and emergency room visits, with the largest treatment affects seen in the smallest infants (<27 weeks' gestation). This suggests that rhSOD did prevent long-term pulmonary injury from ROS in high-risk premature infants. Further therapeutic intervention trials are needed in order to ultimately develop a therapy that can prevent or significantly ameliorate BPD.

Suggested Reading

Attar MA, Donn SM: Mechanisms of ventilator-induced lung injury in premature infants. Semin Neonatol 7:353-360, 2002.

Bancalari E (ed): Bronchopulmonary dysplasia. Semin Perinatol 8:1-92, 2003.

Bancalari E, Sosenko I: Pathogenesis and prevention of neonatal chronic lung disease: Recent developments. Pediatr Pulmonol 8:109-116, 1990.

Davis JM, Parad RB, Michele T, et al: Pulmonary outcome at 1 year corrected age in premature infants treated at birth with recombinant CuZn superoxide dismutase. Pediatrics 111:469-476, 2003.

Davis JM, Rosenfeld W: Bronchopulmonary dysplasia: In Avery GB, Fletcher MA, MacDonald MG (eds): Textbook of Neonatology, 5th ed. Philadelphia, JB Lippincott, 1999, pp 509-532.

Davis JM, Rosenfeld WN, Sanders RJ, Gonenne A: The prophylactic effects of human recombinant superoxide dismutase in neonatal lung injury. J Appl Physiol 74:22-34, 1993.

De Paoli AG, Davis PG, Lemyre B: Nasal continuous positive airway pressure versus nasal intermittent positive pressure ventilation for preterm neonates: A systematic review and meta-analysis. Acta Paediatr 92:70-75, 2003.

Frank L, Groseclose EE: Preparation of birth into an O_2 rich environment: The antioxidant enzymes in the developing rabbit lung. Pediatr Res 18:240-244, 1984.

Jobe AH, Bancalari E: Bronchopulmonary dysplasia. Am J Resp Crit Care Med 163:1723-1729, 2001.

Jobe AH: The new BPD: An arrest of lung development. Pediatr Res 46:641-643, 1999.

Munshi UK, Niu JO, Siddiq MM, Parton LA: Elevation of interleukin-8 and interleukin-6 precedes the influx of neutrophils in tracheal aspirates from preterm infants who develop bronchopulmonary dysplasia. Pediatr Pulmonol 24:331-336, 1997.

Northway WH Jr, Rosan C, Porter DY: Pulmonary disease following respiratory therapy of hyaline-membrane disease. N Engl J Med 76:357-368, 1967.

Pitkanen OM, Hallman M, Andersson SM: Correlation of free oxygen radical–induced lipid peroxidation with outcome in very low birth weight infants. J Pediatr 116:760-764, 1990.

Rojas MA, Gonzalez A, Bancalari E, et al: Changing trends in the epidemiology and pathogenesis of neonatal chronic lung disease. J Pediatr 126:605-610, 1995.

Toce SS, Farrell PM, Leavitt, LA, et al: Clinical and radiographic scoring systems for assessing bronchopulmonary dysplasia. Am J Dis Child 138:581-585, 1984.

Tyson JE, Wright LL, Oh W, et al: Vitamin A supplementation for extremely-low-birth-weight infants. New Engl J Med 340:1962-1968, 1999.

Walsh MC, Wilson-Costello D, Zadell A, et al: Safety, reliability, and validity of a physiologic definition of bronchopulmonary dysplasia. J Perinatol. 23:451-456, 2003.

Walsh MC, Yao Q, Gettner P, et al: Impact of a physiologic definition on bronchopulmonary dysplasia rates. Pediatrics 114:1305-1311, 2004.

Yoon BH, Romero R, Jun JK, et al: Amniotic fluid cytokines (interleukin-6, tumor necrosis factor-alpha, interleukin-1 beta, and interleukin-8) and the risk for the development of bronchopulmonary dysplasia. Am J Obstet Gynecol 177:825-830, 1997.

56

Chronic Lung Disease: Clinical Management

Eduardo Bancalari

I. Rationale: Management of the infant with chronic lung disease (CLD) is aimed at maintaining adequate gas exchange while limiting the progression of the disease. The big challenge is that the supplemental oxygen and mechanical ventilation needed to maintain gas exchange are the main factors implicated in the pathogenesis of the lung damage.

II. Oxygen Therapy

   A. Reduce the FiO_2 as quickly as possible to avoid oxygen toxicity, while maintaining the PaO_2 at a level sufficient to ensure tissue oxygenation and avoid pulmonary hypertension and cor pulmonale.

   B. There is insufficient information to recommend a specific range of oxygen saturation, but there is sufficient evidence that oxygen saturations >95% and PaO_2 >70 mm Hg may be associated with a higher incidence of retinopathy of prematurity and a worse respiratory outcome. Because of this, it is advisable to maintain saturation between 90% and 95% or the PaO_2 between 50 and 70 mm Hg to minimize the detrimental effects of hypo- and hyperoxemia.

   C. After extubation, oxygen can be administered through a hood, or a nasal cannula. In some cases, patients with CLD are discharged home with oxygen therapy.

   D. Adequacy of gas exchange is monitored by arterial blood gas levels.

      1. Blood gas determinations obtained by arterial puncture may not be reliable because the infant responds to pain with crying or apnea.

      2. Transcutaneous PO_2 electrodes are also inaccurate in these infants because they frequently underestimate the true PaO_2.

   E. Pulse oximeters offer the most reliable estimate of arterial oxygenation, are simple to use, and provide continuous information during different behavioral states.

   F. It is important to maintain a relatively normal blood hemoglobin concentration. This can be accomplished with blood transfusions or the administration of recombinant erythropoietin. However, limiting the amount of blood taken for laboratory tests is the most effective and safest measure to prevent anemia.

III. Mechanical Ventilation

   A. Use the lowest settings necessary to maintain gas exchange and limit the duration of mechanical respiratory support to a minimum.

B. Use the lowest peak airway pressure to deliver adequate tidal volumes, (3 to 5 mL/kg).

C. Use short inspiratory times (0.3 to 0.5 seconds).
   1. Avoid shorter inspiratory times and higher flow rates that may exaggerate the maldistribution of the inspired gas.
   2. Longer inspiratory times may increase the risk of alveolar rupture and of negative cardiovascular side effects.

D. Adjust end-expiratory pressure between 2 and 6 cm H_2O so that the minimum oxygen concentration necessary to keep oxygen saturation >90% (PaO_2 >50 mm Hg) is used. Higher PEEP levels (5 to 8 cm H_2O) may help reduce expiratory airway resistance and can improve alveolar ventilation in infants with severe airway obstruction.

E. Limit the duration of mechanical ventilation as much as possible to reduce the risk of ventilator-induced lung injury and infection.

F. Weaning from mechanical ventilation must be accomplished gradually, by reducing peak inspiratory pressures to <15 to 18 cm H_2O and FiO_2 to <0.3 to 0.4.

G. Reduce ventilator rate gradually to 10 to 15 breaths/min to allow the infant to perform an increasing proportion of the respiratory work.

H. The use of patient-triggered ventilation, volume-targeted ventilation, and pressure support of the spontaneous breaths can accelerate weaning and reduce the total duration of mechanical ventilation.

I. During weaning from intermittent positive pressure ventilation (IPPV), it may be necessary to increase the FiO_2 to maintain adequate oxygen saturation levels.

J. Concurrently, the $PaCO_2$ may rise to values of 50 to 60 mm Hg or higher. As long as the pH is within an acceptable range, hypercapnia can be tolerated to wean these patients from the ventilator.

K. Aminophylline or caffeine can be used as respiratory stimulants during the weaning phase.

L. When the patient is able to maintain acceptable blood gas levels for several hours on low ventilator settings (respiratory rate, 10 to 15 breaths/min; peak inspiratory pressure (PIP), 12 to 15 cm H_2O; FiO_2 <0.3 to 0.4) or can be maintained on patient-triggered ventilation at 4 mL/kg V_T, extubation should be attempted.

M. After extubation, it may be necessary to provide chest physiotherapy to prevent airway obstruction and lung collapse caused by retained secretions.

N. In smaller infants, nasal continuous positive airway pressure (CPAP) of 3 to 6 cm H_2O or nasal IPPV can stabilize respiratory function and reduce the need for reintubation and mechanical ventilation.

IV. Fluid Management

A. Infants with CLD tolerate excessive fluid intake poorly and tend to accumulate water in their lungs, and this excess fluid contributes to their poor lung function.

B. Water and salt intake must be limited to the minimum required to provide the necessary fluid intake, and calories should be adequate to meet their metabolic needs and growth.

C. If pulmonary edema persists despite fluid restriction, diuretic therapy can be used successfully. The use of diuretics can produce a rapid improvement in lung compliance and decrease in resistance, but blood gases do not always show improvement.

D. Chronic use of loop diuretics may be associated with hypokalemia, hyponatremia, metabolic alkalosis, hypercalciuria with nephrocalcinosis, hypochloremia, and hearing loss. Some of these side effects may be reduced by using furosemide on alternate days.

E. Because of the side effects and lack of evidence that prolonged use of diuretics changes the incidence or severity of CLD, this therapy is not recommended for routine use and is only indicated for acute episodes of deterioration associated with pulmonary edema.

F. Distal tubular diuretics such as thiazides and spironolactone are also used in infants with CLD, but the improvement with these diuretics is less consistent than with proximal loop diuretics. Side effects such as nephrocalcinosis and hearing loss may be less frequent than with furosemide, and for this reason these diuretics can be used in infants with established CLD who require prolonged diuretic therapy.

V. Bronchodilators

A. Infants with severe CLD frequently have airway smooth muscle hypertrophy and airway hyperreactivity.

B. Because hypoxia can increase airway resistance in these patients, maintenance of adequate oxygenation is important to avoid bronchoconstriction.

C. Inhaled bronchodilators, including beta agonists such as isoproterenol, salbutamol, metaproterenol and isoetharine, and anticholinergic agents such as atropine and ipratropium bromide can reduce airway resistance in infants with CLD. Their effect is short-lived, however, and their use may be associated with cardiovascular side effects such as tachycardia, hypertension, and arrhythmias.

D. Methylxanthines also have been shown to reduce airway resistance in these infants.

1. These drugs have other potential beneficial effects, such as respiratory stimulation anda mild diuretic effect; aminophylline may also improve respiratory muscle contractility.

2. These drugs must be used with caution because of their multiple side effects.

E. There is no evidence that prolonged use of bronchodilators changes the course of CLD in infants, and for this reason their use should be limited to episodes of acute exacerbation of airway obstruction. When indicated, beta agonists are given by inhalation using a nebulizer or a space inhaler connected to a mask or head chamber or inserted in the inspiratory side of the ventilator circuit.

VI. Corticosteroids

A. Many studies have shown rapid improvement in lung function after systemic administration of steroids, facilitating weaning from the ventilator and a reduction in CLD. Steroids may enhance production of surfactant and antioxidant enzymes, decrease bronchospasm, decrease pulmonary and bronchial edema and fibrosis, improve vitamin A status, and decrease the response of inflammatory cells and mediators in the injured lung.

B. Potential complications of prolonged steroid therapy include masking the signs of infection, arterial hypertension, hyperglycemia, increased proteolysis, adrenocortical suppression, somatic and lung growth suppression, and hypertrophic myocardiopathy. Of more concern is the fact that most long-term follow-up studies suggest that infants who received prolonged steroid therapy have a worse neurologic outcome, including an increased incidence of cerebral palsy.

C. Because of the seriousness of the neurologic side effects, specifically when systemic steroids are used early after birth, the use of systemic steroids should only be considered after the first 2 weeks of life in infants who show clear evidence of severe and progressive pulmonary damage and who remain oxygen- and ventilator-dependent.

D. The duration of steroid therapy must be limited to the minimum necessary to achieve the desired effects, usually 3 to 5 days; following the recommendation of the American Academy of Pediatrics, the potential side effects should be discussed with the family before initiating this therapy.

E. Steroids can be administered by nebulization to ventilator-dependent infants. Inhaled steroids may reduce the need for systemic steroids, reducing the side effects associated with prolonged systemic therapy; however, data on effectiveness of topical steroids are not conclusive enough to recommend their routine use.

VII. Nutrition

A. Adequate nutrition is a key aspect of care for the infant with CLD.
   1. Malnutrition can delay somatic growth and the development of new alveoli and can decrease muscle strength, making successful weaning from mechanical ventilation more difficult.
   2. The malnourished infant is more prone to infection and oxygen toxicity.

B. High-calorie formulas and protein supplements are used to maximize the intake of calories and help to restrict fluid intake to prevent congestive heart failure and pulmonary edema.

C. Administration of extra calcium and vitamin D is necessary to prevent rickets.

D. Infants who receive exclusively parenteral nutrition for prolonged periods are more susceptible to developing deficiency of specific nutrients, such as vitamins A and E, and of trace elements, such as iron, copper, zinc, and selenium, all of which play a role in antioxidant function, protection against infection, and lung repair.

E. Infants with severe CLD have been shown to have lower plasma levels of vitamin A, and a deficiency of this vitamin in experimental animals resulted in loss of ciliated epithelium and squamous metaplasia in the airways, changes similar to those observed in infants with severe CLD.

F. Clinical studies in preterm infants with severe respiratory distress syndrome suggest that maintenance of normal plasma levels of vitamin A reduces the incidence and severity of CLD. The use of supplemental vitamin A by intramuscular injection to maintain normal serum levels can reduce CLD, but its use is not widespread because of the reluctance to give repeated intramuscular injections to very small infants.

VIII. Pulmonary Vasodilators

    A. Because pulmonary vascular resistance is extremely sensitive to changes in alveolar PO_2 in infants with CLD, it is important to assure normal oxygenation at all times.

    B. In infants with severe pulmonary hypertension and cor pulmonale, the calcium channel blocker nifedipine has been shown to decrease pulmonary vascular resistance.

        1. This drug is also a systemic vasodilator and can produce a depression of myocardial contractility.

        2. Its safety and long-term efficacy in these infants has not been established.

    C. Inhaled nitric oxide has been administered to infants with CLD in an attempt to improve outcome.

        1. Nitric oxide can improve ventilation-perfusion matching and reduce pulmonary vascular resistance and inflammation.

        2. Although nitric oxide has been shown to improve oxygenation in infants with CLD, there is no clear evidence that this therapy improves long-term outcome, and it should be considered experimental.

    D. Phosphodiesterase inhibitors (sidenafil), prostacyclin (epoprostenol), and endothelin-1 (ET-1) antagonists are potent pulmonary vasodilators that have been used to treat pulmonary hypertension; however, there is not enough information to recommend their routine use in infants with CLD.

Suggested Reading

American Academy of Pediatrics: Postnatal Corticosteroids to treat or prevent chronic lung disease in preterm infants. Pediatrics 109:330-338, 2002.

Aschner JL: New therapies for pulmonary hypertension in neonates and children. Pediatric Pulmonol Suppl 26:132-135, 2004.

Askie LM, Henderson-Smart DJ, Irwig L, Simpson JM: Oxygen-saturation targets and outcomes in extremely preterm infants . N Engl J Med 349:959-967, 2003.

Atkinson SA: Special nutritional needs of infants for prevention of and recovery from bronchopulmonary dysplasia. J Nutr 131:942S-946S, 2001.

Bancalari E (ed): Bronchopulmonary dysplasia. Semin Perinatol 8:1-92, 2003.

Banks BA, Seri I, Ischiropoulos H, et al: Changes in oxygenation with inhaled nitric oxide in severe bronchopulmonary dysplasia. Pediatrics 103:610-618, 1999.

Brunton JA, Saigal S, Atkinson S: Growth and body composition in infants with bronchopulmonary dysplasia up to 3 months corrected age: A randomized trial of a high-energy nutrient-enriched formula fed after hospital discharge. J Pediatr 133:340-345, 1998.

Cole CH, Colton T, Shah BL, et al: Early inhaled glucocorticoid therapy to prevent bronchopulmonary dysplasia. N Engl J Med 340:1005-1010, 1999.

Flynn JT, Bancalari E, Sims E, et al.: A cohort study of transcutaneous oxygen tension and the incidence and severity of retinopathy of prematurity. N Engl J Med 326:1050-1054, 1992.

Greenough A: Update on patient-triggered ventilation. Clin Perinatol 28:533-546, 2001.

Grier DG, Halliday HL: Corticosteroids in the prevention and management of BPD. Semin Neonatol 8:83-91, 2003.

Kao LC, Durand DJ, McCrea RC, et al: Randomized trial of long-term diuretic therapy for infants with oxygen-dependent bronchopulmonary dysplasia. J Pediatr 124:772-781, 1994.

O'Shea TM, Kothadia, JM, Klinepeter KL, et al: Randomized placebo-controlled trial of a 42-day tapering course of dexamethasone to reduce the duration of ventilator dependency in very low birth weight infants: Outcome of study participants at 1-year adjusted age. Pediatrics 104:15-21, 1999.

Reyes Z, Tauscher M, Claure N: Randomized, controlled trial comparing pressure support (PS) + synchronized intermittent mandatory ventilation (SIMV) with SIMV in preterm infants. Pediatr Res 55:466A, 2004.

Tin W: Optimal oxygen saturation for preterm babies. Do we really know? Biol Neonate 85:319-325, 2004.

Tyson JE, Wright LL, Oh W et al: Vitamin A supplementation for extremely-low-birth-weight infants. N Engl J Med 340:1962-1968, 1999.

Yeh TF, Lin YJ, Huang CC, et al: Early dexamethasone therapy in preterm infants: A follow-up study. Pediatrics 101:E7, 1998.

Yeh TF, Lin YJ, Lin HC, et al: Outcomes at school age after postnatal dexamethasone therapy for lung disease of prematurity. N Engl J Med 350:1304-1313, 2004.

57 Long-Term Outcomes of Newborns with Chronic Lung Disease

Saroj Saigal

I. Introduction
   A. Bronchopulmonary dysplasia is defined as a form of chronic lung disease (CLD) that occurs primarily in preterm very low birth weight (VLBW) infants who have received mechanical ventilation and prolonged oxygen supplementation.
   B. First described by Northway, the disease is characterized by airway injury, parenchymal fibrosis, and inflammation. The pattern, prevalence, and pathologic picture of CLD has changed over time with the survival of more and more immature infants who require ventilation and prolonged oxygen at far earlier gestational ages. Also, with the advent of more sophisticated ventilators and improvements in ventilation strategies, the new picture of CLD depicts less fibrosis, but a significant decrease in alveolar and vascular development.
II. Neonatal Morbidity
   A. In most studies, CLD was reported to be associated with significant neonatal morbidity, including intraventricular hemorrhage, hydrocephalus requiring ventricular peritoneal shunts, porencephaly, echodense lesions, periventricular leukomalacia, and retinopathy of prematurity. However, in a large-scale sonographic study at 36 weeks postmenstrual age, CLD was not associated with the occurrence of sonographically defined white matter disease. It is possible that diffuse forms of white matter disease may only be evident on diffusion-weighted MRI.
   B. Infants with CLD have been shown to have higher energy expenditure, which is strongly associated with their respiratory status. Because of their increased respiratory rates and distress, these infants lack adequate protein and energy intake. Their feeding difficulties contribute further to growth failure.
   C. A predictive model using three neonatal morbidities, CLD, brain injury, and retinopathy of prematurity, independently correlated with poor outcomes such as death or neurosensory impairment.
III. Long-Term Outcomes
   A. CLD is associated with significantly greater multisystem adverse outcomes over and above those related to prematurity.

B. The presentation of these problems may vary with the age of the subject.
C. Infancy
  1. Growth failure: Several studies have shown a drop in weight-for-age Z-scores following discharge from the hospital. Long-term growth was also affected, with significantly lower length and weight compared to infants without CLD. Preterm infants with CLD have been shown to have a deficit in mean total body fat and fat-free mass in the first year of life compared to healthy term infants of the same age. Infants with CLD may benefit from a comprehensive postdischarge follow-up to ensure adequate nutritional and energy intake.
  2. Respiratory problems and rehospitalization: A small proportion of infants with CLD are discharged home on low-flow oxygen. Among preterm infants, CLD substantially increased the risk for rehospitalizations for respiratory illnesses during the first year of life.
  3. Mental and motor development: A significant delay in both mental and gross motor performance of infants with CLD has been reported during the first years of life. By 2 years, considerable catch-up occurs, but significant differences in postural control and balance remain, compared to the control group.
  4. Neurosensory impairments: Infants with CLD are at increased risk for cerebral palsy and blindness because of the higher prevalence of intraventricular hemorrhage (IVH) and periventricular leukomalacia (PVL) and the prolonged dependence on oxygen in the neonatal period. However, in some studies, after adjusting for PVL and IVH, the association between CLD and neurologic impairments is no longer apparent.
  5. Postnatal dexamethasone effects: The prevalence of cerebral palsy is higher in infants who received postnatal dexamethasone for CLD. Children who received dexamethasone are also significantly shorter in height and have smaller head circumference and lower cognitive scores than VLBW infants who do not receive postnatal steroids.
D. Mid-childhood
  1. Health: In a recent study, even at the age of 2 to 8 years, VLBW infants with CLD had a higher incidence of respiratory infections and respiratory symptoms provoked by exercise, as well as increased use of inhaled medications and antibiotics, and a higher proportion were receiving physiotherapy and occupational therapy. Overall, the health of the child with CLD continued to have a significant impact and burden on the activities of the other members of the family well beyond the neonatal period.
  2. Growth: In one report, at 8 to 10 years of age, VLBW children with CLD were reported to have significantly lower weight and smaller head circumference but no significant differences in height compared to those without CLD. However, after controlling for confounders, these differences were no longer present. In other studies, both CLD and non-CLD VLBW subjects were reported to be shorter than term controls. Both severity of neonatal illness and recurrent illnesses and hospitalizations were associated with poorer growth. Lean body mass and bone mineral content were also

reported to be lower in the CLD group compared to both preterm non-CLD and term controls.

3. Lung function: At school age, VLBW children who had survived CLD had poorer lung function than non-CLD survivors of similar weight, although few of these abnormalities were in a clinically significant range. At age 7 years, the CLD group had significantly more airway obstruction than non-CLD and term children (significantly reduced forced capacity by 25% to 75%). Bronchial hyperresponsiveness was significantly increased in CLD survivors, and they had lower FEV_1 than the non-CLD preterm group. Overall, at mid-childhood, CLD survivors had long-term airway obstruction and a mild degree of exercise intolerance, whereas preterm children without CLD demonstrated pulmonary function similar to that of term control group.

4. Cognitive and academic consequences (Table 57-1): VLBW CLD survivors demonstrated significant deficits compared to non-CLD VLBW and term children in IQ scores rating reading and mathematics, with differences of up to 6 to 8 points in these measures. Impaired psychoeducational performance was noted particularly in language abilities and reading skills. A higher

TABLE 57-1 Cognitive, Academic, and Motor Outcomes for VLBW CLD and non-CLD and Term Controls at Age 8 Years*

Parameter	VLBW CLD (n = 98)	VLBW non-CLD (n = 75)	Term (n = 99)	P
WISC III, full-scale IQ (mean [SD])	83 (20)	92 (16)	102 (15)	.001[†‡§]
Woodcock Johnson calculation (mean [SD])	85 (23)	94 (18)	106 (19)	.001[†‡§]
Bruininks-Oseretsky test of motor proficiency (mean [SD])	43 (15)	51 (13)	58 (12)	.001[†‡§]
Special education (%)	54	37	25	.01[†‡]
ADHD diagnosis (%)	15	7	4	.01[†‡]
Occupational therapy (%)	52	11	5	.001[†‡]
Physical therapy (%)	50%	13%	2%	.001[†‡§]

*Except for attention-deficit/hyperactivity disorder, these differences persisted even among the neurologically intact group.
[†]CLD group differed from VLBW group.
[‡]CLD group differed from term group.
[§]VLBW group differed from term group.
CLD, chronic lung disease; VLBW, very low birth weight .
Adapted from Short EJ, Klein NK, Lewis BA, et al: Cognitive and academic consequences of bronchopulmonary dysplasia and very low birth weight: 8-year-old outcomes. Pediatrics 12:e359, 2003.

proportion of CLD subjects had full-scale and performance IQ scores <70 (2 SD below mean). These differences persisted after adjustment for confounding social and biologic factors. CLD children were more likely to be enrolled in special educational classes compared with both comparison groups. Even with a neurologically intact sample of CLD children, significant differences were found for many outcome measures in comparison with non-CLD and term controls. CLD and duration of oxygen predicted poor school performance. Once again, in every instance, CLD children who received steroids did worse than the non-steroid CLD group.

5. Motor performance: VLBW CLD children had poorer gross and fine motor skills and poorer coordination and visual motor integration skills. These neuromotor deficits were not associated with the degree of prematurity, but rather with the severity of the lung disease. A higher proportion of the CLD cohort was receiving occupational therapy and physiotherapy than its non-CLD counterpart.

E. Adolescence
   1. Respiratory function: Only two studies are found in the literature on CLD infants at adolescence, and both focused on lung function abnormalities. In the first study of 17 children between ages 8 and 15 years, airflow obstruction and airway hyperresponsiveness were shown to persist but did not get worse with age.
   2. In the second study, 46 adolescent CLD survivors with a mean age of 17.7 years had a substantially decreased FEV_1, increased bronchial hyperresponsiveness, and other markers of age-related decline in lung function, suggesting the potential for early-onset chronic obstructive pulmonary disease in children with CLD.

IV. Summary
   A. A review of the current literature suggests that CLD has consequences far beyond prematurity, which are manifested in growth failure, recurrent infections, and hospitalization, impaired psychoeducational performance, motor deficits, and abnormal lung function as late as adolescence.
   B. Families of infants with CLD suffer a significant burden in their lifestyle and limitations in routine activities.
   C. Early postnatal dexamethasone therapy has been shown to lead to additional substantial adverse effects on neuromotor and cognitive function.

Suggested Reading

Gray PH, O'Callaghan MJ, Rogers YM: Psychoeducational outcome at school age of preterm infants with bronchopulmonary dysplasia. J Pediatr Child Health 40:114-120, 2004.

Halvorsen T, Skadberg BT, Eide GE, et al: Pulmonary outcome in adolescents of extreme preterm birth: A regional cohort study. Acta Paediatr 2004;93:1294-1300, 2004.

Huysman WA, de Ridder M, de Bruin NC, et al: Growth and body composition in preterm infants with bronchopulmonary dysplasia. Arch Dis Child Fetal Neonatal Ed 88:F46-F51, 2003.

Korhonen P, Koivisto AM, Ikonen S, et al: Very low birthweight, bronchopulmonary dysplasia and health in early childhood. Acta Paediatr 88:1385-1391, 1999.

Short EJ, Klein NK, Lewis BA, et al: Cognitive and academic consequences of bronchopulmonary dysplasia and very low birth weight: 8-year-old outcomes. Pediatrics 12:e359, 2003.

Yeh TF, Lin YJ, Lin HC, et al: Outcomes at school age after postnatal dexamethasone therapy lung disease of prematurity. N Engl J Med 350:1304-1313, 2004.

Weaning and Extubation

58

Steven M. Donn and Sunil K. Sinha

I. General Concepts
   A. Weaning
      1. Definition: The process of shifting work of breathing from ventilator to patient by decreasing the level of support.
      2. Generally heralded by:
         a. Improvement in gas exchange
         b. Improving spontaneous drive
         c. Greater assumption of work of breathing by the patient
   B. Imposed work of breathing
      1. Endotracheal tube (ETT) resistance
      2. Ventilator circuit
      3. Demand valve
      4. Estimated to require tidal volume (V_T) of 4 mL/kg to overcome imposed work of breathing
   C. Physiologic essentials for weaning
      1. Respiratory drive
         a. Must be adequate to sustain alveolar ventilation
         b. Assessment
            (1) Observation
            (2) Measurement of V_T
            (3) Trial
               (a) Low intermittent mandatory ventilation (IMV) rate
               (b) Endotracheal continuous positive airway pressure (CPAP)
               (c) Minute ventilation (MV) (see later)
      2. Reduced respiratory system load
         a. Respiratory system load: Forces required to overcome the elastic and resistive properties of the lungs and airways.
         b. Part of total pressure generated by the respiratory muscles must overcome elasticity to change lung volume, whereas the remainder must overcome resistive properties in order to generate gas flow.
         c. Time constant
            (1) Product of compliance and resistance.
            (2) Describes how quickly gas moves in and out of the lung.
            (3) Determines whether there is adequate time to empty lung and avoid gas trapping and inadvertent peak end-expiratory pressure (PEEP).

3. Maintenance of MV
   a. Product of V_T and rate.
   b. Normal range, 240 to 360 mL/kg/min.
   c. Inadequate alveolar ventilation can result from inadequate V_T, rate, or both.
D. Elements of weaning
   1. V_T determinants
      a. Amplitude (ΔP) is the difference between peak inspiratory pressure (PIP) and PEEP
      b. Inspiratory time (T_I)
      c. Gas flow rate
      d. Compliance
   2. Frequency (respiratory rate)
      a. Impacts CO_2 removal.
      b. If too rapid, may lead to hypocarbia and decreased spontaneous drive.
   3. MV
      a. Measure V_T and rate.
      b. Assess spontaneous versus mechanical components.
   4. Work of breathing
      a. The force or pressure necessary to overcome forces that oppose volume expansion and gas flow during respiration.
      b. Product of pressure and volume, or the integral of the pressure-volume loop.
      c. Proportional to compliance.
      d. Additional components
         (1) Imposed work
         (2) Elevated resistance
      e. Indirect measure is energy expenditure (oxygen consumption).
   5. Nutritional aspects
      a. Inadequate calories may preclude successful weaning by not providing sufficient energy.
      b. Prevent catabolism.
      c. Avoid excess non-nitrogen calories, which increase CO_2 production.
II. Weaning Strategies
   A. General principles
      1. Decrease the potentially most harmful parameter first.
      2. Limit changes to one parameter at a time.
      3. Avoid changes of large magnitude.
      4. Document the patient's response to all changes.
   B. Oxygenation
      1. Primary determinants
         a. FiO_2
         b. Mean airway pressure
            (1) PIP
            (2) PEEP
            (3) Inspiratory time (T_I)
      2. Sequence
         a. Try to decrease FiO_2 to 0.4.

   b. If PaO_2 is high and $PaCO_2$ is normal, decrease PIP,
      PIP and PEEP, or T_I.
   c. If PaO_2 is high and $PaCO_2$ is low, decrease PIP and/or rate (if IMV).
   d. If PaO_2 and $PaCO_2$ are high, decrease PEEP or T_I and/or
      increase rate.
3. Practical hints
   a. If FiO_2 >0.4, maintain Hb >15 g/dL.
   b. Weaning is facilitated by continuous pulse oximetry.
   c. Avoid "flip-flop" by making small FiO_2 changes early in
      disease course.
   d. Avoid a mean airway pressure (Pāw) that is too low to maintain
      adequate alveolar volume.
C. Ventilation
   1. Primary determinants
      a. Amplitude (ΔP) = PIP − PEEP
      b. Rate (frequency [f])
      c. MV = $V_T \times f$
      d. Expiratory time (T_E) (or I:E [inspiration:expiration] ratio)
   2. Sequence
      a. If $PaCO_2$ is low and PaO_2 is high, decrease PIP or rate (if IMV).
      b. If $PaCO_2$ is low and PaO_2 is normal, decrease rate (if IMV) or T_E.
      c. If $PaCO_2$ and PaO_2 are low, increase PEEP or decrease T_E
         (longer I:E ratio), or decrease rate (if IMV).
   3. Practical hints
      a. Try to maintain normal MV.
      b. Keep V_T in range of 4 to 8 mL/kg.
      c. Avoid overdistention but maintain adequate lung volumes.
      d. Low $PaCO_2$ diminishes spontaneous respiratory drive.
      e. Avoid pre-extubation fatigue by weaning below an adequate
         level of support to overcome the imposed work of breathing.
D. Specific modes of ventilation
   1. Assist/control (A/C)
      a. Decrease PIP (decreases in rate have no effect if spontaneous
         rate is higher than control rate).
      b. Maintain sufficient ΔP to achieve adequate ventilation.
      c. Provide adequate V_T to avoid tachypnea.
      d. Alternative strategy: Slowly increase assist sensitivity to increase
         patient effort and condition respiratory musculature.
      e. Extubate from A/C or consider switching to synchronous
         intermittent mandatory ventilation (SIMV).
   2. SIMV
      a. Decrease SIMV rate.
      b. Decrease PIP.
      c. Maintain MV.
      d. Alternative: Increase assist sensitivity.
   3. IMV
      a. Decrease PIP (lower Pāw) for O_2.
      b. Decrease rate for CO_2.
      c. Maintain MV and adequate V_T.

    4. SIMV/pressure support
      a. Decrease SIMV rate.
      b. Decrease pressure support level.
      c. Extubate when $V_T = 4$ mL/kg.
    5. High-frequency ventilation (see Chapters 33 to 35)
III. Adjunctive Treatments for Weaning
  A. Methylxanthines (theophylline, aminophylline, caffeine)
    1. Mechanisms of action
      a. Increase diaphragmatic contractility and decrease fatigability.
      b. Are direct stimulants of respiratory center.
      c. Reset CO_2 responsiveness.
      d. Have a diuretic effect.
    2. Indications
      a. Periextubation support
      b. Apnea or periodic breathing
    3. Complications
      a. Gastric irritation, vomiting
      b. Tachycardia
      c. CNS irritation, seizures
    4. Comments
      a. Monitor serum concentrations.
      b. Periextubation support is usually discontinued 48 to 72 hours postextubation.
  B. Diuretics
    1. Mechanism of action: Treat pulmonary edema.
    2. Indications
      a. Pulmonary edema
      b. Patent ductus arteriosus
      c. Chronic lung disease (CLD)
    3. Complications
      a. Electrolyte disturbances
      b. Contraction alkalosis
      c. Nephrolithiasis/nephrocalcinosis (furosemide)
    4. Comments
      a. Monitor serum electrolytes.
      b. May need supplemental Na, K, Cl.
      c. Long-term furosemide therapy is not advised; spironolactone and chlorothiazide are preferred.
  C. Bronchodilators
    1. Mechanism of action: Relaxation of bronchial smooth muscle
    2. Indication: Bronchospasm or reactive airways leading to increased airway resistance
    3. Complications
      a. Tachyphylaxis
      b. Tachycardia
      c. Hypertension
    4. Comments
      a. Document efficacy before continuing.
      b. May be given systemically or by inhalation.

       c. If inhalational route, use spacer.

D. Corticosteroids
  1. Mechanisms of action
    a. Anti-inflammatory
    b. Decrease edema
  2. Indications
    a. Upper airway edema
    b. Pulmonary edema
    c. CLD
  3. Complications
    a. Hypertension
    b. Hyperglycemia
    c. Increased risk of infection
    d. Gastric bleeding
    e. Myocardial hypertrophy (long-term use)
    f. Decreased growth velocity (long-term use)
  4. Comments
    a. Several dosing regimens have been suggested (see Chapter 61).
    b. Used for short duration.
    c. Be aware of need for stress doses for infection, surgery, etc.
    d. Inhalational route may be effective.
    e. May wish to administer concomitant histamine$_2$ blocker such as ranitidine.

IV. Impediments to Weaning
A. Infection (especially pulmonary)
  1. Increased caloric expenditure
  2. Inflammation
  3. Edema
  4. Decreased pulmonary blood flow
  5. Myocardial depression
B. Neurologic dysfunction or neuromuscular disease
  1. Decreased respiratory drive
  2. Neuromuscular incompetence
  3. Alveolar hypoventilation
  4. Examples
    a. Significant intraventricular hemorrhage (IVH)
    b. Posthemorrhagic hydrocephalus
    c. Periventricular leukomalacia (PVL)
C. Electrolyte disturbances
  1. Chronic diuretic therapy
  2. Renal tubular dysfunction
  3. Excess free water intake
  4. Total parenteral nutrition (TPN)
D. Metabolic alkalosis
  1. Infant may hyperventilate.
  2. Correct underlying abnormality.
E. Congestive heart failure
  1. Pulmonary edema
  2. Impaired gas exchange

3. Organ hypoperfusion
4. May require high PEEP
F. Anemia
   1. Decreased oxygen-carrying capacity
   2. High circulatory demands and excessive energy expenditure
   3. Apnea
G. Pharmacologic agents
   1. Sedatives may depress respiratory drive.
   2. Prolonged use of paralytics may lead to atrophy of respiratory musculature.
H. Nutritional
   1. Inadequate caloric intake
   2. Too many non-nitrogen calories, resulting in excess CO_2 production
V. Extubation and Postextubation Care
   A. Extubation
      1. Assessment
         a. Reliable respiratory drive and ability to maintain adequate alveolar ventilation
         b. Low ventilatory support
         c. No contraindications
      2. Extubation
         a. The stomach should be empty. If infant was recently fed, aspirate stomach contents.
         b. Suction endotracheal tube and nasopharynx.
         c. When heart rate and SaO_2 are normal, quickly remove ETT.
         d. Provide FiO_2 as needed.
   B. Postextubation CARE
      1. Nasal CPAP (see Chapter 24)
         a. Clinical trials showed mixed results. Some clinicians prefer to extubate directly to nasal CPAP to maintain continuous distending pressure and decrease work of breathing.
         b. Use 4 to 6 cm H_2O.
         c. May be useful to maintain upper airway patency in infants with stridor.
      2. Nasal cannula
         a. Can provide necessary FiO_2.
         b. Can provide gas flow to help overcome nasal resistance.
         c. Allows most patient freedom.
      3. Oxygen hood
         a. Can provide necessary FiO_2.
         b. More confining than nasal cannula but easier to regulate specific FiO_2.
      4. Prone positioning
         a. Stabilizes chest wall.
         b. Improves diaphragmatic excursion by allowing abdominal viscera to fall away from diaphragm, and thus decreases work of breathing.
         c. Umbilical catheters should be removed.

5. Stridor
   a. May result from subglottic edema or laryngotracheomalacia.
   b. Treatment options
      (1) FiO$_2$/humidity
      (2) CPAP
      (3) Inhalational sympathomimetics (e.g., racemic epinephrine)
      (4) Corticosteroids
   c. If persistent, consider reintubation or airway evaluation (see Chapter 23).
   d. Subglottic stenosis may require tracheostomy.
6. Methylxanthines
   a. Some studies have suggested efficacy in the periextubation setting.
   b. Duration of treatment is 24 to 96 hours (longer if respiratory control irregularities occur).
   c. Recommended serum theophylline concentration is 8 to 12 µg/mL.
7. Ongoing assessments
   a. Blood gas assessment: Assure adequate gas exchange.
   b. Chest radiograph: Not routinely necessary unless there is clinical evidence of respiratory distress.
   c. Weight gain: If inadequate, may indicate excessive caloric expenditure for respiratory work.

Suggested Reading

Balsan MJ, Jones JG, Watchko JF, Guthrie RD: Measurements of pulmonary mechanics prior to the elective extubation of neonates. Pediatr Pulmonol 9:238-243, 1990.

Barrington KJ, Finer NN: A randomized, controlled trial of aminophylline in ventilatory weaning of premature infants. Crit Care Med 21:846-850, 1993.

Baumeister BL, El-Khatib M, Smith PG, Blumer JL: Evaluation of predictors of weaning from mechanical ventilation in pediatric patients. Pediatr Pulmonol 24:344-352, 1997.

Bernstein G, Mannino FL, Heldt GP, et al: Randomized multicenter trial comparing synchronized and conventional intermittent mandatory ventilation in neonates. J Pediatr 128:453-463, 1996.

Chan V, Greenough A: Comparison of weaning by patient triggered ventilation or synchronous intermittent mandatory ventilation in preterm infants. Acta Paediatr 83:335-337, 1994.

Davis P, Jankow R, Doyle L, Henschke P: Randomised, controlled trial of nasal continuous positive pressure in the extubation of infants weighing 600 to 1250 g. Arch Dis Child 79:F54-F57, 1998.

Dimitriou G, Greenough A, Laubscher B: Lung volume measurements immediately after extubation by prediction of "extubation failure" in premature infants. Pediatr Pulmonol 21:250-254, 1996.

Donn SM, Sinha SK: Controversies in patient-triggered ventilation. Clin Perinatol 25:49-61, 1998.

El-Khatib MF, Baumeister B, Smith PG, et al: Inspiratory pressure/maximal inspiratory pressure: Does it predict successful extubation in critically ill infants and children? Intensive Care Med 22:264-268, 1996.

Fiastro JF, Habib MP, Quan SF: Pressure support compensation for inspiratory work due to endotracheal tubes and demand continuous positive airway pressure. Chest 93:499-505, 1988.

Gillespie LM, White SD, Sinha SK, Donn SM: Usefulness of the minute ventilation test in predicting successful extubation in newborn infants: A randomized clinical trial. J Perinatol 23:205-207, 2003.

McIntyre NR, Leatherman NE: Mechanical loads on the ventilatory muscles. Am Rev Respir Dis 139:968-972, 1989.

Robertson NJ, Hamilton PA: Randomised trial of elective continuous positive airway pressure (CPAP) compared with rescue CPAP after extubation. Arch Dis Child 79:F58-F60, 1998.

Sheth RD, Pryse-Phillips WEM, Riggs JE, Bodensteiner JB: Critical illness neuromuscular disease in children manifested as ventilator dependence. J Pediatr 126:259-261, 1995.

Sillos EM, Veber M, Schulman M, et al: Characteristics associated with successful weaning in ventilator-dependent preterm infants. Am J Perinatol 9:374-377, 1992.

Sinha SK, Donn SM: Weaning newborns from mechanical ventilation. Semin Neonatol 7:421-428, 2002.

Sinha SK, Donn SM, Gavey J, McCarty M: A randomised trial of volume-controlled versus time-cycled, pressure-limited ventilation in preterm infants with respiratory distress syndrome. Arch Dis Child 77:F202-F205, 1997.

Tapia JL, Cancalari A, Gonzales A, Mercado ME: Does continuous positive airway pressure (CPAP) during weaning from intermittent mandatory ventilation in very low birth weight infants have risks or benefits? A controlled trial. Pediatr Pulmonol 19:269-274, 1995.

Veness-Meehan, Richter S, Davis JM: Pulmonary function testing prior to extubation in infants with respiratory distress syndrome. Pediatr Pulmonol 9:2-6, 1990.

Wilson BJ Jr, Becker MA, Linton ME, Donn SM: Spontaneous minute ventilation predicts readiness for extubation in mechanically ventilated preterm infants. J Perinatol 18:436-439, 1998.

Adjunctive Therapies

Nutritional Management of the Ventilated Infant

59

Gilberto R. Pereira

I. Introduction
   A. Respiratory distress is a leading cause of neonatal morbidity and mortality, and mechanical ventilation remains the most common therapeutic modality applied in neonatal intensive care units.
   B. The neonate receiving mechanical ventilation is at risk for developing nutritional deficiencies for a variety of reasons, including:
      1. Inadequate nutritional intake
      2. Higher energy requirements
      3. Altered nutrient requirement
      4. Intolerance to enteral feeding
      5. Development of feeding disorders.
   C. The purpose of this chapter is to review the different methods of providing nutritional support to neonates receiving mechanical ventilation with the goal of optimizing the infant's nutritional status, growth, and development.
   D. Initially, most newborns receiving mechanical ventilation are supported exclusively by parenteral nutrition, later by a combination of parenteral and enteral nutrition and subsequently by enteral nutrition alone. The practical aspects of providing energy and nutrient requirements of neonates during parenteral and enteral nutrition are reviewed. In addition, a significant number of infants treated with mechanical ventilation develop chronic lung disease and associated feeding disorders that have a major adverse effect on their subsequent growth and development. Some strategies to minimize and treat these complications are discussed.

II. Energy Requirements
   A. Energy requirements are well established during the newborn period and are known to vary according to gestational age, mode of alimentation, and environmental factors. Table 59-1 describes the various components and the total energy requirements of premature and term infants.
   B. Energy requirements are greater in premature infants compared with those of full-term infants because of their faster growth rate and increased energy losses in stools.
   C. Energy requirements are lower during parenteral nutrition as compared to enteral nutrition because energy is neither utilized for the thermic effect of feeding nor malabsorbed in stools.

TABLE 59-1. Energy Requirements for Neonates (Cal/kg)

	Full-Term	Premature
Resting expenditure	50	50
Physical Activity*	20	15
Cold Stress†	10	10
Thermic Effect of Feeding‡	8	8
Fecal Losses*‡	7	12
Growth*	15	25
Total	110	120

Modified from the American Academy of Pediatrics Committee on Nutrition: Nutritional needs of premature infants. In Kleinman RE (ed): Pediatric Nutrition Handbook. Elk Grove Village, Ill., 2004, pp 23-54.
*Significant differences between full-term and premature infants.
†Increased if outside neutral thermal environment.
‡Not required during parenteral nutrition.

  D. In addition, energy requirements may vary if the infant is kept outside neutral thermal zone. The maintenance of heat balance in the neonate is commonly practiced in contemporary intensive care units by the routine use of servo-controlled incubators, radiant warmers, and close monitoring of the environmental and infant's skin temperature.
  E. Energy requirements during mechanical ventilation also vary with the patient's condition and the mode of ventilation.
    1. Pediatric patients treated with mechanical ventilation have been shown to be hypermetabolic, with increased resting energy expenditure. Conclusive studies on this topic are lacking in neonates because of inaccuracies in measuring indirect calorimetry in intubated neonates.
    2. It is estimated that infants with severe respiratory distress who receive sedation or skeletal muscle relaxants have lower energy requirements than those who are breathing spontaneously and remain physically active.
    3. In general, a total energy intake varying from 90 to 100 kcal/kg/day is sufficient for most neonates receiving mechanical ventilation as long as they are sedated, normothermic, and receiving parenteral nutrition. Additional intakes ranging from 10 to 20 kcal/kg/day are indicated for infants who are premature, physically active, or receiving full enteral feedings.
III. Parenteral Nutrition
  A. Parenteral nutrition is the main mode of alimentation for critically ill neonates receiving mechanical ventilation, especially during the immediate postnatal period when many infants are enterally fasting.

B. Parenteral nutrition is usually continued until enteral feedings are providing sufficient calories to support growth.

C. Parenteral nutrition solutions should supply all necessary nutrients at maintenance rates, including electrolytes and minerals to correct the common biochemical abnormalities that occur during the neonatal period.

1. Amino acids should be provided at amounts to meet requirements for full-term infants (2 g/kg/day) and premature infants (3 to 4 g/kg/day), with the higher value used for the most immature infants. In one study, early commencement of amino acids, at intakes as low as 1.15 g/kg/day, was shown to be extremely beneficial in maintaining positive nitrogen retention and preventing protein catabolism. These data suggest the presence of avid amino acid retention during the immediate postnatal period. Similar studies confirmed this finding and showed improvement in plasma aminograms without evidence of aminoacidemia or azotemia.

2. Nonprotein calories should provide comparable amounts of calories derived from carbohydrates and fat emulsions. Although the administration of dextrose and/or glucose is essential for maintaining normal glucose serum levels, rates of infusion exceeding 8 to 10 mg/kg/min may result in hyperglycemia, especially if fast advancements are performed in premature infants.

   a. During fetal life and the early postnatal period, the secretion of insulin depends on the plasma concentrations of amino acids such as leucine and arginine as well as serum glucose concentrations. Therefore, the administration of amino acids influences glucose homeostasis.

   b. The intravenous administration of insulin in conjunction with dextrose has been shown to improve glucose tolerance, calorie intake, and weight gain in premature infants who are glucose-intolerant during parenteral nutrition. The administration of continuous insulin infusions, however, requires close monitoring of glucose serum levels and insulin doses.

3. Fat emulsions should be quickly advanced to 3 g/kg/day over the first 2 to 3 days of life as long as serum triglycerides are not elevated and hyperlipedemia is avoided. Early studies showed that the administration of lipid emulsions at high infusion rates, such as 1 g/kg/ over 4 hours, resulted in hyperlipidemia and in a transient decrease in oxygenation. These complications can be minimized by the current practice of administering lipid emulsions over longer infusion times, usually over a 24-hour period. A significant justification for the use of fat emulsions is to provide essential fatty acids and to reduce glucose loads. The oxidation of fat produces less CO_2 for the same amount of oxygen consumed. This reduction in CO_2 production and its elimination may be beneficial for patients with compromised lung function.

4. Premature infants receiving parenteral nutrition are at risk of developing vitamin A deficiency because of their low hepatic stores

and low serum-binding proteins level at birth. There are also significant losses of vitamin A into the delivery system used for parenteral nutrition.

    a. As of 2005, the largest randomized, controlled trial was performed in 807 premature infants with a birth weight of less than 1 kg who received 5000 IU of vitamin A intramuscularly three times a week for the first month of life.

    b. The results of this trial showed a modest but beneficial effect of vitamin A supplementation in reducing the incidence of chronic lung disease.

IV. Enteral Nutrition

  A. The types of enteral feedings and supplements recommended for newborn infants are summarized in Table 59-2.

  B. Human milk is the preferred type of feeding for premature and term newborns.

    1. For preterm infants, human milk should be fortified routinely once feeding tolerance is established. Fortification is recommended to increase the levels of protein, energy, minerals, and vitamins, which results in improved growth of premature infants.

    2. In the absence of human milk, the choice of formulas is dependent on the gestational age of the infant (e.g., term versus preterm infant formulas).

      a. Standard infant formulas for term infants contain cow's milk protein, lactose, vegetable oils, and minerals and vitamins to supply the requirements of the growing infant. If iron-fortified preparations are used, no additional supplementation is needed.

      b. Premature infant formulas contain protein as hydrolyzed whey, 50% of the fat as medium-chain triglycerides, and a reduced lactose load by the supplementation of glucose polymers. In addition, these formulas contain a higher concentration of minerals, vitamins, and trace elements than those of formulas for term infants.

      c. Premature infant formulas are available at concentrations of 20 kcal/oz for initial feedings and at 24 kcal/oz after full enteral feedings are achieved.

      d. These formulas are also available with and without iron fortification, and their use requires no additional vitamin supplementation when taken at full volume.

      e. Postdischarge formulas are indicated for small premature infants after hospital discharge or at 40 weeks post-conceptual age in the event that the infant remains hospitalized after that age. These formulas provide the preterm infant with a nutrient intake that is between that of a preterm and a full-term formula. Postdischarge formulas are recommended for 9 months after hospital discharge for the purpose of promoting growth and bone mineralization. Because these preparations are iron- and vitamin-fortified, no supplements are needed.

    3. Concentrated formulas with a calorie density varying from 24 up to 30 kcal/30 mL may be given to infants older than 1 month who are

TABLE 59-2. Enteral Feedings and Supplements for Newborn Infants

Feedings	Indications	Special Composition	Comments	Supplements
Mature human milk	Full-term infants with intact GI function	High nutrient bioavailability; immune factors; hormones; growth factors; low osmolality	Preferred feeding; model for composition of formulas; psychological and immunologic benefits; low cost	Vitamin D, 200 IU/day; Fe, 2 mg/kg/day (?)
Standard infant formulas: Similac, Enfamil, Gerber, Carnation GS, Similac PM 60:40, Lactofree	Full-term infants with intact GI function	Cow's milk protein: casein or whey predominant*; lactose only carbohydrate (except Lactofree); fat blend with predominance of LCTs; low renal solute load*	Alternative to human milk; promote adequate growth; Similac PM 60:40 commonly used for patients with cardiac-renal disease	Fluoride, depending on local water supply, after 6 mo; Fe, 2 mg/kg/day if formula is not Fe-fortified
Preterm human milk	Premature infants (<37 wk gestation)	Higher protein, calories, and NaCl compared to mature human milk; immune factors; growth factors; hormones; low osmolality	Preferred feeding; special compositional differences persist during first month of lactation; psychological and immunologic benefits	Liquid fortifier, 1 mL:1 mL; powder fortifier, 1 packet: 25 mL; Poly-Vi-Sol, 0.5 mL/day (with liquid fortifier); Fe, 2 mg/kg/day by 2 weeks of age
Premature infant formulas: Similac Special Care, Enfamil Premature	Premature infants (<37 wk gestation)	Whey-predominant protein; reduced lactose load; 50% fat as MCTs; high concentration of minerals and vitamins; available as 20 or 24 kcal/oz; available with and without Fe fortification†‡	Alternative to fortified preterm human milk; enhances digestion and nutrient absorption by premature infants	Fe, 2 mg/kg/day by age 2 weeks, if formula is not Fe-fortified; Poly-Vi-Sol, 0.5-1 mL/day when intake is less than 170 mL/day† or 151 mL/day ‡
Postdischarge infant formulas: Enfacare, Neosure	Premature infants with Birth weight <1800 g; for use post hospital discharge	Intermediate composition between standard and premature infant formulas; increased levels of protein, minerals, vitamins, trace elements; available as 22 kcal/oz; Fe-fortified	Increased growth and bone mineralization when used for 9 mo post hospital discharge	Fluoride, depending on local water supply, after 6 mo

*Similac PM 60:40.
†Similac Special Care.
‡Enfamil Premature.
GI, gastrointestinal; LCTs, long-chain triglycerides; MCTs, medium-chain triglycerides.

TABLE 59-3. Energy Supplements for Newborn Infants

	Weight/Volume	Calorie Density
Glucose polymers	1 g	3.8 kcal
MCT oil	1 g (1.1 mL)	8.3 kcal
Microlipid	1 mL	4.5 kcal
Duocal	1 g	4.9 kcal

MCT, medium-chain triglyceride.

    still receiving mechanical ventilation, if fluid restriction becomes necessary for cardiorespiratory management.

4. The calorie density of formulas can be increased by the addition of calorie supplements. Table 59-3 describes the commercially available supplements that contain carbohydrates, lipids, or a combination of these substrates. The choice of calorie supplements depends on the infant's medical condition. Carbohydrate supplements are preferred for infants with cholestatic jaundice or fat malabsorption, whereas fat supplements are preferred for infants with preserved intestinal function but severe chronic lung disease in order to reduce CO_2 production and elimination. Calorie supplements should be used with caution: the total calorie intake of the feeding must not be disproportionate to the contents of protein and other nutrients that are necessary for growth.

C. The initiation of enteral feedings in the ventilated newborn should not be delayed for periods >1 week, unless they are strongly contraindicated by the presence of hemodynamic instability, use of vasopressors, intestinal obstruction, symptomatic patent ductus arteriosus, septic ileus, or necrotizing enterocolitis.

1. Early initiation of enteral feedings prevents the adverse effects of prolonged starvation on the developing gastrointestinal tract, such as shortening of the intestinal villi, loss of mucosal DNA, decrease in protein content, and reduction in enzymatic activity.

2. The administration of "minimal" enteral feedings while the infant is receiving parenteral nutrition has been well studied in multiple clinical trials, all of which showed positive effects, including:
   a. Improved feeding tolerance
   b. Shorter time to achieve full enteral nutrition
   c. Shorter duration of parenteral nutrition
   d. Increased gastrointestinal motility
   e. Increased weight gain
   f. Shorter length of hospitalization.

3. None of these studies showed an increased incidence of necrotizing enterocolitis in infants receiving minimal enteral feedings.

D. During mechanical ventilation, enteral feedings are routinely provided by nasogastric tube.
  1. Gastric gavage is the preferred method to provide enteral feedings in intubated patients. Gastric feedings supply nutrients at lower risk, lower cost, and in a more physiologic manner than feedings that bypass the stomach.
  2. Transpyloric feedings are not recommended for routine use because they bypass the stomach, an important site of protein and fat digestion in the neonate.
  3. The activity of lingual lipase and gastric lipase is well developed at birth, resulting in the digestion of more than 30% of ingested triglycerides.
  4. Transpyloric feedings have been associated with complications such as:
    a. Decreased fat and potassium absorption
    b. Bacterial colonization of the upper gastrointestinal tract
    c. Intestinal perforation, the risk of which can be minimized by the use silicone or silastic feeding tubes.
  5. In practice, transpyloric feedings are considered the second method of choice for intubated infants receiving mechanical ventilation. Transpyloric feedings are indicated in patients who are intolerant to gastric feedings because of:
    a. Delayed gastric emptying
    b. Severe gastroesophageal reflux (GER)
    c. High risk for aspiration.
  6. There is considerable debate about whether the infant with respiratory failure should receive gastric feedings intermittently or continuously.
    a. Intermittent gastric feedings are considered more physiologic, easier to administer, and more practical for monitoring gastric residuals. For these reasons, intermittent gastric feedings have been considered the method of choice for feeding the ventilated neonate. See Table 59-4.
    b. The administration of continuous gastric feedings results in less adverse effects on respiratory pattern, pulmonary function tests (minute ventilation, dynamic compliance, and pulmonary resistance), and control of breathing compared with intermittent gastric feedings and should be considered the first method of choice for patients with severe respiratory distress. Continuous gastric feedings should also be used in patients who are intolerant to intermittent gastric feedings.
  7. Traditionally, enteral feedings are initiated and advanced at rates approximating 20 mL/kg/day, taking about 7 days to achieve full enteral nutrition.
    a. More recently, two randomized controlled trials comparing slow feeding advancement (20 mL/kg/day) with fast advancement (35 and 30 mL/kg/day) reported beneficial effects of faster rates, including shorter time to achieve full feedings and shorter duration of parenteral nutrition.

TABLE 59-4. Methods of Feeding the Ventilated Infant

	Indications	Complications	Management
Intermittent gastric (gavage)	Preferred method for intubated infants	Vomiting and aspiration	Measure gastric residuals prior to each feeding, abdominal girth q6-8h
Continuous gastric	Severe respiratory distress; intolerance to intermittent feedings	Vomiting and aspiration; difficulty in assessing significant residuals	Measure gastric residuals q6-8h, abdominal girth q6-8h
Jejunal feedings	Intolerance to gastric feedings; severe GER; delayed gastric emptying; aspiration pneumonia	GI perforation; decreased fat absorption; dumping syndrome	Use only silartic feeding tubes; use formula with MCTs; avoid hyperosmolar feedings

GER, gastroesophageal reflux; GI, gastrointestinal; MCT, medium-chain triglycerides.

      b. These studies also showed comparable rates of feeding intolerance and necrotizing enterocolitis whether the infants received fast or slow feeding advancements.

V. Chronic Lung Disease (CLD)

  A. Infants who develop CLD after a prolonged course of mechanical ventilation often exhibit growth failure and require special nutritional management.

  B. Several studies have reported increased energy requirements in infants with CLD compared to age-matched healthy controls.

    1. The differences in energy expenditure ranged from 11 to 24 kcal/kg/day. These studies concluded that high metabolic demands could be explained by increased work of breathing from altered pulmonary mechanics. Also, stress and inflammation, need for catch-up growth, and the use of medications such as caffeine, theophylline, and beta agonists may contribute to the increased energy expenditure in infants with CLD.

    2. Failure to recognize these differences in energy expenditure is one of the causes contributing to growth failure in these infants.

  C. Infants with CLD often require fluid restriction and diuretic therapy as part of their respiratory management.

    1. Although the effectiveness of diuretic therapy for chronic lung disease remains controversial, the use of these medications continue to be a common method for treating pulmonary edema.

    2. Infants receiving diuretics for prolonged periods may require additional supplements of sodium, chloride, potassium, and calcium to compensate for increased renal losses. Chronic depletion of these minerals may impair growth and bone mineralization.

    3. Concentrated feedings (24, 27, and even 30 kcal/30 mL) are frequently recommended with the purpose of providing appropriate calorie intake during fluid restriction. Highly concentrated feedings may not be well tolerated during the first month of life, and slow increments in concentration are recommended.

  D. Two randomized controlled trials evaluated the use of nutrient-enriched formulas in infants with chronic lung disease, compared with standard formulas.

    1. These studies demonstrated beneficial effects of concentrated feedings, including improvement in growth, protein status, lean body mass, and whole body bone mineral content.

    2. The use of highly concentrated feedings can cause problems such as delayed gastric emptying and exacerbation of GER, as well as severe irritation if feedings are accidentally aspirated.

  E. Vitamin A has a role as an antioxidant and as a key nutrient for maintaining lung epithelial cell integrity. A meta-analysis by Darlow and Graham (2004) evaluated the effect of supplemental vitamin A in premature infants <1500 g on the incidence of death or on the need for supplemental oxygen at 1 month or 36 weeks corrected gestational age. The combined sample included a total of 1251 patients who received placebo or vitamin A injections three times a week. The results showed a modest reduction in death or oxygen supplementation at 1 month and at 36 weeks among infants receiving supplemental vitamin A.

VI. Feeding Disorders

    A. Feeding disorders may develop in infants treated with mechanical ventilation, impairing long-term growth, nutritional status, and developmental outcome.

    B. In general, feeding disorders are first recognized after the patient is extubated and then fails multiple attempts to be orally fed.

    C. Oropharyngeal hypersensitivity, defined as a pathologic aversion to oral stimulation, is evidenced by an avoidance behavior to the introduction of any type of oral feeding.

        1. This disorder results from prolonged endotracheal intubation, frequent oral and nasal pharyngeal suctioning, prolonged use of nasal and oral gastric feeding tubes, and the use of nasal cannula oxygen at high flows.

        2. Delay in the critical time to learn how to feed may result in the loss of rooting and sucking reflexes and contribute to the feeding problem.

        3. The treatment of oropharyngeal hypersensitivity includes a program of desensitization of the infant's oral pharynx with positive stimulation and attempts to minimize negative stimulation. The latter implies replacement of nasogastric and orogastric feeding tubes with gastrostomy tubes and the use of tracheostomy instead of continuing endotracheal intubation if mechanical ventilation needs to be continued.

    D. Swallowing disorders affecting the three phases may also be observed after prolonged courses of mechanical ventilation.

        1. These disorders may affect the three phases of swallowing: oral, pharyngeal, and esophageal.

        2. Swallowing disorders can be seen in association with congenital anomalies such as micrognathia, choanal atresia, cleft lip and palate, tracheoesophageal fistulas, and laryngeal clefts. They can also be acquired and observed in infants with severe CLD, laryngotracheomalacia, and neurologic insults that result in cerebral palsy.

        3. Assessment of swallow dysfunction includes a comprehensive history, physical examination, and evaluation of neurologic, pulmonary, and gastrointestinal status. Videofluoroscopy is the radiologic evaluation of choice to detect abnormalities in the different phases of swallowing and the risk of aspiration.

        4. Treatment depends on the symptoms, etiology, and feeding history and usually requires special therapy in five categories: positioning, oral sensory normalization, modification of food consistency, adaptation of feeding devices, and oral feeding exercises.

    E. Pathologic GER may also be seen in infants who received mechanical ventilation, especially in those who develop CLD, neurologic insults resulting in cerebral palsy, and tracheomalacia or subglottic stenosis resulting from prolonged endotracheal intubation.

1. The clinical presentation of pathologic GER includes the presence of frequent gastric residuals, episodes of vomiting, failure to thrive, and aspiration pneumonia.
2. Medical management with antacids, H_2 receptor antagonists, proton pump inhibitors, or when GER symptoms are life-threatening or persistent; jejunal feedings may be necessary.
3. In severe cases of GER that are refractory to medical management, Nissen fundoplication may be indicated.

Suggested Reading

American Academy of Pediatrics Committee on Nutrition: Nutritional needs of premature infants. In Kleinman RE (ed): Pediatric Nutrition Handbook. Elk Grove Village, Ill., 2004, pp 23-54.

Binder ND, Raschko PK, Benda GI, et al: Insulin infusions with parenteral nutrition in extremely low birthweight infants with hyperglycemia. J Pediatr 114:223-230, 1989.

Blondheim O, Abbasi S, Fox WW, Bhutani V: Effect of enteral feeding rate on pulmonary functions of very low birth weight infants. J Pediatr 122:751-755, 1993.

Caple J, Armentrout D, Huseby V, et al: Randomized controlled trial of slow versus rapid feeding volume advancement in preterm infants. Pediatrics 114:1597-1600, 2004.

Chen JW, Wong PWK: Intestinal complications of naso-jejunal feeding in low birth weight infants. J Pediatr 85:109-110, 1974.

Coss-Bu JA, Jefferson LS, Walding D, et al: Resting energy expenditure and nitrogen balance in critically ill pediatric patients on mechanical ventilation. Nutrition 14:649-652, 1998.

Darlow BA, Graham PJ: Vitamin A supplementation for preventing morbidity and mortality in very low birthweight infants. Cochrane Database of Systematic Reviews (4):CD000501, 2004.

Hamosh M: Fat digestion in the newborn. The role of lingual lipase and pre-duodenal digestion. Pediatr Res 13:615-622, 1979.

Kuzner SI, Garg M, Bautista DB, et al: Growth failure in bronchopulmonary dysplasia: Elevated metabolic rates and pulmonary mechanics. J Pediatr 112:73-80, 1988.

Pereira GR, Fox WW, Stanley CA, et al: Decreased oxygenation and hyperlipemia during intravenous fat emulsions in premature infants. Pediatrics 66:26-30, 1980.

Puangco MA, Schandler RJ: Clinical experience in enteral support for premature infants with bronchopulmonary dysplasia. J Perinatol 20:87-91, 2000.

Rayys SF, Ambalavanan N, Wright L: Randomized trial of slow vs fast feed advancement on the incidence of NEC in VLBW infants. J Pediatr 134:293-297, 1999.

Schandler R, Shulman RJ, Lau C, et al: Randomized trial of gastrointestinal priming and tube feeding method. Pediatrics 103:434-438, 1999.

Tyson JE, Wright LL, Oh W, et al: Vitamin A supplementation for extremely low-birth-weight infants. National Institute of Child Health and Human Development Neonatal Research Network. N Engl J Med 340:1962-1968, 1999.

Van Goudoever JB, Colen T, Wattimena JL, et al: Immediate commencement of amino acid supplementation in preterm infants: Effect on serum amino acid concentrations and protein kinetics on the first day of life. J Pediatr 127:458-465, 1995.

Yunis RA, Oh W: Effects of intravenous glucose loading on oxygen consumption, carbon dioxide production, and resting energy expenditure in infants with bronchopulmonary dysplasia. J Pediatr 115:127-132, 1989.

60 Surfactant Replacement Therapy

Thierry Lacaze-Masmonteil

I. Introduction
   A. Pulmonary surfactant, a multicomponent complex of several phospholipids, neutral lipids, and specific proteins, is synthesized and secreted into alveolar spaces by type II epithelial cells.
   B. Pulmonary surfactant reduces the collapsing force in the alveolus, confers mechanical stability to the alveoli, and maintains the alveolar surface relatively free of liquid.
   C. Administration of a natural animal-derived surfactant to a surfactant-deficient preterm animal or human newborn decreases the minimum pressure required to open the lung, increases the maximal lung volume, and prevents lung collapse at low pressure.
II. Structure and Function
   A. Surfactant is primarily composed of phospholipids (85%) and proteins (10%). Most of the phospholipids consist of phosphatidylcholine (PC), and one particular PC molecule, DPPC (dipalmitoyl phosphatidylcholine), is the most prevalent component. The structure of DPPC is suited to form a stable monolayer generating the low surface tension required to prevent alveolar collapse at end-expiration.
   B. Phospholipids alone do not exhibit all the biophysical properties of pulmonary surfactant.
      1. These properties include the ability to:
         a. Generate low minimum surface tension on dynamic compression,
         b. Absorb from the subphase to the interface,
         c. Respread when collapse occurs after condensation,
         d. Vary surface tension during expansion and compression at each respiratory cycle.
      2. The contribution of low-molecular-weight SP-B and SP-C to both structural organization and functional durability is essential.
   C. SP-B and SP-C: These proteins promote the rapid absorption of phospholipids at the air-liquid interface and account for the sustained low surface-tension activity after dynamic compression.
      1. Lethal respiratory failure occurs at birth in homozygous mice harboring an SP-B gene inactivated after homologous recombination. SP-B deficiency, inherited as an autosomal recessive

condition, has been identified in full-term newborn infants exhibiting severe and fulminant respiratory failure.

  2. SP-C dramatically enhances the spread of phospholipids. Whereas SP-C knocked-out animals do not manifest any respiratory symptoms at birth, SP-C–deficient adult animals develop pneumonitis and emphysema. Dominantly inherited mutations in the SP-C gene of siblings with interstitial lung disease have recently been described, suggesting that either inadequate SP-C synthesis or the accumulation of an abnormal SP-C precursor may account for some forms of chronic interstitial lung disease in childhood.

  D. SP-A and SP-D: SP-A and SP-D belong to the collection family, a subgroup of the lectin superfamily. They are marginally involved in the surface tension–lowering ability of pulmonary surfactant and play an important role in the innate lung defense barrier against pathogenic organisms.

III. Exogenous Surfactants: Exogenous surfactants are currently classified into two families (Table 60-1).

  A. Mammalian surfactant preparations (natural surfactant) are purified and extracted with organic solvents from either lung minces or lung lavages. Their phospholipid concentration is >80%, and all contain the low-molecular-weight hydrophobic proteins SP-B and SP-C, but not SP-D. There are several significant differences in the composition of these preparations. For instance, the porcine minced lung extract poractant (Curosurf) undergoes an additional purification step that removes neutral lipid, whereas free fatty acids and DPPC are added to the bovine minced lung extract beractant (Survanta). Moreover, SP-B concentration is lower in the lung minced preparation compared with lung lavage extracts.

  B. The entirely synthetic surfactant preparations are composed mainly of DPPC. For almost 20 years, Exosurf has been the most widely used synthetic protein-free surfactant. Recently, a new generation of synthetic surfactants has been developed that contains phospholipids and chemically or genetically engineered peptide analogues of SP-B or SP-C. Lucinactant (Surfaxin) is composed of DPPC, palmitoyloleoyl phosphatidylglycerol (POPG), and palmitic acid, combined with a synthetic peptide (Sinapultide) whose spatial structure resembles one of the domains of SP-B. Another synthetic surfactant composed of DPPC, POPG, palmitic acid, and recombinant SP-C obtained by expression in a prokaryotic system has been developed and is currently under evaluation.

IV. Efficacy

  A. Evidence for the efficacy of either prophylactic (treatment within the first 30 minutes after birth, regardless the respiratory status) or rescue (treatment usually after 2 hours, when signs of respiratory failure are present) administration in the treatment of RDS comes from overviews and meta-analyses of more than 40 trials, in which nearly 10,000 infants have been enrolled. These meta-analyses demonstrate the following:

TABLE 60-1. Surfactants Currently Available

Surfactant	Origin	Characteristics	Protein	First Dose mg/kg (mL/kg)	Additional Doses (maximal number) mg/kg (mL/kg)
Natural Surfactants					
Infasurf	Calf lung lavage	Chloroform/methanol extracted	SP-B/SP-C	105 (3)	max 2 doses at least q12h;105 (3)
BLES	Cow lung lavage	Chloroform/methanol extracted	SP-B/SP-C	135 (5)	max 2 doses at least q6h; 135 (5)
Survanta	Minced bovine lung extract	Enriched with DPPC, tripalmitoylglycerol, and free fatty acids	SP-C/low SP-B content	100 (4)	max 3 doses at least q6h; 100 (4)
Curosurf	Minced porcine lung extract	No neutral lipids (liquidgel chromatography)	SP-B/SP-C	100-200 (1.25-2.5)	max 2 doses at least q6h; 100 (1.25)
Synthetic Surfactants					
Exosurf*	Synthetic preparation	DPPC + hexadecanol (9%) + tyloxapol (6%)	0	67 (5)	max 2 doses at least q12h; 67 (5)
Surfaxin	Synthetic preparation	DPPC/POPG 3/1 + free fatty acids (palmitic acid)	Sinapultide (3%)	175 (5.8)	max 2 doses at least q6h; 175 (5.8)

*Not available in North America.
BLES, bovine lipid extract surfactant; DPPC, dipalmitoyl phosphatidylcholine; POPG, palmitoyloleoyl phosphatidylglycerol.

   1. There is a consistent 40% reduction in the odds of neonatal death after surfactant treatment, either natural or synthetic, administered as a prophylactic or rescue treatment.
   2. Both types of surfactant and both treatment strategies have also resulted in a significant reduction of 30% to 50% in the risk for of pulmonary air leaks (interstitial emphysema, pneumothorax).
   3. Because the increase in survival is mainly observed among extremely premature infants, the incidence of chronic lung disease (CLD) has not been significantly reduced despite the widespread use of surfactant.
B. Instilling surfactant before the onset of respiratory distress syndrome (RDS) has been shown to partially avoid barotrauma and vascular injury resulting from mechanical ventilation.
   1. An overview of prophylactic versus rescue strategies in controlled studies demonstrates that prophylactic administration of surfactant results in a reduction in mortality and is associated with a reduction in the risk for of pneumothorax.
   2. Because systematic surfactant administration in the delivery room will result in a large number of infants being submitted to an unnecessary treatment, as well as the potential side effects of endotracheal intubation (hypoxia and trauma), prophylaxis is usually limited to the most immature babies.
   3. No national guidelines addressing the timing of surfactant administration are currently available. In many centers across North America, infants born at or <26 weeks are eligible for prophylactic treatment.
C. Several trials have been recently conducted to assess the benefit of an "early rescue" strategy (early administration to symptomatic infants before 2 hours of life) compared to the classic rescue treatment.
   1. Meta-analyses of these trials demonstrate that early selective surfactant administration is associated with a decreased risk of neonatal mortality and results in a significant reduction in the incidence of pneumothorax.
   2. Infants born at >26 weeks and <32 weeks of gestation should receive surfactant without delay if they require supplemental oxygen with FiO_2 >0.3 on nasal continuous positive airway pressure (CPAP) or mechanical ventilation at 90 minutes of life.
   3. Ideally, early rescue surfactant should be administered before 2 hours of life in this population.
   4. In practice, it is the responsibility of each center to develop an institutionally approved surfactant treatment protocol.
D. Many randomized trials have compared the efficacy of natural surfactant to synthetic, protein-free surfactant.
   1. A meta-analysis shows a significant reduction in the incidence of pneumothorax and mortality.
   2. Because considerable attention is currently being given to strategies that minimize lung injury, most institutions are using predominantly natural preparations with rapid onset of action. In this respect, infants treated with calf lung surfactant extract

(Infasurf) or poractant (Curosurf) have a swifter improvement in oxygenation and reduced ventilatory requirements compared with infants treated with beractant (Survanta).

E. Two recent randomized clinical trials have compared Surfaxin to Exosurf, Survanta, and Curosurf.

1. There were more survivors without CLD in the Surfaxin group than in the Exosurf group.

2. There was no significant difference in the incidence of survival without BPD between the three protein-containing surfactants. (Exosurf is no longer available in North America.)

V. Other Indications

A. Inactivation of surfactant by several compounds is often involved in the pathogenesis of various respiratory disorders, including meconium aspiration syndrome (MAS), pneumonia, and sepsis. These disorders may represent potential targets for surfactant therapy. Most of the experimental or clinical studies reported so far have been carried out with natural surfactant, mainly because surfactant proteins improve resistance of phospholipids to inactivation.

B. The physiopathologic mechanisms of hypoxemia in MAS include airway obstructions, chemical pneumonitis, persistent pulmonary hypertension of the newborn with right-to-left extrapulmonary shunting, and surfactant dysfunction.

1. Surfactant is inhibited by meconium in vitro and in vivo.

2. Meta-analysis of two randomized, controlled trials confirmed the benefit of natural surfactant in MAS; the administration of several doses of a natural preparation improved oxygenation and reduced the need for extracorporeal membrane oxygenation (ECMO).

3. Bronchoalveolar lavage with dilute surfactant seems to be a promising approach for the treatment of severe MAS.

4. Based on these results, a phase 3 clinical trial is presently underway in the U.S. to assess both the efficacy and the safety of bronchoalveolar lavage with dilute lucinactant (Surfaxin) in severe MAS.

C. In a retrospective review of a large series of preterm and term infants with respiratory failure associated with group B streptococcal sepsis, improved oxygenation and decreased ventilatory requirements were observed after administration of natural surfactant. However, there is insufficient evidence that surfactant treatment improves the long-term outcome in septic newborns with respiratory failure.

VI. Administration and Practical Concerns

A. Manufacturer's recommended doses are indicated in Table 60-1. All natural surfactants require warming to room temperature before administration. Surfaxin requires a warming step at 111.2 °F (44 °C) in a heating block for 15 minutes before administration. Surfactant treatment should be accomplished after clinical ascertainment of proper endotracheal tube (ETT) placement. Performing a chest radiograph prior to giving surfactant is indicated only when conditions such as pneumothorax need to be ruled out.

B. Administration

    1. Dosing is usually divided into two aliquots and administered via a 5-Fr catheter passed in the ETT.

    2. The infant is manually ventilated during administration to ensure maximal dispersion.

    3. Each half-dose is injected over 1 to 2 minutes via a sideport adaptor, the infant's head and torso being placed in a position rotated 30 to 45 degrees to the right for the first half-dose and 30 to 45 degrees to the left for the second half-dose.

    4. Transient oxygen desaturation and mild bradycardia are frequently observed during administration and may require adjustment of the ventilation and FiO_2 or interruption of surfactant administration.

    5. Curosurf can also be administered in one bolus over 1 minute via a dual-lumen ETT without positioning, interruption of mechanical ventilation, or bagging.

  C. The improvement in gas exchange after administration is usually rapid (within a few minutes), and ventilation pressure and volume must be adjusted after administration by observing chest expansion and monitoring tidal volume and PCO_2.

    1. Because oxygenation improves rapidly, continuous monitoring of O_2 saturation during and after administration is mandatory.

    2. Around one third of treated infants still require mechanical ventilation with FiO_2 >0.3, 6 hours after the first dose; these infants are eligible for retreatment (see Table 60-1).

    3. There is no proven benefit to more than two additional doses.

Suggested Reading

Bancalari E, Claure N, Sosenko IRS: Bronchopulmonary dysplasia: Changes in pathogenesis, epidemiology, and definition. Semin Neonatol 8:63-71, 2003.

Griese M: Pulmonary surfactant in health and human lung diseases: State of the art. Eur Respir J 13:1455-1476, 1999.

Jobe AH: Surfactant and mechanical ventilation. In Marini JJ, Slutsky AS (eds): Physiological Basis of Ventilatory Support. New York, Marcel Dekker, 1998, pp 209-230.

Lacaze-Masmonteil T: Exogenous surfactant therapy: newer developments. Semin Perinatol 8:433-440, 2003.

Moya F, Gadzinowski J, Bancalari E, et al: A multicenter, randomized, masked comparison trial of lucinactant, colfosceril palmitate, and beractant for the prevention of respiratory distress syndrome among very preterm infants. Pediatrics 115:1018-1029, 2005.

Sinha SK, Lacaze-Masmonteil T, Valls I Soler A, et al: A randomized, controlled trial of lucinactant versus poractant alfa among very premature infants at high risk for respiratory distress syndrome. Pediatrics 115:1030-1038, 2005.

Soll RF, Dargaville P: Surfactant for meconium aspiration syndrome in full term infants. Cochrane Database Syst Rev (2):CD002054, 2000.

Soll RF, Morley CJ: Prophylactic versus selective use of surfactant in preventing morbidity and mortality in preterm infants. Cochrane Database Syst Rev (2):CD000510, 2001.

Weaver TE, Conkright JJ: Function of surfactant proteins B and C. Annu Rev Physiol 63:555-578, 2001.

Whitsett JA, Weaver TE: Hydrophobic surfactant proteins in lung function and disease. N Engl J Med 347:2141-2148, 2002.

Yost CC, Soll RF: Early versus delayed selective surfactant treatment for neonatal respiratory distress syndrome. Cochrane Database Syst Rev (2):CD001456, 2000.

61 Pharmacologic Agents

Sam W. J. Richmond

I. Analgesics
  A. Fentanyl
    1. A short-acting opioid analgesic used for perioperative pain relief. The short action is mainly a function of rapid redistribution into fat and muscle depots because the elimination half-life is actually quite long—4 hours in the adult and probably twice as long in the newborn. Morphine may be a better alternative for sustained pain relief.
    2. Dosage: Anesthetic doses of 5 to 10 μg/kg IV will provide good pain relief for about 1 hour in the newborn. Respiratory drive will usually be abolished and artificial ventilation will be needed. Respiratory depression may also occur unexpectedly, presumably following redistribution from fat or muscle depots. Continuous infusions of 3 μg/kg/hr are effective for a period, but tolerance develops rapidly and, if the infusion is continued for more than 4 to 5 days, serious withdrawal symptoms may follow discontinuation.
  B. Morphine
    1. This is the best studied opiate analgesic for use in the newborn period. Respiratory depression, urinary retention, and constipation can occur with normal doses, and hypotension, bradycardia, and seizures with overdose.
    2. Dosage
      a. For relief of severe pain, such as in necrotizing enterocolitis or following surgery, a loading dose of 240 μg/kg followed by an infusion of 20 μg/kg/hr is probably required. This dose will cause respiratory depression, and artificial ventilation will be needed.
      b. For sedation of a ventilated baby, a loading dose of 120 μg/kg and an infusion of 10 μg/kg/hr will usually be sufficient. For less severe pain in the nonventilated baby, a dose of 100 μg/kg every 12 hr may be sufficient.
      c. For the treatment of opiate withdrawal, oral doses of 40 μg/kg (sometimes more than this in babies of heavy users) initially every 4 hours are advised, with increases in dosage interval resulting in withdrawal over 6 to 10 days.
      d. For elective intubation, give a dose of 120 to 200 μg/kg at least 2 minutes and preferably 5 minutes before intubation. This is

best followed by a sedative (e.g., midazolam) and perhaps a muscle relaxant (e.g., atracurium). This dose may produce apnea.

C. Acetaminophen (paracetamol)

1. Analgesic and antipyretic with no anti-inflammatory properties. Acetaminophen is well absorbed by mouth and, less predictably, rectally. It is conjugated in the liver and excreted in urine. Half-life is about 4 hours.

2. Dosage: Oral loading dose is 24 mg/kg followed by a maintenance dose of 12 mg/kg orally every 4 hours (every 8 hours in babies <32 weeks gestational age [GA]). Consider measuring plasma levels if regular dosage is continued at this level for more than 24 hours (pain relief requires a level of 12 to 24 mg/L). Rectal administration is less predictable, but a loading dose of 36 mg/kg followed by a maintenance dose of 24 mg/kg every 8 hours is suitable for a term baby.

II. Bronchodilators and Respiratory Stimulants

A. Aminophylline/theophylline

1. An effective remedy for apnea of prematurity, although caffeine is easier and safer to use. Toxic effects include tachycardia, hyperactivity, and seizures. Therapeutic ranges for treatment of apnea of prematurity are 7 to 12 µg/mL and for treatment of bronchospasm in older infants are 10 to 20 µg/mL.

2. Dosage: A loading dose of 6 mg/kg followed by 2.5 to 3.5 mg/kg IV every 12 hours will generally abolish apnea of prematurity in most babies. Treatment can be continued with oral theophylline. A loading dose of 9 mg/kg is followed by 4 mg/kg every 12 hours.

B. Caffeine

1. Caffeine is the drug of choice for the treatment of apnea of prematurity for many clinicians. It has a wider safe therapeutic range than the theophyllines, is well absorbed by mouth, and only needs to be given once daily. It is most commonly given as caffeine *citrate,* 1 mg of which is equivalent to 0.5 mg of caffeine *base.* Doses are usually quoted as doses of the citrate.

2. Dosage: Give a loading dose of 20 mg/kg of caffeine citrate orally or IV, followed by a once-daily dose of 5 mg/kg. Both the loading dose and the maintenance dose can be safely doubled if necessary.

C. Albuterol (U.S.)/salbutamol (U.K.)

1. Selective β_2-adrenergic agonist, bronchodilator. Half-life in adults is 6 hours. Side effects include tachycardia, tremor, and irritability. It is well absorbed orally.

2. Dosage: 100 to 500 µg/kg nebulized 4 to 8 times daily, or 100 to 300 µg/kg orally 3 to 4 times daily.

D. Ipratropium: An anticholinergic bronchodilator synergistic with β-agonists. This is a synthetic derivative of atropine, given as 125 µg nebulized, every 6 to 8 hours.

E. Epinephrine (for stridor)

1. Direct-acting sympathomimetic agent with a more marked effect on β-adrenoreceptors than on α-adrenoreceptors.

      2. Can be used (nebulized) to treat stridor.

      3. Dosage: 50 to 100 µg/kg prn.

III. Diuretics

  A. Bumetanide (U.K.)

      1. Loop diuretic more potent than furosemide and with similar mechanism of action.

      2. Causes significant urinary losses of sodium, chloride, calcium, and bicarbonate.

      3. Half-life in newborns is 2 to 6 hours.

      4. Dosage: 5 to 50 µg/kg q6h IV, IM, or orally.

  B. Chlorothiazide

      1. Benzothiazide diuretic usefully combined with spironolactone for additional effect. This is probably the safest diuretic combination for long-term control of fluid retention in congestive cardiac failure and chronic lung disease (CLD) in the newborn, although it can result in considerable urinary calcium losses.

      2. Dosage: 10 mg/kg (usually combined with 1 mg/kg of spironolactone) orally twice daily. This dose can be safely doubled and even quadrupled (with careful monitoring). Potassium supplements usually are not needed if both drugs are given together.

  C. Furosemide

      1. A loop diuretic which inhibits active chloride reabsorption in the loop of Henle and the distal tubule, resulting in reduced passive sodium reabsorption and diuresis. Side effects include significant urinary losses of sodium, chloride, potassium, bicarbonate, and calcium. Furosemide stimulates renal synthesis of prostaglandin E_2 and may increase the risk of patent ductus arteriosus. It is ototoxic and enhances the ototoxic effect of aminoglycosides. Chronic use may cause nephrolithiasis or nephrocalcinosis. There is some evidence for a direct effect improving lung function in CLD if nebulized furosemide is given.

      2. Dosage

        a. 1 mg/kg IV or 2 mg/kg orally given once or twice a day. Patients on long-term treatment should receive potassium chloride to prevent hypokalemia.

        b. In renal failure, a single 5 mg/kg dose may help to reduce ischemic tubular damage.

        c. In infants with CLD, 1 mg/kg of the IV preparation diluted in 2 mL of 0.9% saline and given by nebulizer once every 6 hours may improve pulmonary compliance without affecting renal function.

  D. Spironolactone

      1. Competitive inhibitor of aldosterone, resulting in potassium-sparing diuresis. Spironolactone usually is used in combination with a thiazide diuretic such as chlorothiazide.

      2. Dosage: 1 mg/kg orally twice daily (combined with chlorothiazide, 10 mg/kg twice daily). Up to 4 mg/kg every 24 hours may be safely used, if necessary, but should be closely monitored.

IV. Inotropes (see also hydrocortisone)
   A. Dobutamine
      1. A synthetic inotropic catecholamine with primarily β_1-adrenergic activity, but in high doses it exhibits both α and β_2 effects. It stimulates myocardial contractility and increases cardiac output. Because it has less effect than dopamine on systemic vascular resistance, dobutamine has less effect in raising blood pressure (however, effectively increasing tissue perfusion is likely to be a more important goal than reaching a specific blood pressure target). Tachycardia may occur at high dosage, and tissue ischemia may occur if the infusion infiltrates.
      2. Dosage: Start with a dose of 5 µg/kg/min by continuous IV infusion, increasing to 10 to 20 µg if needed. Do not give bicarbonate or other alkaline solutions through the same line, as this will inactivate dobutamine. Never administer through an arterial catheter.
   B. Dopamine
      1. A naturally occurring catecholamine precursor of noradrenaline
      2. Dosage: Generally speaking, at low doses (2 to 5 µg/kg/min), dopamine causes coronary, mesenteric, and renal vasodilation (although it is questionable whether this is of clinical significance), whereas at high doses (6 to 15 µg/kg/min) it causes vasoconstriction. It is best given via a central vein and it is inactivated by bicarbonate and other alkaline solutions. Never administer through an arterial catheter.
   C. Milrinone
      1. A selective phosphodiesterase inhibitor that seems to work by increasing cyclic AMP concentration. It acts as an inotrope but also has some vasodilator action, resulting in increased cardiac output. Use only for short periods, because long-term oral use in adults was associated with an unexplained increase in mortality. The volume of distribution in infancy is much higher than in adults; thus it is necessary to use a loading dose.
      2. Dosage: A standard regime is 60 µg/kg IV over 15 minutes, followed by 0.5 µg/kg/min for 15 minutes, followed by 0.25 µg/kg/min for up to 2 days. Coinjection with furosemide will cause precipitation.
   D. Noradrenaline (norepinephrine)
      1. Sympathomimetic vasoconstrictor. Mainly causes increase in cardiac contractility, heart rate, and myocardial oxygen consumption (β_1 stimulation). High-dose infusion can also increase peripheral vasoconstriction (α_1 stimulation), resulting in significantly increased cardiac after-load and a decrease in cardiac output.
      2. Dosage calls for careful judgment. Give 0.1 µg/kg/min of noradrenaline base via a central vein. This may be increased to a maximum of 1.5 µg/kg/min as long as limb perfusion and urine output are carefully monitored. Never administer through an arterial catheter.

    E. Adrenaline (epinephrine)
      1. Direct-acting sympathomimetic agent with a more marked effect on β-adrenoceptors than on α-adrenoceptors. Adrenaline is used in the treatment of cardiac arrest secondary to electromechanical dissociation or as an infusion to treat serious hypotension (although this may cause significant vasoconstriction and is likely to affect renal perfusion).
      2. Dosage
        a. For cardiac arrest: 10 to 100 μg/kg IV, given by intracardiac, intratracheal, or intraosseous route.
        b. For hypotension: 0.1 to 0.3 μg/kg/min (maximum 1.5 μg/kg/min) IV.

V. Skeletal Muscle Relaxants
    A. Atracurium
      1. Atracurium besylate is a nondepolarizing competitive antagonist of acetylcholine at the motor end plate of voluntary muscle. Its effect can be reversed by anticholinesterases such as neostigmine. A major advantage is that it does not depend on either renal or hepatic function for degradation.
      2. Dosage: 500 μg/kg IV will cause complete paralysis lasting about 20 minutes. For sustained paralysis, give an infusion of 400 μg/kg/hr. Babies older than 1 month of age may require 500 μg/kg/hr.
    B. Pancuronium
      1. Pancuronium is a nondepolarizing competitive antagonist of acetylcholine similar to atracurium. This effect extends to autonomic cholinergic receptors as well as those in skeletal muscle. It is partially metabolized in the liver and excreted by the kidneys and has a variable duration of action in the newborn of the order of 2 to 4 hours. Its effects can be reversed with atropine and neostigmine.
      2. Dosage: Give 100 μg/kg to produce complete paralysis within a couple of minutes and adjust repeat doses (50 to 150 μg/kg), based on the duration of the observed effect.
    C. Suxamethonium (succinylcholine)
      1. Suxamethonium acts as a depolarizing competitive agonist of acetylcholine. Brief muscle contraction is seen before paralysis occurs. These contractions have been reported as painful by adults.
      2. Dosage: 2 mg/kg will provide paralysis for 5 to 10 minutes. A dose of atropine (15 μg/kg) is often given before any dose of suxamethonium and should certainly be given before a second dose.
    D. Vecuronium
      1. A nondepolarizing competitive antagonist of acetylcholine similar to pancuronium. It is metabolized by the liver and excreted in urine.
      2. Dosage: 30 to 150 μg/kg bolus will cause complete paralysis lasting 1 to 2 hours.

VI. Steroids
  A. Betamethasone
    1. A potent glucocorticoid given to mothers with threatening preterm birth prior to 34 weeks GA in order to encourage fetal lung development.
    2. Dosage: Give the mother 12 mg IM and repeat once after 24 hours.
  B. Dexamethasone
    1. A potent glucocorticoid similar to betamethasone. It is used in similar fashion to encourage fetal lung development, although some evidence suggests that it is less effective at enhancing fetal lung development. Although it appears to be beneficial in treating severe cases of CLD, the ideal treatment regimen has not yet been established, and high-dose treatment in the neonatal period appears to be associated with high levels of cerebral palsy in survivors. Treatment of babies with dexamethasone causes increased protein catabolism, which affects growth. Hypercalcuria, hypertension, hyperglycemia, gastrointestinal hemorrhage, left ventricular outflow tract obstruction, hypokalemia, and increased risk of infection are other well-recognized adverse effects.
    2. Dosage
      a. Traditional regimen: 250 µg/kg base orally or IV twice daily for 7 days, followed if necessary by a 9-day course of tapering dosage.
      b. Durand regimen: 100 µg/kg orally or IV twice daily for 3 days, then 50 µg/kg twice daily for 4 days.
      c. DART Trial regimen: 60 µg/kg orally or IV twice daily on days 1 to 3, then 40 µg/kg twice daily on days 4 to 6, 20 µg/kg twice daily on days 7 and 8, and 8 µg/kg on days 9 and 10.
      d. Postintubation airway edema: 200 µg/kg orally or IV at 8-hour intervals starting 4 hours before extubation.
  C. Hydrocortisone
    1. Glucocorticoid with minimal mineralocorticoid effect. It is used primarily for physiologic replacement but can also be useful in the treatment of acute hypotension.
    2. Dosage
      a. Standard replacement treatment requires a dose of 6 to 9 mg/m^2/day. Three times this dose may be needed during acute illness. Start with 1 to 2 mg orally every 8 hours.
      b. Doses of 2 mg/kg IV followed by 1 mg/kg IV every 8 to 12 hours are effective in treating hypotension.
VII. Sedatives
  A. Chloral hydrate
    1. Well absorbed orally, metabolized in the liver, and excreted in urine. This sedative acts within 30 minutes; half-life of active metabolite is 36 hours.
    2. Dosage
      a. 45 mg/kg as a single dose. Higher doses (75 mg/kg) have been used for sedation for imaging but can produce hypoxemia.

       b. 30 mg/kg orally every 6 hours can be helpful in babies with cerebral irritability. Drug accumulation may occur if used for more than 48 hours.

  B. Midazolam

    1. Benzodiazepine anxiolytic and sedative. Midazolam is metabolized in the liver and excreted in urine. Drug accumulation may occur with repeated doses. IV infusion or rapid bolus dosage has been reported to produce seizures in some babies.

    2. Dosage

      a. 150 µg/kg IV, IM, or intranasally produces rapid sedation and can be used for induction of anesthesia. (Midazolam does not relieve pain.)

      b. 100 µg/kg IV may be used for sedation prior to elective intubation (together with morphine for pain relief and atracurium for paralysis).

      c. 10 to 60 µg/kg/hr IV can be used for sedation of ventilated babies for 3 to 4 days. This dose should be halved after the first day for babies <33 weeks GA to prevent accumulation.

VIII. Pulmonary Vasodilators

  A. Nitric oxide

    1. Given as a gas by inhalation. Nitric oxide acts on receptors within the muscle of blood vessel walls to produce vasodilation. It is *rapidly* inactivated by hemoglobin, producing methemoglobin. Half-life is <5 seconds. Vasodilator effect is therefore limited to the pulmonary circulation. Methemoglobin levels need to be monitored and kept below 2.5%.

    2. Dosage: In term babies and those more than 34 weeks GA, start at 20 parts per million (ppm). If this produces a rise in postductal PaO_2 of at least 20 mm Hg (3 kPa) with no alteration in ventilator settings, reduce the concentration to the lowest compatible with a sustained response, usually 5 ppm. Stop treatment quickly if there is no response. Once started on nitric oxide, babies are extremely sensitive to any interruption in supply.

  B. Tolazoline

    1. Vasodilator affecting both pulmonary and systemic vessels with an α-adrenergic-blocking effect. Tolazoline seems to work best when severe acidosis has been corrected. It is cardiotoxic in high dosage and accumulates in renal failure.

    2. Dosage

      a. 1 to 2 mg/kg given as a rapid bolus ideally into a *peripheral or central vein that drains into the superior vena cava*. If a positive response is seen, an infusion of 200 µg/kg/hr may be helpful. May result in severe systemic hypotension.

      b. 200 µg/kg given as an intratracheal bolus instillation has been reported anecdotally to be effective.

    3. No longer available in the U.S.

Suggested Reading

Hey E (ed): Neonatal Formulary, 4th ed. London, BMJ Books, 2003. (www.neonatalformulary.com)

Young TE, Mangum OB (eds): A Manual of Drugs Used in Neonatal Care, 11th ed. Raleigh, NC, Acorn Publishing, 1998.

62

Sedation and Analgesia

Elaine M. Boyle and Neil McIntosh

I. Definitions
  A. Stress: Normal adaptive physiologic response generated by certain external stimuli. There may be no conscious awareness and thus no associated suffering.
  B. Distress: Suffering or maladaptive behavior resulting from emotional effects of excessive stress that may be affected by past experience. In newborn infants, an observer infers this from behavioral cues (Table 62-1).
  C. Pain: Particular form of distress, related by the adult as a hurtful experience or emotion.
  D. Nociception: Behavioral and physiologic effects of a noxious stimulus independent of associated psychological and emotional responses. This most accurately describes neonatal "pain".
II. Indicators of Pain in the Newborn
  A. Behavioral
    1. Cry (not applicable to intubated infants)
    2. Facial expression (brow bulge, eye squeeze, nasolabial furrowing, mouth or lip purse, tongue tautness, chin quiver)
    3. Withdrawal of affected limb
    4. Changes in tone (general increase in activity, flexion of trunk and extremities, "fetal" posturing or arching, leg extension, finger splaying, or fisting)
    5. Sleep cycle disturbances accompanied by twitches, jerks, irregular breathing, grimaces, or whimpers
    6. Self-regulatory or comforting behaviors such as lowered behavioral state, postural changes, hand-to-mouth movements, sucking, and expression of "focused alertness"
  B. Physiologic
    1. Increase in heart rate
    2. Increase in blood pressure
    3. Changes in respiratory rate
    4. Changes in oxygenation
    5. Fluctuations in skin color and temperature
    6. Increase in palmar sweating after 37 weeks' gestation
    7. Swings in cerebral circulation and intracranial pressure
    8. Gastrointestinal disturbances
III. Assessment of Pain or Distress
  A. General

TABLE 62-1. Potential Causes of Distress in the Newborn Infant

1. Ventilation

Endotracheal intubation

Presence of endotracheal tube and fixation devices

Distress of mandatory ventilator breaths

Restriction of movement and posture required for ventilation

2. Repeated Acute Invasive Procedures

Endotracheal suctioning

Arterial/venous/capillary blood sampling

Venipuncture

3. Minor Surgical Procedures

Chest drain insertion

Suprapubic aspiration of urine

Lumbar puncture

Ventricular tap

4. Coexisting Infective/Inflammatory Conditions

Necrotizing enterocolitis

Osteomyelitis

Meningitis

Generalized sepsis

5. Complications of Necessary Procedures

Cellulitis or abscess from infiltrated intravenous infusion

Cutaneous probe burns

6. Postoperative Following Major Surgery

Patent ductus arteriosus ligation

Laser therapy for retinopathy of prematurity

Bowel repair/resection following perforation or necrotizing enterocolitis

7. Disruptive Handling

Positioning for radiographs

(Continued)

TABLE **62-1.** Potential Causes of Distress in the Newborn Infant–Cont'd

Ultrasound scans
General caregiving procedures
8. Environmental Stress
Excessive light, either daylight or from phototherapy
Excessive and distressing sound of monitor alarms, incubator doors, etc.
Unfamiliar tactile environment without physical containment
9. Physiologic Stress
Drug withdrawal
Respiratory insufficiency/air hunger
Nutritional (i.e., hunger)
10. Repeated Relatively Noninvasive Procedures
Transcutaneous gas monitoring probe changes
Bolus feeds
Drug administration
Blood pressure measurement using inflatable cuff

    1. Acute distress: Based largely on behavioral or physiologic measures
    2. Subacute distress: Difficult to assess
        a. Increased activity or "thrashing"
        b. "Frozen" or withdrawn behavior
  B. Specific
    1. Clinical tools (Table 62-2)
        a. Neonatal facial coding system
        b. Premature infant pain profile
    2. Research tools
        a. Neuroendocrine markers (cortisol, adrenaline, endorphins)
        b. Metabolic-biochemical markers of catabolism (3-methylhistidine)
        c. Computerized analysis of physiologic data (e.g., vagal
           tone changes)
  C. Pain assessment in ventilated or preterm infants
    1. Behavioral responses are modified by:
        a. Prematurity
        b. State of arousal
        c. Severity of illness.
    2. Habituation to subacute pain or stress occurs.
    3. True audible cry is not possible.

Table 62-2. Validated Pain Assessment Scores for Use in the Newborn

I. Neonatal Facial Coding System (NFCS) (Grunau and Craig, 1987)

Facial response to heel-stick (i.e., acute and obvious pain) in different sleep-wake states. The following 10 features are scored:
1. Brow bulge
2. Eye squeeze
3. Nasolabial furrow
4. Open lips
5. Vertical stretch mouth
6. Horizontal mouth
7. Lip purse
8. Tongue taut
9. Chin quiver
10. Tone exaggeration with startling or twitching

II. Premature Infant Pain Profile (PIPP) (Stevens et al, 1996)

Process	Indicator	0	1	2	3	Score
Chart	Gestational age	≥36 wk	32-35 wk	28-31 wk	≤28 wk	
Observe infant for 15 sec	Behavior/state	Active/awake Eyes open Facial movements	Quiet/awake Eyes open No facial movements	Active/asleep Eyes closed Facial movements	Quiet/asleep Eyes closed No facial movements	
Observe baseline heart rate	Heart rate Max ___	0-4 BPM Increase	5-14 BPM Increase	15-24 BPM Increase	≥25 BPM Increase	
Observe baseline SaO$_2$	SaO$_2$ Min ___	0-2.4% Decrease	2.5-4.9% Decrease	5.0-7.4% Decrease	≥7.5% Increase	
Observe infant for 30 sec	Brow bulge	None 0-9% of time	Minimum 10-39% of time	Moderate 49-69% of time	Maximum 70% of time or more	
	Eye squeeze	None 0-9% of time	Minimum 10-39% of time	Moderate 49-69% of time	Maximum 70% of time or more	
	Nasolabial furrow	None 0-9% of time	Minimum 10-39% of time	Moderate 49-69% of time	Maximum 70% of time or more	

4. Endotracheal tube or other respiratory support alters facial expression.
5. Monitoring and infusions change posture and restrict movement.
6. Agitation or distress may be secondary to a process other than pain (e.g., respiratory insufficiency, drug withdrawal).

IV. Aims of Management
   A. Sedation (Table 62-3)
   B. Analgesia
   C. Physiologic stability
   D. Decrease in ventilator asynchrony in ventilated infants

V. Nonpharmacologic Interventions
   A. Environmental measures
     1. Control of light, temperature, and noise
     2. Positioning and physical containment
   B. Behavioral measures
     1. Non-nutritive sucking
     2. Sucrose
       a. Effects mediated by sweet taste
       b. Only effective by oral route
       c. Administer 2 minutes before procedure
       d. Dose: 0.5 to 1 mL sucrose (24%)

VI. Pharmacologic Interventions
   A. Opioids
     1. Reduce endocrine stress response.
     2. Reduce asynchronous respiration during ventilation (sedative effect).
     3. Produce physiologic stability.
     4. Side effects
       a. Hypotension
       b. Respiratory depression
       c. Bronchospasm (theoretical)
       d. Decreased gut motility
       e. Chest wall rigidity (caused by stimulation of excitatory pathways in spinal cord; give boluses slowly)
       f. Withdrawal: Wean gradually if given for more than 5 days. Late rebound respiratory depression may occur from enterohepatic recirculation or release from fat stores.
     5. Specific agents
       a. Morphine sulfate
         (1) Most widely used
         (2) Loading dose: 100 to 150 μg/kg over 30 minutes
         (3) Maintenance: 10 to 20 μg/kg/hr
         (4) Dose for procedures: 50 to 100 μg/kg over 30 minutes (higher doses may be needed)
       b. Fentanyl
         (1) Less histaminic effect than morphine
         (2) Tends to reduce pulmonary vascular resistance; may be preferable in persistent pulmonary hypertension of the newborn (PPHN), congenital diaphragmatic hernia (CDH), and chronic lung disease (CLD)

TABLE 62-3. Use of Analgesics and Sedatives

Relatively Minor Procedures		
Procedure	Comment	Suggested Approach
Heel prick	Affected by technique and heel perfusion; EMLA is not effective	Automated lances; pacifier/sucrose; avoid EMLA
Vein and arterial puncture		Pacifier/sucrose; topical anesthetic cream
Suprapubic urine aspiration		Pacifier/sucrose; topical anesthetic cream
Insertion of nasogastric tube	Discomfort with gag, vagal reflex	Insert slowly

Moderate/Major Procedures		
Procedure	Issues	Suggested Approach
Lumbar puncture	Pain or skin puncture Stress of restraint	Pacifier/sucrose; topical anesthetic Correct positioning/technique; lidocaine infiltration of skin (avoid deep infiltration because of risk of spinal injection); consider opiate if infant is ventilated
Chest drain insertion	Skin, muscle, pleural pain	Opiate—slow bolus; lidocaine infiltration of skin and pleura—if time
Chest drain (in situ)		Opiate infusion if infant is distressed
Ventricular tap	Pain of skin penetration	Topical anesthetic; consider opiate if infant is ventilated
Elective intubation	Discomfort; gag/cough; vagal reflex	Opiate—slow bolus with muscle relaxant
Laser/cryotherapy for retinopathy of prematurity	Discomfort/restraint Eyeball pain Vagal reflex (Reestablish full monitoring before procedure)	Ventilation Oxybuprocaine eye drops Topical anesthesia Opiate loading and infusion or inhaled anesthetic before intubation Muscle relaxant to abolish eye and other movements (after intubation) Atropine to prevent bradycardia (intubation, oculocardiac reflex)

EMLA, eutectic mixture of lidocaine and prilocaine as 5% cream.

415

and during extracorporeal membrane oxygenation (ECMO)
- (3) Large doses are tolerated without adverse hemodynamic effects
- (4) Chest wall rigidity if given quickly
- (5) Loading dose: 5 to 15 μg/kg over 30 minutes
- (6) Maintenance: 1 to 5 μg/kg/hr

6. Weaning
  a. Depends on duration of treatment.
  b. Signs of withdrawal
     (1) Irritability
     (2) Inconsolable cry
     (3) Tachypnea
     (4) Jitteriness
     (5) Hypertonicity
     (6) Vomiting
     (7) Diarrhea
     (8) Sweating
     (9) Skin abrasions
     (10) Seizures
     (11) Yawning
     (12) Nasal stuffiness
     (13) Sneezing
     (14) Hiccups
  c. If treatment has been given for:
     (1) <48 hours, stop without weaning.
     (2) 3 to 7 days, reduce maintenance dose by 25% to 50% daily.
     (3) >7 days, reduce by dose by 10% to 20% every 6 to 12 hours as tolerated.

B. Nonopioids
  1. Acetaminophen (paracetamol)
     a. Analgesic and antipyretic. Analgesia is additive to opioid effect.
     b. Newborns are relatively resistant to liver toxicity with no respiratory or cardiovascular depression, gastrointestinal irritation, or platelet dysfunction.
     c. Is useful in inflammatory pain.
     d. Dosage
        (1) Oral: 10 to 15 mg/kg q4-6hr (may load with 24 mg/kg)
        (2) Rectal: 20 to 25 mg/kg q4-6hr (maximum daily dose 60 mg/kg)
  2. Ibuprofen
     a. Nonsteroidal anti-inflammatory drug (NSAID)
     b. Recommended dose as for ductal closure (no information available regarding analgesic dose): 10 mg IV/PO, then 5 to 10 mg q24hr

C. Sedative drugs
  1. Adjuvants to analgesic, but no pain relief
  2. Useful for long-term ventilation

3. Useful when tolerance to opioids develops
4. May allow weaning from opioids
5. May help older babies with severe CLD
6. Specific agents
   a. Midazolam
     (1) Benzodiazepine
     (2) IV bolus for procedures, infusion for background sedation
     (3) Respiratory depression and hypotension; synergistic with opioids
     (4) Withdrawal (agitation, abnormal movements, depressed sensorium) after prolonged use
     (5) Loading dose: 0.15 to 0.2 mg/kg over 30 minutes
     (6) Maintenance: 0.4 μg/kg/hr
   b. Chloral hydrate
     (1) Causes generalized neuronal depression
     (2) Does not appear to produce respiratory depression
     (3) May be given orally or rectally
     (4) Onset of action in 30 minutes, duration 2 to 4 hours
     (5) Slow development of tolerance
     (6) Dosage
       (a) Sedation: 25 to 50 mg/kg
       (b) Hypnosis: Up to 100 mg/kg

D. Local anesthetics
  1. Lidocaine
    a. Infiltrates skin/mucous membranes.
    b. 0.5% solution; maximum dose is 1.0 mL/kg.
    c. With overdosage, systemic absorption may cause sedation, cardiac arrhythmia, cardiac arrest, and seizures.
  2. Topical anesthetic creams
    a. Apply pea-sized amount of lidocaine with occlusive dressing 30 to 60 minutes before procedure.
    b. An alternative is EMLA (eutectic mixture of lidocaine and prilocaine as 5% cream).
     (1) Vasoconstrictor
     (2) Minimal risk of methemoglobinemia
    c. Amethocaine (Ametop) (less vasoconstriction)

VII. Experience of Pain in the Newborn
  A. The preterm infant
    1. Increased sensitivity to pain (reduced pain threshold)
    2. Development of hypersensitivity as a result of repeated tissue damage
    3. Hyperalgesia
     a. More pain neurotransmitters in spinal cord
     b. Delayed expression of inhibitory neurotransmitters
    4. Higher plasma concentrations of analgesic and anesthetic agents are required to obtain clinical effects, compared with older age groups
    5. Nonpainful handling (e.g., caregiving) may activate pain pathways and be experienced as chronic pain (wind-up)

B. Sources of pain and distress
  1. Painful conditions
    a. Necrotizing enterocolitis
      (1) Low threshold for analgesia
      (2) Intravenous treatment needed
      (3) NSAIDs contraindicated (gastrointestinal side effects)
    b. Meningitis/osteomyelitis
      (1) Consider morphine if baby is distressed.
      (2) Acetaminophen/paracetamol to relieve pain, fever
  2. Ventilation
    a. Use environmental and behavioral measures.
    b. Generally consider morphine only if baby is still obviously distressed or for painful procedures.
    c. Beware of hypotension with morphine use in extremely preterm infants.
  3. Medical/surgical procedures (see Table 62-3)
C. Short-term consequences of pain and inadequate analgesia
  1. Acute pain
    a. Behavioral and physiologic changes (see Sections IIA and IIB) to limit the duration of "protest" against painful experience.
    b. These changes involve great energy expenditure.
  2. Continuing (i.e., chronic) pain: The body reorients its behavioral and physiologic expression of pain to conserve energy and expresses "despair."
    a. Passivity
    b. Little or no body movement
    c. Expressionless face
    d. Decreased variability in heart rate and respiration
    e. Decreased oxygen consumption
VIII. Clinical Implications of Pain or Inadequate Analgesia
  A. Responses to pain may be extreme enough to have an adverse effect on clinical state. Some experimental evidence:
    1. Short-term consequences
      a. Frequent invasive procedures soon after birth in the extremely immature infant may contribute to physiologic instability.
      b. Cardiac surgery causes extreme metabolic responses. Clinical outcome can be improved by analgesia—there is a reduced incidence of postoperative sepsis, metabolic acidosis, disseminated intravascular coagulation, and death.
      c. Circumcision without analgesia in term baby boys causes increased irritability, decreased attentiveness and orientation, poor regulation of behavioral state and motor patterns, and altered sleep and feeding patterns lasting for up to 7 days.
      d. Babies born at 28 weeks' gestation, compared with those born at 32 weeks' gestation, show reduced behavioral and increased cardiovascular responsiveness at 4 weeks of age. The magnitude of the changes correlates with the total number of invasive procedures experienced.

  2. Long-term consequences
     a. Neonatal circumcision results in increased behavioral responses
        to vaccination at 4 to 6 months of age, which can be attenuated
        by the use of anesthetics.
     b. Stressful conditions at birth are associated with an increased
        cortisol response to vaccination at 4 to 6 months of age.
     c. Increased behavioral reactivity to heelstick sampling in term
        newborns correlates with increased distress to immunizations
        at 6 months of age.
     d. Ex-preterm infants showed increased somatization at $4\frac{1}{2}$ years
        of age. The strongest predictor was the duration of stay in
        neonatal intensive care.
B. Therapeutic interventions and outcome
  1. Analgesia
     a. Acute physiologic and behavioral changes can be attenuated
        with opioid analgesia.
     b. The routine use of morphine as "background" analgesia in
        preterm infants does not reduce, and may increase, the
        occurrence of intraventricular hemorrhage.
  2. Individualized developmental care
     a. Aims to minimize stress and pain and support
        neurobehavioral development.
     b. Has been suggested to reduce the incidence of intraventricular
        hemorrhage and lead to improved developmental outcomes,
        but further investigation is required.

Suggested Reading

Anand KJS, Hall RW, Desai N, et al: Effects of morphine analgesia in ventilated preterm neonates:
    Primary outcomes from the NEOPAIN randomised trial. Lancet 363:1673-1682, 2004.
Anand KJS, Menon G, Narsinghani U, McIntosh N: Systemic analgesic therapy. In Anand KJS,
    McGrath PJ (eds): Pain in Neonates, 2nd revised and enlarged edition. Pain Research and
    Clinical Management, Vol. 10. Amsterdam, Elsevier Science, 2000, pp 159-188.
Grunau RV, Johnston CC, Craig KD: Neonatal facial and cry responses to invasive and
    non-invasive procedures. Pain 42:295-305, 1990.
Johnston CC, Stevens B, Craig KD: Developmental changes in pain expression in premature,
    full-term, two and four month old infants. Pain 52:201-208, 1993.
Stevens B, Johnston C, Gibbins S: Pain assessment in neonates In Anand KJS, McGrath PJ (eds):
    Pain in Neonates, 2nd revised and enlarged edition. Pain Research and Clinical Management,
    Vol. 10. Amsterdam, Elsevier Science, 2000, pp 101-134.
Stevens B, Ohlsson A: Sucrose for analgesia in newborn infants undergoing painful procedures.
    Cochrane Database Syst Rev CD001069, 2000.

63

Inhaled Nitric Oxide Therapy

John P. Kinsella

I. Introduction
   A. Inhaled nitric oxide (iNO) therapy for the treatment of newborns with hypoxemic respiratory failure and pulmonary hypertension has dramatically changed management strategies for this critically ill population.
   B. iNO therapy causes potent, selective, and sustained pulmonary vasodilation and improves oxygenation in term newborns with severe hypoxemic respiratory failure and persistent pulmonary hypertension.
   C. Multicenter randomized clinical studies have demonstrated that iNO therapy reduces the need for extracorporeal membrane oxygenation (ECMO) treatment in term neonates with hypoxemic respiratory failure.
   D. The potential role of iNO in the preterm newborn is currently controversial and its use remains investigational in this population.

II. Rationale for iNO Therapy
   A. The physiologic rationale for iNO therapy in the treatment of neonatal hypoxemic respiratory failure is based upon its ability to achieve potent and sustained pulmonary vasodilation without decreasing systemic vascular tone.
   B. Persistent pulmonary hypertension of the newborn (PPHN) is a syndrome associated with diverse neonatal cardiac and pulmonary disorders that are characterized by high pulmonary vascular resistance (PVR) causing extrapulmonary right-to-left shunting of blood across the ductus arteriosus and/or foramen ovale (see Chapter 51).
   C. Extrapulmonary shunting from high PVR in severe PPHN can cause critical hypoxemia, which is poorly responsive to inspired oxygen or pharmacologic vasodilation.
   D. Vasodilator drugs administered intravenously, such as tolazoline and sodium nitroprusside, are often unsuccessful because of systemic hypotension and an inability to achieve or sustain pulmonary vasodilation.
   E. The ability of iNO therapy to selectively lower PVR and decrease extrapulmonary venoarterial admixture accounts for the acute improvement in oxygenation observed in infants with PPHN.
   F. Oxygenation can also improve during iNO therapy in some newborns who do not have extrapulmonary right-to-left shunting. Hypoxemia in these cases is primarily the result of intrapulmonary shunting caused by continued perfusion of lung units that lack ventilation (e.g., atelectasis), with variable contributions from ventilation-perfusion

(V/Q) inequality. Low-dose iNO therapy can also improve oxygenation by redirecting blood from poorly aerated or diseased lung regions to better-aerated distal airspaces ("microselective effect").

G. The clinical benefits of low-dose iNO therapy may include reduced lung inflammation and edema, as well as potential protective effects on surfactant function, but these effects remain clinically unproven.

H. The diagnostic value of iNO therapy is also important in that failure to respond to iNO raises important questions about the specific mechanism of hypoxemia. Poor responses to iNO should lead to further diagnostic evaluation for "unsuspected" anatomic cardiovascular or pulmonary disease.

III. Evaluation of the Cyanotic Term Newborn for iNO Therapy

A. History

1. Assess the primary cause of hypoxemia. Marked hypoxemia in the newborn can be caused by lung parenchymal disease with intrapulmonary shunting, pulmonary vascular disease causing extrapulmonary right-to-left shunting, or anatomic right-to-left shunting associated with congenital heart disease.

2. Assessment of risk factors for hypoxemic respiratory failure

a. Prenatal ultrasound studies

(1) Lesions such as diaphragmatic hernia and cystic adenomatoid formation are frequently diagnosed prenatally.

(2) Although many anatomic congenital heart diseases can be diagnosed prenatally, vascular abnormalities (e.g., coarctation, anomalous pulmonary venous return) are more difficult to diagnose.

(3) In the newborn with cyanosis, a history of a structurally normal heart on fetal ultrasonography should be confirmed with echocardiography.

3. Maternal historical information

a. History of severe and prolonged oligohydramnios causing pulmonary hypoplasia.

b. Prolonged fetal brady- and tachyarrhythmias and marked anemia (caused by hemolysis, twin-twin transfusion, or chronic hemorrhage) may cause congestive heart failure, pulmonary edema, and respiratory distress.

c. Maternal illness (e.g., diabetes mellitus), medications (e.g., aspirin causing premature constriction of the ductus arteriosus, association of Ebstein anomaly with maternal lithium use), and drug use may contribute to disordered transition and cardiopulmonary distress in the newborn.

d. Risk factors for infection causing sepsis/pneumonia should also be considered, including premature or prolonged rupture of membranes, fetal tachycardia, maternal leukocytosis, uterine tenderness, and other signs of intra-amniotic infection.

4. Events at delivery

      a. If positive pressure ventilation is required in the delivery room, the risk of pneumothorax increases.

      b. History of meconium-stained amniotic fluid, particularly if meconium is present below the cords, should raise the suspicion of meconium aspiration syndrome (MAS) (see Chapter 50).

      c. Birth trauma (e.g., clavicular fracture and phrenic nerve injury) or acute fetomaternal/fetoplacental hemorrhage may also cause respiratory distress in the newborn.

B. Physical examination

  1. The initial physical examination provides important clues to the etiology of cyanosis (see Chapter 11).

  2. Marked respiratory distress in the newborn (retractions, grunting, nasal flaring) suggests the presence of pulmonary parenchymal disease with decreased lung compliance.

  3. Recognize that airways disease (e.g., tracheobronchomalacia) and metabolic acidemia can also cause severe respiratory distress.

  4. In contrast, the newborn with cyanosis alone ("nondistressed tachypnea") typically has cyanotic congenital heart disease (most commonly transposition of the great vessels) or idiopathic PPHN.

C. Interpretation of pulse oximetry measurements

  1. Right-to-left shunting across the ductus arteriosus causes postductal desaturation.

  2. Interpretation of preductal (right hand) and postductal (lower extremity) saturation by pulse oximetry provides important clues to the etiology of hypoxemia in the newborn.

  3. If the measurements of pre- and postductal SaO_2 are equivalent, this suggests either that the ductus arteriosus is patent and pulmonary vascular resistance is subsystemic (i.e., the hypoxemia is caused by parenchymal lung disease with intrapulmonary shunting or cyanotic heart disease with ductal-dependent pulmonary blood flow), or that the ductus arteriosus is closed (precluding any interpretation of pulmonary artery pressure without echocardiography).

  4. It is exceptionally uncommon for the ductus arteriosus to close in the first hours of life in the presence of suprasytemic pulmonary artery pressures.

  5. When the postductal SaO_2 is lower than preductal SaO_2 (>5%), the most common cause is suprasystemic pulmonary vascular resistance in infants with PPHN, causing right-to-left shunting across the ductus arteriosus (associated with MAS, surfactant deficiency/dysfunction, congenital diaphragmatic hernia [CDH], pulmonary hypoplasia, or idiopathic).

  6. Duct-dependent systemic blood flow lesions (hypoplastic left heart syndrome, critical aortic stenosis, interrupted aortic arch, and coarctation) may also present with postductal desaturation.

  7. Anatomic pulmonary vascular disease (alveolar-capillary dysplasia, pulmonary venous stenosis, and anomalous venous return with obstruction) can cause suprasystemic pulmonary vascular

resistance with right-to-left shunting across the ductus arteriosus
and postductal desaturation.

8. The unusual occurrence of markedly lower preductal SaO_2
   compared with postductal measurements suggests one of two
   diagnoses: transposition of the great vessels with pulmonary
   hypertension or transposition with coarctation of the aorta.

D. Laboratory and radiologic evaluation

1. One of the most important tests to perform in the evaluation
   of the newborn with cyanosis is the chest radiograph.

2. The chest radiograph can demonstrate the classic findings
   of respiratory distress syndrome (RDS) (air bronchograms, diffuse
   granularity, and underinflation), MAS, and CDH.

3. The important question to ask when viewing the chest radiograph
   is whether the severity of hypoxemia is out of proportion to the
   radiographic changes. Marked hypoxemia despite supplemental
   oxygen in the absence of severe pulmonary parenchymal disease
   radiographically suggests the presence of an extrapulmonary right-
   to-left shunt (idiopathic PPHN or cyanotic heart disease).

4. Other essential measurements include an arterial blood gas to
   determine the blood gas tensions and pH, a complete blood
   count to evaluate for signs of infection, and blood pressure
   measurements in the right arm and a lower extremity to determine
   aortic obstruction (interrupted aortic arch, coarctation).

E. Response to supplemental oxygen (100% oxygen by hood, mask, or
endotracheal tube)

1. Marked improvement in SaO_2 (increase to 100%) with
   supplemental oxygen suggests an intrapulmonary shunt
   (lung disease) or reactive PPHN with vasodilation.

2. The response to mask continuous positive airway pressure (CPAP)
   is also a useful discriminator of severe lung disease and other causes
   of hypoxemia.

3. Most infants with PPHN have at least a transient improvement in
   oxygenation in response to interventions such as high inspired
   oxygen and/or mechanical ventilation. If the preductal SaO_2 never
   reaches 100%, the likelihood of cyanotic heart disease is high.

F. Echocardiography (see Chapter 22)

1. The definitive diagnosis in newborns with cyanosis and hypoxemic
   respiratory failure often requires echocardiography (Fig. 63-1).

2. The initial echocardiographic evaluation is important to rule out
   structural heart disease causing hypoxemia (e.g., coarctation of the
   aorta, total anomalous pulmonary venous return).

3. It is critically important to diagnose congenital heart lesions for
   which iNO treatment would be contraindicated.

4. Additional congenital heart diseases that can present with
   hypoxemia unresponsive to high inspired oxygen concentrations
   (e.g., dependent on right-to-left shunting across the ductus
   arteriosus) include critical aortic stenosis, interrupted aortic arch,
   and hypoplastic left heart syndrome. Decreasing PVR with iNO in

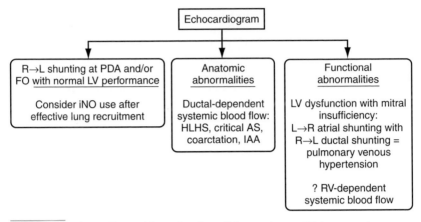

FIGURE 63-1. Echocardiographic evaluation of the newborn with hypoxemic respiratory failure. AS, aortic stenosis; FO, foramen ovale; HLHS, hypoplastic left heart syndrome; IAA, interrupted aortic arch; iNO, inhaled nitric oxide; L→R, left-to-right; LV, left ventricular; R→L, right-to-left; RV, right ventricle.

     these conditions could lead to systemic hypoperfusion and delay definitive diagnosis.

5. PPHN is defined by the echocardiographic determination of extrapulmonary venoarterial admixture (right-to-left shunting at the foramen ovale and/or ductus arteriosus), not simply by evidence of increased PVR.

6. Doppler measurements of atrial and ductal level shunts provide essential information when managing a newborn with hypoxemic respiratory failure.

7. Left-to-right shunting at the foramen ovale and ductus with marked hypoxemia suggests predominant intrapulmonary shunting, and interventions should be directed at optimizing lung inflation.

8. In the presence of severe left ventricular dysfunction and pulmonary hypertension, pulmonary vasodilation alone may be ineffective in improving oxygenation. The echocardiographic findings in this setting include right-to-left ductal shunting (caused by suprasystemic PVR) and mitral insufficiency with left-to-right atrial shunting.

IV. Candidates for iNO Therapy

    A. Several pathophysiologic disturbances contribute to hypoxemia in the newborn infant, including cardiac dysfunction, airway and pulmonary parenchymal abnormalities, and pulmonary vascular disorders (Fig. 63-2).

        1. In some newborns with hypoxemic respiratory failure, a single mechanism predominates (e.g., extrapulmonary right-to-left shunting in idiopathic PPHN), but more commonly, several of these mechanisms contribute to hypoxemia.

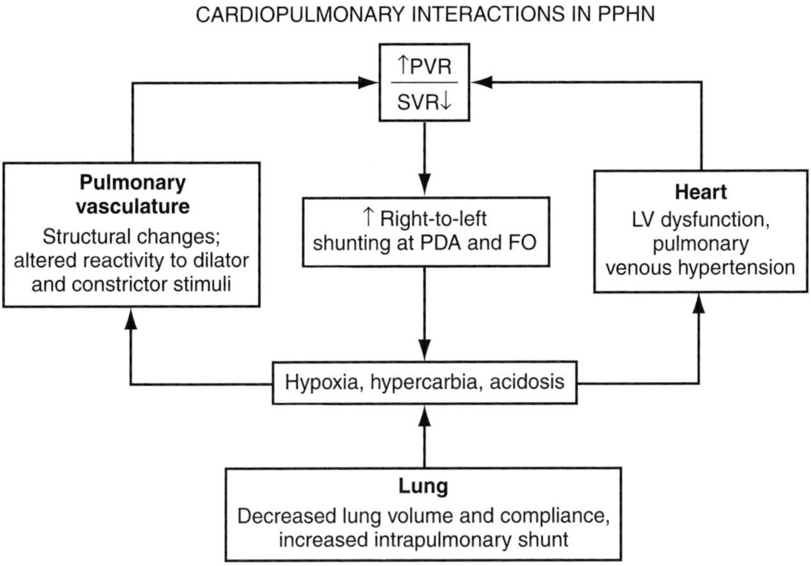

CARDIOPULMONARY INTERACTIONS IN PPHN

FIGURE 63-2. Cardiopulmonary interactions in persistent pulmonary hypertension of the newborn (PPHN). FO, Foramen ovale; LV, left ventricular; PDA, patent ductus arteriosus; PVR, pulmonary vascular resistance; SVR, systemic vascular resistance.

2. MAS represents the "perfect storm" of cardiopulmonary pathophysiology. Meconium may obstruct some airways, decreasing V/Q ratios and increasing intrapulmonary shunting. Other lung segments may be overventilated relative to perfusion and cause increased physiologic dead space. Moreover, the same patient may have severe pulmonary hypertension with extrapulmonary right-to-left shunting at the ductus arteriosus and foramen ovale, and left ventricular dysfunction.

3. The effects of iNO may be suboptimal when lung volume is decreased in association with pulmonary parenchymal disease. Atelectasis and airspace disease (pneumonia, pulmonary edema) will decrease effective delivery of iNO to its site of action in terminal lung units.

4. The effects of iNO on V/Q matching appear to be optimal at low doses (<20 ppm).

5. In cases complicated by homogeneous (diffuse) parenchymal lung disease and underinflation, pulmonary hypertension may be exacerbated because of the adverse mechanical effects of underinflation on PVR. In this setting, effective treatment of the underlying lung disease is essential (and sometimes sufficient) to cause resolution of the accompanying pulmonary hypertension.

B. Clinical criteria

1. Gestational and postnatal age
   a. Available evidence from clinical trials supports the use of iNO in near-term (>34 weeks' gestation) and term newborns.
   b. The use of iNO in infants <34 weeks' gestation remains investigational (see later).
   c. Clinical trials of iNO in newborns have incorporated ECMO treatment as an end point. Therefore, most patients have been enrolled in the first few days of life.
   d. Although one of the pivotal studies used to support a new drug application for iNO therapy included as an entry criterion a postnatal age up to 14 days, the average age at enrollment in that study was 1.7 days.
   e. Currently, clinical trials support the use of iNO before treatment with ECMO, usually within the first week of life.
   f. Clinical experience suggests that iNO may be of benefit as an adjuvant treatment after ECMO therapy in patients with sustained pulmonary hypertension (e.g., CDH). Postnatal age alone should not define the duration of therapy in cases in which prolonged treatment could be beneficial.
2. Severity of illness
   a. Studies support the use of iNO in infants who have hypoxemic respiratory failure with evidence of PPHN requiring mechanical ventilation and high inspired oxygen concentrations.
   b. The most common criterion employed has been the oxygenation index (OI). Although clinical trials commonly allowed for enrollment with an OI >25, the mean level at study entry in multicenter trials approximated 40.
   c. There is no evidence that starting iNO therapy at a lower OI (i.e., <25) reduces the need for treatment with ECMO.
   d. Current multicenter studies suggest that indications for treatment with iNO may include an OI >25 with echocardiographic evidence of extrapulmonary right-to-left shunting.

V. Treatment Strategies
   A. Dosage
      1. The first studies of iNO treatment in term newborns reported initial doses that as high as 80 ppm. Early laboratory and clinical studies established the boundaries of iNO dosing protocols for subsequent randomized clinical trials in newborns.
      2. Recommended starting dose for iNO in the term newborn is 20 ppm.
      3. Increasing the dose to 40 ppm does not generally improve oxygenation in infants who do not respond to the lower dose of 20 ppm.
      4. Although brief exposures to higher doses (40 to 80 ppm) appear to be safe, sustained treatment with 80 ppm of iNO increases the risk of methemoglobinemia.
   B. Duration of treatment
      1. In multicenter clinical trials, the typical duration of iNO treatment has been <5 days, which parallels the clinical resolution of persistent pulmonary hypertension.

2. Individual exceptions occur, particularly in cases of pulmonary hypoplasia.

3. If iNO is required for >5 days, investigations into other causes of pulmonary hypertension should be considered (e.g., alveolar capillary dysplasia), particularly if discontinuation of iNO results in suprasystemic elevations of pulmonary artery pressure by echocardiography.

4. Discontinue iNO if the FiO_2 is <0.60 and the PaO_2 is >60 mm Hg without evidence of rebound pulmonary hypertension or a >15% increase in FiO_2 after iNO withdrawal.

C. Weaning

1. After improvement in oxygenation occurs with the onset of iNO therapy, strategies for weaning the iNO dose become important.

2. Numerous approaches have been employed, and few differences have been noted until final discontinuation of iNO treatment.

3. In one study, iNO was reduced from 20 to 6 ppm after 4 hours of treatment without acute changes in oxygenation. In another trial, iNO was reduced in a stepwise fashion to as low as 1 ppm without changes in oxygenation.

D. Monitoring

1. Early experience suggested that careful monitoring of NO and NO_2 levels should be carried out using chemiluminescence devices.

2. It has now become clear that NO_2 levels remain low at delivered iNO doses within the recommended ranges.

3. The currently available systems use electrochemical cells and appear to be reliable when used appropriately.

4. Methemoglobinemia occurs after exposure to high concentrations of iNO (80 ppm). This complication has not been reported at lower doses of iNO (<20 ppm).

5. Because methemoglobin reductase deficiency may occur unpredictably, it is reasonable to measure methemoglobin levels by co-oximetry within 4 hours of starting iNO therapy, and subsequently at 24-hour intervals.

E. Ventilator management

1. Along with iNO treatment, other therapeutic strategies have emerged for the management of the term infant with hypoxemic respiratory failure.

2. Considering the important role of parenchymal lung disease in specific disorders included in the syndrome of PPHN, pharmacologic pulmonary vasodilation alone should not be expected to cause sustained clinical improvement in many cases.

3. Patients not responding to iNO can show marked improvement in oxygenation with adequate lung inflation alone.

4. In newborns with severe lung disease, high-frequency oscillatory ventilation (HFOV) is frequently used to optimize lung inflation and minimize lung injury.

5. In clinical pilot studies using iNO, the combination of HFOV and iNO caused the greatest improvement in oxygenation in some newborns who had severe pulmonary hypertension complicated by

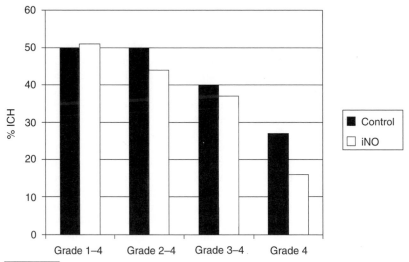

FIGURE 63-3. Incidence of intracranial hemorrhage (ICH) by grade in premature infants enrolled in a randomized, controlled trial of nitric oxide (iNO).

diffuse parencyhmal lung disease and underinflation (e.g., RDS, pneumonia).

6. A randomized, multicenter trial demonstrated that treatment with HFOV + iNO was often successful in infants with severe pulmonary hypertension who failed to respond to HFOV or iNO alone, and differences in responses were related to the specific disease associated with the various complex disorders (see Figure 63-2).

VI. The Preterm Newborn: Preliminary studies in human preterm infants with severe hypoxemic respiratory failure support the potential role of low-dose iNO as adjuvant therapy.

A. A pilot trial of iNO in preterm infants showed acute improvement in oxygenation after 60 minutes of treatment.

B. Survival to discharge was 52% in the iNO group and 47% in controls. Total ventilator days for survivors was less for the iNO group.

C. In contrast to uncontrolled pilot studies, there was no difference in the incidence of intracranial hemorrhage between the control and iNO treated groups (Fig. 63-3).

D. Low-dose iNO caused acute improvement in oxygenation in preterm newborns with severe hypoxemic respiratory failure, without increasing the risk of bleeding.

E. Currently, several multicenter clinical trials are underway to test the safety and efficacy of iNO in preterm newborns with respiratory failure.

F. At the present time, the use of iNO in preterm infants remains investigational.

Suggested Reading

Antunes MJ, Greenspan JS, Holt WJ, et al: Assessment of lung function pre-nitric oxide therapy: A predictor of response? Pediatr Res 35:212A, 1994.

Clark RH: High-frequency ventilation. J Pediatr 124:661-670, 1994.

Clark RH, Kueser TJ, Walker MW, et al: Low-dose inhaled nitric oxide treatment of persistent pulmonary hypertension of the newborn. N Engl J Med. 342:469-474, 2000.

Davidson D, Barefield ES, Kattwinkel J, et al: Inhaled nitric oxide for the early treatment of persistent pulmonary hypertension of the term newborn: A randomized, double-masked, placebo-controlled, dose-response, multicenter study. Pediatrics 101:325-334, 1998.

Davidson D, Barefield ES, Kattwinkel J, et al: Safety of withdrawing inhaled nitric oxide therapy in persistent pulmonary hypertension. Pediatrics 104:231-236, 1999.

Drummond WH, Gregory G, Heymann MA, Phibbs RA: The independent effects of hyperventilation, tolazoline, and dopamine on infants with persistent pulmonary hypertension. J Pediatr 98:603-611, 1981.

Gerlach H, Rossaint R, Pappert D, Falke KJ: Time-course and dose-response of nitric oxide inhalation for systemic oxygenation and pulmonary hypertension in patients with adult respiratory distress syndrome. Eur J Clin Invest 1993; 23:499-502, 1993.

Gersony WM: Neonatal pulmonary hypertension: Pathophysiology, classification and etiology. Clin Perinatol 11:517-524, 1984.

Goldman AP, Tasker RC, Haworth SG, et al: Four patterns of response to inhaled nitric oxide for persistent pulmonary hypertension of the newborn. Pediatrics 98:706-713, 1996.

Hallman M: Molecular interactions between nitric oxide and lung surfactant. Biol Neonate 71:44-48, 1997.

Kinsella JP, Abman SH: Efficacy of inhalational nitric oxide therapy in the clinical management of persistent pulmonary hypertension of the newborn. Chest 105:92S-94S, 1994.

Kinsella JP, Abman SH: Recent developments in the pathophysiology and treatment of persistent pulmonary hypertension of the newborn. J Pediatr 126:853-864, 1995.

Kinsella JP, Abman SH: Clinical approach to the use of high frequency oscillatory ventilation in neonatal respiratory failure. J Perinatol 16:S52-S55, 1996.

Kinsella JP, Abman SH: Clinical approach to inhaled nitric oxide therapy in the newborn. J Pediatr 136:717-726, 2000.

Kinsella JP, Neish SR, Ivy DD, et al: Clinical responses to prolonged treatment of persistent pulmonary hypertension of the newborn with low doses of inhaled nitric oxide. J Pediatr 123:103-108, 1993.

Kinsella JP, Neish SR, Shaffer E, Abman SH: Low-dose inhalational nitric oxide in persistent pulmonary hypertension of the newborn. Lancet 340:819-820, 1992.

Kinsella JP, Truog WE, Walsh WF, et al: Randomized, multicenter trial of inhaled nitric oxide and high frequency oscillatory ventilation in severe persistent pulmonary hypertension of the newborn. J Pediatr 131:55-62, 1997.

Kinsella JP, Walsh WF, Bose CL, et al: Inhaled nitric oxide in premature neonates with severe hypoxaemic respiratory failure: A randomised controlled trial. Lancet 354:1061-1065, 1999.

Levin DL, Heymann MA, Kitterman JA, et al: Persistent pulmonary hypertension of the newborn. J Pediatr 89:626, 1976.

Neonatal Inhaled Nitric Oxide Study Group: Inhaled nitric oxide in full-term and nearly full-term infants with hypoxic respiratory failure. N Engl J Med 336:597-604, 1997.

Roberts JD, Fineman JR, Morin FC, et al: Inhaled nitric oxide and persistent pulmonary hypertension of the newborn. N Engl J Med 336:605-610, 1997.

Roberts JD, Polaner DM, Lang P, Zapol WM: Inhaled nitric oxide in persistent pulmonary hypertension of the newborn. Lancet 340:818-819, 1992.

Rossaint R, Falke KJ, Lopez F, et al: Inhaled nitric oxide for the adult respiratory distress syndrome. N Engl J Med 328:399-405, 1993.

Stevenson DK, Kasting DS, Darnall RA, et al: Refractory hypoxemia associated with neonatal pulmonary disease: The use and limitations of tolazoline. J Pediatr 95:595-599, 1979.

Wessel DL, Adatia I, Van Marter LJ, et al: Improved oxygenation in a randomized trial of inhaled nitric oxide for persistent pulmonary hypertension of the newborn. Pediatrics 100:e7, 1997.

64

Extracorporeal Membrane Oxygenation

Robert E. Schumacher

I. Description
   A. Extracorporeal membrane oxygenation (ECMO) is a means whereby an infant (usually term) with reversible lung failure is afforded a period of "lung rest" by use of an artificial lung. Such a period of rest may allow lung recovery and ultimately survival of the infant.
   B. Oxygen delivery is determined by oxygen content and cardiac output. Venovenous (VV) ECMO increases oxygen content. Venoarterial (VA) ECMO increases oxygen content and can increase cardiac output (pump flow).
   C. Ventilation is determined by gas flow though the artificial lung.
II. ECMO Circuit
   A. For VA bypass, venous blood is passively drained via the right atrium and passed via a roller pump to a venous capacitance reservoir (bladder box), membrane lung, heat exchanger, and arterial perfusion cannula. The right internal jugular vein and common carotid artery are used as access points and are often ligated as part of the bypass procedure.
   B. For VV bypass, a double lumen cannula is used. In this isovolemic procedure, blood is removed from and returned to the right atrium; the remainder of the circuit is the same as in VA ECMO.
   C. To prevent thrombotic complications while on ECMO, the infant is treated with systemic heparinization.
III. Patient Selection
   A. For "standard" neonatal ECMO, the infant should:
      1. Be at least 35 weeks' gestational age (intracranial hemorrhage remains a significant concern for premature infants).
      2. Have a cranial sonogram with no intraventricular hemorrhage (IVH) higher than grade I.
      3. Have no major bleeding problem.
      4. Have reversible respiratory failure.
      5. Be failing conventional medical management.
   B. Failure of conventional medical management is a definition that should be "individualized" for each ECMO center.
      1. Guidelines (based on experience with populations) are used, but the ultimate decision is up to those caring for the individual infant. Cutpoint values (i.e., ECMO/no ECMO) should be chosen, taking into account probabilities for mortality and long-term morbidity.

Because different disease processes have different outcome probabilities, it is rational to take this into consideration when applying criteria. General criteria provide guidance.

2. Oxygenation index (OI) criteria

   a. The OI is based on the following equation:

   $$OI = \frac{\text{Mean airway pressure (P\bar{a}w)}}{PaO_2 \text{ (postductal)}} \times FiO_2 \times 100$$

   b. After stabilization, if the OI is 40 on three of five occasions (each value separated by >30 minutes and <60 minutes) ECMO criteria have been met (University of Michigan "absolute"criteria).

   c. VV ECMO may not provide the same cardiac support as VA ECMO.

      (1) Infants with severe cardiac compromise may not tolerate VV ECMO. How to identify such patients is difficult.

      (2) Because the risk of carotid artery ligation is not present, consideration for VV ECMO is made at lower OI values (25 to 40).

3. Other criteria include A-aDO$_2$, acute deterioration, intractable air leaks, and "unresponsive to medical management."

IV. Management

   A. Initial bypass problems

      1. Hypotension

         a. Hypovolemia: The ECMO circuit has high blood capacitance; treat this with volume. The technician should have packed red blood cells (PRBCs) or colloid available from the circuit priming procedure.

         b. Sudden dilution of vasopressors, especially with VV ECMO: Correct by having separate pressor infusion pumps to infuse into circuit.

         c. Hypocalcemia from stored blood: Circuit can be primed with calcium to prevent this.

      2. Bradycardia from vagal stimulation by catheter(s).

      3. Consequences of catheter misplacement: Correct catheter placement should be documented radiographically.

   B. Initial management

      1. VA bypass: Wean ventilator rapidly (10 to 15 minutes) to "rest" settings (FiO$_2$, 0.3; pressure, 25/4 cm H$_2$O; rate, 20 breaths/minute; inspiratory time [T$_I$], 0.5 to 1.0 second). Use SvO$_2$ as guide. Continuous positive airway pressure (CPAP)/high positive end-expiratory pressure (PEEP) (10 to 12 cm H$_2$O) may shorten bypass time. Inotropes can usually be quickly discontinued.

      2. VV bypass: Wean with caution. The infant is still dependent on innate myocardial function for O$_2$ delivery. SvO$_2$ is useful only for trends at the same pump flow rate. The innate lung still provides gas exchange. High CPAP with VV ECMO may impede cardiac output; if desired, use end-tidal carbon dioxide (ETCO$_2$) to optimize PEEP. Inotropes must be weaned with caution.

3. Infants have self-decannulated; restraints are mandatory.
4. Head position is critical; if the head is turned too far left, the left jugular vein will be occluded (right is already ligated). Such a scenario may lead to CNS venous hypertension.
5. Analgesia and sedation usually are required. A narcotic used for analgesia; if additional sedation is needed, benzodiazepines or phenobarbital is a reasonable choice.
6. Heparin management
   a. Prior to cannulation, the loading dose is 100 U/kg.
   b. Drip concentration is 60 U/mL (6 mL [1000 U/mL] heparin in 94 mL D_5W).
   c. Usual consumption is 20 to 40 U/kg/hr. This is affected by blood-surface interactions in the circuit, the infant's clotting status, and heparin elimination (renal excretion).
   d. Titrate heparin to keep activated clotting time (ACT) in the desired range (usually 160 to 180 seconds).
C. Daily management, patient protocols, problems
   1. Chest radiograph: Daily.
   2. Cranial sonogram: Obtain the first day after cannulation, after every change in neurologic status, and minimally every third day.
      a. Brain hemorrhage includes both typical and atypical (including posterior fossa) hemorrhages. If hemorrhage is seen and the infant is able to be taken off ECMO, do so. If the infant is likely to die if removed from bypass, has stable hemorrhage, or is neurologically stable, consider keeping the infant on bypass with strict attention to lower ACT values (160 to 180 seconds), and keeping platelet counts higher (e.g., 125,000 to 200,000/mm³).
      b. Cranial sonography is not as good as CT for demonstrating peripheral/posterior fossa lesions.
   3. Fluids: Monitor I/O, weight; the membrane lung provides an additional area for evaporative losses.
      a. Total body water (TBW) is high: This is a common occurrence; etiology is probably multifactorial. A problem arises when TBW is high but intravascular volume is low (capillary leak); vigorous attempts at diuresis in this instance will not help and can be harmful. Aggressive diuresis may allow greater caloric intake. Some argue that vigorous attempts at diuresis can hasten lung recovery; others state that diuresis is a marker for improvement and attempts to hasten it are of no avail. If diuresis is deemed advisable, use diuretics first, hemofilter last (furosemide in combination with theophylline may be helpful). Expect decreased urine output when a hemofilter is used.
      b. Potassium: Serum values often low and require replacement; check for alkalosis. (Low K^+ may be related to the use of washed red blood cells.)
      c. Pump is primed with banked blood; ionized Ca^{2+} can be low. Checking and correcting the circuit can prevent this.

4. Hemostasis/hemolysis
   a. Obtain daily assay of fibrinogen, fibrin split products, serum hemoglobin, and platelet count.
   b. Clots are common, especially in the venous capacitance reservoir (bladder). Pre-lung clots are usually left alone. Post-lung clots are handled by the ECMO technician. When clots appear, review platelet/heparin consumption, fibrin split products, etc.
   c. Bleeding
      (1) From neck wound: Treat with cannula manipulation, light pressure, or fibrin glue.
      (2) Hemothorax/pericardium will present with decreased pulse pressure and decreased pump filling. Treated by drainage first.
      (3) A more common problem if previous surgery has been done (e.g., congenital diaphragatic hernia [CDH], thoracostomy tube).
      (4) Treat with blood replacement; keep platelet counts high (>150,000/mm^3), lower acceptable ACT values.
5. Total parenteral nutrition (TPN): A major benefit of ECMO can be immediate provision of TPN and adequate caloric/low volume intake (use high dextrose concentrations).
6. Blood products
   a. Minimize donor exposures; give only when indicated.
   b. Excessive PRBC administration without increasing pump flow leads to lower aortic PO_2 but similar to greater oxygen delivery.
7. Hypertension is a known complication. The final mechanism by which it is achieved is usually high TBW. It is almost always transient and resolves near the end of a run. A working definition is mean arterial pressure (MAP) >75 mm Hg. Initial treatment is with diuretics.
8. White blood cell (WBC) count often is low, probably from peripheral migration of WBCs.
9. Infection is not a common problem. Suspect infection if unanticipated increasing ECMO support is required. Fungal infection is a concern.
10. Bilirubin can be elevated, especially with sepsis or long ECMO runs. A cholestatic picture is typical; plastic tubing may be hepatotoxic. Hepatosplenomegaly is common.
11. Cardiac stun: Once on ECMO, a dramatic decrease in cardiac performance is seen in up to 5% of infants. Seen more frequently in infants on VA ECMO, it may be ECMO-induced from increased afterload. The stun phenomenon usually resolves, but infants with it do have higher overall mortality rates. Treatment is supportive.
D. Circuit problems (more common problems)
   1. Air in circuit: Treatment depends on location; often can be aspirated.
   2. Pump
      a. Pump cutouts: Kinked tube, malposition, low volume, low filling pressure (pneumothorax, hemopericardium), agitated infant.
      b. Electric failure: Pump can be cranked by hand.

   c. Occlusion set too loose: falsely high flow readings; too tight: hemolysis.
   3. Lung pathophysiology: The membrane lung can get "sick" (can have pulmonary embolus, edema, etc.). Treatment depends upon the specific problem.
E. Weaning
   1. SvO$_2$ is the easiest measure to follow; wean by preset parameters.
   2. Chest radiograph is very helpful.
      a. Usually shows initial complete opacification.
      b. Starts to clear prior to "reventilating" the lungs and serves as a marker for lung recovery. Anticipate "trial off" with this early sign.
   3. Pulmonary mechanics tests: Compliance becomes poor hours after starting bypass, and improvement is an early marker of lung recovery.
   4. ETCO$_2$: Increasing expired CO$_2$ is indicative of return of lung function.
F. Trial off
   1. Lung conditioning: Lungs are periodically (hourly) inflated using a long (5-second) sustained inflation.
   2. Turning up the ventilator FiO$_2$ and monitoring SvO$_2$ will give a feel for whether there is effective pulmonary gas exchange.
   3. Increased ventilator settings to achieve adequate tidal volumes 30 to 60 minutes before trial off appears to allow recruitment of lung units.
   4. VA: Obtain blood gas values every 10 minutes. Wean FiO$_2$ aggressively. Because the infant is still on bypass but with no effective gas exchange through the membrane, use venous line SvO$_2$ to wean FiO$_2$, as it is now a true venous saturation. Residual O$_2$ in the membrane lung may falsely elevate O$_2$ content for 20 to 30 minutes.
   5. A successful trial off depends upon the individual infant. In general, the infant should be stable on FiO$_2 = 0.4$, with standard ventilator settings.
G. Inability to wean from ECMO (non-CDH) with prolonged need for bypass (e.g., 7 days) and little or no improvement, an underlying "rare" lung disease must be considered. Bronchoscopy and lavage and or biopsy may allow the diagnosis of rare lung disease (e.g., surfactant protein B deficiency, alveolar capillary dysplasia).
H. Decannulation
   1. Notify surgeon as soon as possible.
   2. Administer a skeletal muscle relaxant.
   3. The need for surgical repair of the carotid artery or jugular vein is controversial.
V. Post-ECMO Follow-Up
   A. Neck: Sutures are removed in 7 days.
   B. Platelets will continue to fall post-ECMO. Serial counts are necessary until infant is stable (24 to 48 hours).
   C. CNS
      1. EEG is a sensitive screening test for acute functional CNS problems.
      2. CT/MRI: Obtained because of relative insensitivity of sonography to posterior fossa and lateral parenchymal lesions.
      3. Brainstem audiometric evoked responses (BAER): Because of high incidence of sensorineural hearing loss with persistent pulmonary

hypertension of the newborn (PPHN), hearing screening is recommended. Delayed-onset hearing loss has been described and repeated screening is advised.

D. Airway: Vocal cord paresis seen in approximately 5% of infants post ECMO; acute respiratory deterioration has occurred. If persistent stridor is noted, flexible bronchoscopy is recommended. Hoarseness has always resolved clinically (days to months).

E. Long-Term Follow-Up:
   1. Neurodevelopmental follow-up should be provided: 10% to 20% of infants have major problems.
   2. Medical problems include lower respiratory tract infections.

Suggested Reading

Bartlett RH: Extracorporeal life support for cardiopulmonary failure. Curr Prob Surg 27:621-705, 1990.

Elbourne D, Field D, Mugford M: Extracorporeal membrane oxygenation for severe respiratory failure in newborn infants. Cochrane Database Syst Rev (1):CD001340, 2002.

Glass P, Wagner AE, Papero PH, et al: Neurodevelopmental status at age five years of neonates treated with extracorporeal membrane oxygenation. J Pediatr 127:447-557, 1995.

Kim ES, Stolar CJ: ECMO in the newborn. Am J Perinatol 17:345-356, 2000.

Schumacher RE, Baumgart S: Extracorporeal membrane oxygenation 2001: The odyssey continues. Clin Perinatol 28:629-653, 2001.

Zwischenberger JB, Steinhorn RH, Bartlett RH (eds): ECMO: Extracorporeal Cardiopulmonary Support in Critical Care, 2nd ed. Ann Arbor, Extracorporeal Life Support Organization, 2000.

65

Liquid Ventilation for Neonatal Respiratory Failure

Stefano Tredici, Rupa Seetharamaiah,
David S. Foley, and Ronald B. Hirschl

I. Description: Liquid ventilation is the process of enhancing pulmonary function through the instillation of perfluorocarbon (PFC) liquid into the lungs.
   A. Partial liquid ventilation (PLV): The achievement of gas exchange through the delivery of gas tidal volumes to lungs that have been filled with PFC liquid.
   B. Total liquid ventilation (TLV): The achievement of gas exchange through the delivery of tidal volumes of PFC liquid to the lungs using a specialized mechanical liquid ventilator.
II. Physiology of PFC Ventilation
   A. PFCs are inert liquids that are produced by the fluorination of common organic hydrocarbons. The carbon chain length and any additional atom give unique properties to each PFC molecule.
   B. Physical properties of PFCs
      1. Density: Denser than hydrocarbon counterparts with levels approaching twice that of water (1.75 to 1.95 g/mL at 25° C).
      2. Surface tension: Weak intermolecular forces and remarkably low surface tensions (15 to 20 dynes/cm at 25° C).
      3. Respiratory gas solubility: Solubilities of the respiratory gases in PFCs are significantly greater than their corresponding solubilities in water or nonpolar solvents.
         a. O_2 solubility at 37° C = 44 to 55 mL gas/100 mL liquid.
         b. CO_2 solubility at 37° C = 140 to 210 mL gas/100 mL liquid.
      4. An ideal PFC for respiratory application should have the properties of high gas solubility and moderate vapor pressure and viscosity. These properties, however, may not be found in a single pure PFC. Thus, recent studies are focusing on PFC combinations that may optimize the fluid properties to better suit a particular application.
      5. Vapor pressure: PFCs are relatively volatile (vapor pressure ranges from 11 to 85 mm Hg at 37° C). This property is important because it governs the evaporation rate of PFCs from the lungs during and after both PLV and TLV; high vapor pressure liquid would need more frequent supplementation than a low vapor pressure liquid.

C. Basis for the use of liquid ventilation in neonatal ventilator-dependent respiratory failure
  1. Gas exchange
     a. The dependent portion of the lungs tends to be collapsed or filled with inflammatory exudate during severe pulmonary inflammation, leading to ventilation-perfusion (V/Q) mismatching and hypoxemia.
     b. The high densities of PFC liquids facilitate their distribution to the dependent portions of the lungs where the atelectatic lung appears to be recruited.
     c. PFCs have also been shown to redistribute pulmonary blood flow to the better-inflated, nondependent segments.
     d. These effects, combined with the high respiratory gas solubilities of PFCs, lead to improvements in ventilation-perfusion matching and arterial oxygenation.
  2. Pulmonary compliance
     a. PFCs lead to an increase in pulmonary compliance secondary to their density-related recruiting effect on collapsed, inflamed alveoli. However, during PLV, an increase in the PFC dose can be associated with a reduction in compliance. This is related to the heterogeneous distribution of the gas in the partly liquid-filled lungs.
     b. PFCs act as an artificial surfactant and increase the stability of small airways.
     c. The regions of the lung that are filled with PFC liquid (all regions for TLV, the dependent regions for PLV) exhibit a reduction of the gas-liquid interface in the distal airway, which also reduces surface active forces favoring alveolar collapse.
     d. The result of these effects is enhanced alveolar recruitment at lower inflation pressures.
  3. Reduction of lung injury
     a. Effects may relate to improved alveolar inflation and better displacement and lavage of inflammatory mediators and debris from the affected portions of the lungs or to a limitation of excessive ventilator pressures as the result of improvements in compliance.
     b. PFCs have been shown to have in vitro anti-inflammatory activities, such as reduction in neutrophil chemotaxis and nitric oxide production, as well as decreased lipopolysaccharide (LPS)-stimulated macrophage production of cytokines. Neutrophil infiltration also appears to be reduced following lung injury in liquid-ventilated animals. In vivo evaluation has shown a reduction in the release of tumor necrosis factor alpha (TNFα), interleukin (IL)-1, and IL-6 in human alveolar macrophages in PFC-exposed lungs.
D. Uptake, biodistribution, elimination, and toxicology
  1. Uptake: PFCs are absorbed in small quantities from the lungs during liquid ventilation, reaching a steady state at 15 to 30 minutes of liquid breathing.

2. Biodistribution: PFCs have preferential distribution to tissues with high lipid content. These compounds are cleared most quickly from vascular, lipid-poor tissues such as muscle.

3. Elimination: PFCs do not undergo significant biotransformation or excretion. They are eliminated primarily by evaporation from the lungs and are scavenged by macrophages in the lungs and other tissues.

4. Toxicology: Pulmonary, metabolic, hematologic, and clinical effects of liquid ventilation have been studied extensively in laboratory animals, with no significant pulmonary or systemic toxicity noted. Clinical studies have identified transient hypoxemia during PFC dosing and the development of pneumothorax as potential short-term complications of PLV in humans.

III. Partial Liquid Ventilation (PLV)

A. PLV is a hybrid method of gas exchange, achieved through the delivery of conventional gas tidal volumes to PFC-filled lungs.

   1. Methods

     a. Lungs are filled to an estimated fraction of FRC (approximately 5 to 30 mL/kg, depending on disease process, age, and weight) with PFC liquid, and conventional ventilation is superimposed to achieve gas exchange.

     b. Adequate filling of the lungs is judged by the presence of a fluid meniscus in the endotracheal tube at zero positive end-expiratory pressure (PEEP), by the opacification of the dependent portions of the lungs on lateral chest radiography, and by the adequacy of gas tidal volumes. Fluid may be added or withdrawn.

   2. Theoretical basis for use of PLV in respiratory distress syndrome (RDS)

     a. PLV has relative simplicity, because the need for a complex mechanical liquid ventilator is eliminated.

     b. The presence of dense PFC fluid in the dependent regions of the lungs allows the recruitment of severely inflamed airways for the purpose of gas exchange. Oxygenation during PLV can occur either by the gas ventilation of these airways directly or by the oxygenation of the liquid as it equilibrates with the inspired gas.

     c. CO_2 elimination is enhanced by increased gas tidal volumes.

     d. Compliance is enhanced secondary to alveolar recruitment and the surfactant-like activity of the PFCs. Because the gas-liquid interface is not completely eliminated during PLV, compliance improvement is not as dramatic as that seen during TLV and can actually deteriorate if the lungs are overfilled with PFC liquid.

B. Clinical studies of PLV in neonatal ventilator-dependent respiratory failure.

   1. Leach et al (1996) reported significantly improved gas exchange and pulmonary compliance during PLV in 13 premature infants (24 to 34 weeks' gestation at birth) with refractory RDS as part of a multicenter, non-controlled trial. Significant complications occurring during the trial were limited to the development of grade IV intraventricular hemorrhage (IVH) in one patient.

Of the 10 patients completing at least 24 hours of PLV, survival to a corrected gestational age of 36 weeks was 60%.

2. Pranikoff et al (1996) evaluated the use of PLV in four newborn patients maintained with extracorporeal life support (ECLS) for respiratory failure secondary to congenital diaphragmatic hernia (CDH). During 5 to 6 days of PLV therapy, patients exhibited significant increases in arterial oxygen tension and static pulmonary compliance compared with pretreatment values. The therapy was well tolerated and significant complications were limited to the development of pulmonary hemorrhage in one patient 4 days after the final dose of PFC.

3. Migliori et al (2004) evaluated the use of high-frequency partial liquid ventilation in two infants with chronic lung disease and severe respiratory failure. Both patients showed improved gas exchange with reduction in oxygen indices.

IV. Total Liquid Ventilation (TLV)
   A. In TLV, lungs are completely filled with PFC, and a liquid tidal volume is perfused into and drained from the lungs for the purpose of gas exchange using a specialized mechanical liquid ventilator.
   B. Clinical studies of TLV
      1. The feasibility and potential of liquid ventilation as treatment for severe respiratory distress was reported in 1990 by Greenspan et al.
      2. Liquid ventilation was performed in three preterm neonates in whom conventional treatment had failed.
      3. Improvement of pulmonary mechanics without hemodynamic impairment was reported in all infants.
      4. The severity of pulmonary injury before the initiation of liquid ventilation precluded a successful outcome.

V. PFC-Induced Lung Growth
   A. Different studies have demonstrated the effectiveness of PFC to induce lung growth in neonates with CDH on ECLS.
   B. A multicenter, prospective, randomized pilot study showed better survival for the group treated with PFC to induce lung growth (75%) compared with patients treated with conventional ventilation (40%), although the number of patients in the study was very small.

VI. Conclusion: At present, liquid ventilation is not yet an approved therapy for clinical use and remains investigational.

Suggested Reading

Furhman BP, Paczan PR, DeFancisis M: PFC-assisted gas exchange. Crit Care Med 19:712-722, 1991.

Greenspan JS, Wolfson MR, Rubenstein SD, et al: Liquid ventilation of human preterm neonates. J Pediatr 117:106-111, 1990.

Hirschl RB, Croce M, Gore D, et al: Prospective, randomized controlled pilot study of partial liquid ventilation in adult acute respiratory distress syndrome. Am J Respir Crit Care Med 165:781-787, 2002.

Hirschl RB, Pranikoff T, Gauger P, et al: Liquid ventilation in adults, children and neonates. Lancet 346:1201-1202, 1995.

Ivascu FA, Hirschl RB: New approaches to managing congenital diaphragmatic hernia. Semin Perinatol 28:185-198, 2004.

Leach CL, Greenspan JS, Rubenstein SD, et al: Partial liquid ventilation with perflubron in infants with severe respiratory distress syndrome. New Engl J Med 335:761-767, 1996.

Migliori C, Bottino R, Angeli A, et al: High frequency partial liquid ventilation in two infants. J Perinatol 24:118-120, 2004.

Pranikoff T, Gauger P, Hirschl RB: Partial liquid ventilation in newborn patients with congenital diaphragmatic hernia. J Pediatr Surg 31:613-618, 1996.

Shaffer TH, Douglas PR, Lowe CA, et al: The effects of liquid ventilation on cardiopulmonary function in preterm lambs. Pediatr Res 17:303-306, 1983.

Shaffer TH, Moskowitz GD: Demand-controlled liquid ventilation of the lungs. Appl Physiol 36:208-213, 1974.

Shaffer TH, Wolfson MR, Clark C: Liquid ventilation (state of the art review). Pediatr Pulmonol 14:102-109, 1992.

Tredici S, Komori E, Funakubo A, et al: A prototype of a liquid ventilator using a novel hollow fiber oxygenator in a rabbit model. Crit Care Med 32:2104-2109, 2004.

Wolfson MR, Shaffer TH: Liquid ventilation during early development: Theory, physiologic processes and application. J Appl Physiol 1990; 13:1-12, 1990.

Wolfson MR, Shaffer TH: Liquid ventilation: An adjunct for respiratory management. Paediatr Anaesthes 14:15-23, 2004.

Wolfson MR, Tran N, Bhutani VK, et al: A new experimental approach for the study of cardiopulmonary physiology during early development. J Appl Physiol 65:1436-1443, 1998.

Complications Associated with Mechanical Ventilation

Thoracic Air Leaks

66

Steven M. Donn and C. Fred Baker

I. Description: Thoracic air leak refers to a collection of gas outside the pulmonary space. A variety of disorders are included in this category, including pneumothorax, pneumomediastinum, pneumopericardium, pulmonary interstitial emphysema (PIE), pneumoperitoneum, and subcutaneous emphysema.

II. Incidence and Risk Factors: Estimates of the overall incidence of air leak in normal term infants range from 0.07% to 1%.
  A. Estimates of the incidence vary, depending on:
    1. Degree of perinatal hypoxemia
    2. Technique of resuscitation
    3. Concomitant respiratory disease
    4. Type and style of assisted ventilation
    5. Quality of radiographs and their interpretation
  B. The likelihood of pneumothorax being symptomatic without underlying lung disease is small and many go undetected.
  C. Several disease states increase the risk of pulmonary air leaks:
    1. Respiratory distress syndrome (RDS), incidence 5% to 20%
    2. Meconium aspiration syndrome (MAS), incidence 20% to 50%
    3. Pulmonary hypoplasia
    4. PIE

III. Pathophysiology: Air leak syndromes arise by a common pathway that involves damage of the respiratory epithelium, usually by high transpulmonary pressures. Damaged epithelium allows air to enter the interstitium, causing PIE. With continued high transpulmonary pressures, air dissects toward the visceral pleura and/or hilum via the peribronchial or perivascular spaces.
  A. Pneumothorax occurs when the pleural surface is ruptured, resulting in the leakage of air into the pleural space.
  B. Pneumomediastinum results when air, following the path of least resistance, enters the mediastinum.
  C. Pneumopericardium results, as above, when air dissects into the pericardium.
  D. Subcutaneous emphysema occurs when air from the mediastinum egresses into the fascial planes of the neck and skin.
  E. Pneumoperitoneum results from the dissection of retroperitoneal air, from pneumomediastinal decompression, into the peritoneum. (It can also occur from a ruptured abdominal viscus.)

IV. Air Leak Syndromes
   A. Pneumothorax often results from high inspiratory pressures and uneven ventilation.
      1. Etiology
         a. Spontaneous pneumothoraces (seen in up to 1% of normal term infants around the time of birth; only about 10% of these are symptomatic).
         b. Lung diseases such as MAS, congenital bullae, and pulmonary hypoplasia, which result in uneven lung compliance and alveolar overdistention.
         c. Direct injury by suctioning through the endotracheal tube is a rare cause of pneumothorax.
         d. Respiratory support
            (1) Prolonged inspiratory time (T_I) (I:E $\geq$1:1)
            (2) High mean airway pressure (Pāw) (>12 cm H_2O)
            (3) Low inspired gas temperature (<36.5° C). This is especially true for infants weighing <1500 g and is thought to result from decreased mucociliary clearance precipitating airway obstruction at lower temperatures and lower humidity.
            (4) Poor patient-ventilator interaction (dyssynchrony—i.e., infants who actively expire during part or all of the positive pressure plateau).
      2. Diagnosis is made based on clinical signs, physical examination, arterial blood gases, transillumination, and radiography.
         a. Clinical signs of pneumothorax include those of respiratory distress—e.g., tachypnea, grunting, flaring, and retractions. Cyanosis, decreased breath sounds over the affected side, chest asymmetry, episodes of apnea and bradycardia, shift in cardiac point of maximal impulse, and hypotension also may occur.
         b. Arterial blood gases may show respiratory or mixed acidosis and hypoxemia.
         c. Transillumination may reveal an increased transmission of light on the involved side.
         d. Chest radiography remains the gold standard for diagnosis of pneumothorax.
      3. Treatment of pneumothorax is discussed later.
      4. Prevention
         a. Fast-rate ventilation (>60 breaths/minute) may reduce active expiration, a precursor of pneumothorax. This is done in an attempt to provoke more synchronous respiration. If this fails, the infant may require sedation and/or paralysis to reduce active expiration. High-frequency ventilation may also provide better ventilation and oxygenation while decreasing the incidence of pneumothorax.
         b. Patient-triggered ventilation reduces the incidence of air leak by synchronizing respiration. Using this mode of ventilation, the infant's respiratory efforts trigger the delivery of the positive pressure inflation. When synchronous respiration is

achieved, the development of pneumothorax is lessened. Flow-cycling enables complete synchronization even during expiration.

    c. Suppression of respiratory activity by patient paralysis may be an important means of preventing pneumothoraces in patients who are actively exhaling or "fighting" the ventilator.

B. PIE occurs most often in ventilated, preterm infants with RDS. Interstitial air can be localized or widespread throughout one or both lungs. PIE alters pulmonary mechanics by decreasing compliance, increasing residual volume and dead space, and increasing V/Q mismatch. It also impedes pulmonary blood flow.

    1. Diagnosis is made based on clinical signs, transillumination, and chest radiography.

        a. Clinical signs of PIE include profound respiratory acidosis and hypoxemia. Because air is interstitial instead of intra-alveolar, proper gas exchange does not occur, decreasing ventilation. Trapped gas reduces pulmonary perfusion by compression of blood vessels resulting in hypoxemia.

        b. Transillumination of a chest with diffuse and widespread PIE results in increased transmission of light, similar to that seen in a pneumothorax.

        c. Chest radiography may reveal a characteristic cystic appearance or may be more subtle, with rounded, nonconfluent microradiolucencies in earlier stages. In later stages of PIE, radiography may show large bullae formation with hyperinflation in the involved portions of lung.

    2. Management

        a. Generalized management of PIE is focused on reducing or preventing further barotrauma to the lung.

           (1) Decrease peak inspiratory pressure (PIP) to the minimum required to attain acceptable arterial blood gases (PaO_2, 45 to 50 mm Hg or 6 to 6.7 kPa; PCO_2, <60 mmHg or 8 kPa).

           (2) Reduction in positive end-expiratory pressure (PEEP) may also help decrease PIE.

           (3) High-frequency jet ventilation (HFJV) is a successful means of ventilation for infants with PIE. This mode results in improved ventilation at lower peak and mean airway pressures with more rapid resolution of PIE.

        b. Localized PIE may resolve spontaneously or may persist for several weeks with a sudden enlargement and deterioration in the infant's condition. Progressive overdistention of the affected area can cause compression of the adjacent normal lung parenchyma.

V. Pneumothorax

    A. Nitrogen washout is a controversial but sometimes effective way of eliminating a small pneumothorax.

        1. Technique

           a. Infant is placed in a 1.0 FiO_2 oxygen hood for 12 to 24 hours.

    b. Vital signs including oxygen saturation, heart rate, and blood pressure are continuously monitored.

  2. Precautions

    a. Do not use in preterm infant.

    b. Do not use if pneumothorax is under tension.

B. Needle aspiration can be used to treat a symptomatic pneumothorax. It frequently is curative in infants who are not mechanically ventilated and may be a temporizing treatment in infants who are mechanically ventilated.

  1. Technique

    a. Attach a 23-gauge butterfly needle to a 50-cc sterile syringe by way of a three-way stopcock.

    b. Locate the second or third intercostal space in the mid-clavicular line on the affected side.

    c. Prepare the area with antiseptic solution.

    d. Under sterile conditions, if possible, locate the intercostal space *above* the rib (to avoid lacerating intercostal vessels located on the inferior surface of the rib). Insert the needle through the skin and into the pleural space while applying continuous suction with the syringe as the needle is inserted. A rush of air is usually experienced when the pleural space has been entered.

    e. Once the pleural space has been entered, stop advancing the needle to avoid risk of puncturing the lung.

    f. Apply slow, steady suction to the syringe until resistance is felt, indicating that no more air remains in the area surrounding the needle.

    g. Air is evacuated from the syringe by turning off the stopcock to the infant and evacuating air from the side port.

    h. Once all possible air is evacuated, remove the needle and dress the site, if necessary.

  2. Complications

    a. Infection

    b. Laceration of intercostal vessels

    c. Incomplete evacuation of air leak

    d. Lung puncture

    e. Damage to other intrathoracic structures (e.g., phrenic nerve, thoracic duct)

    f. Recurrence of air leak

C. Chest tube drainage (thoracostomy) is usually needed for continuous drainage of pneumothoraces that develop in infants receiving positive pressure ventilation, because the air leak may be persistent under these conditions.

  1. Technique

    a. Select a chest tube of appropriate size. For very small infants, 10-Fr chest tubes are adequate; for larger infants, 12-Fr chest tubes are better. Be sure that the trocar is freely mobile inside the chest tube.

b. Locate the fifth intercostal space in the anterior axillary line on the affected side.

c. Prepare the site with antibacterial solution.

d. Administer analgesic to the infant.

e. Cover the site with sterile drapes.

f. Inject the area with a small amount of 1% lidocaine solution.

g. Make a small incision (approximately 1 cm) *directly over* the sixth rib. Avoid breast tissue and the nipple.

h. With a curved hemostat, dissect subcutaneous tissue above the rib. Make a subcutaneous track to the third or fourth interspace.

i. Applying continuous, firm pressure, enter the pleural space with the closed hemostat. Widen the opening by spreading the tips of the hemostat.

j. Carefully insert the chest tube. If a trocar is used, insert it only 1.0 to 1.5 cm to avoid puncturing the lung. Advance the chest tube a few centimeters to the desired location while withdrawing the trocar. The anterior pleural space is usually the most suitable for infants in a supine position. Be certain that the side ports of the chest tube are within the pleural space. Vapor is usually observed in the chest tube if it is in the pleural space.

k. Attach the chest tube to an underwater drainage system under low (-10 to -20 cm H_2O) continuous suction.

l. Suture the chest tube in place and close the skin incision using 3-0 or 4-0 silk. The chest tube is best held in place with a "purse string" stitch encircling it. Taping the tube is also recommended.

m. Cover the area with sterile petrolatum gauze and a sterile, clear plastic surgical dressing.

n. Confirm proper chest tube placement radiographically. If residual air remains, the chest tube may need to be readjusted, or a second tube placed until air is evacuated or no longer causing compromise.

2. Pigtail catheter technique

a. Less dissection is required compared with straight chest tube placement.

b. 8.5-Fr preassembled kits are available.

c. Prepare site with antibacterial solution.

d. Administer analgesia.

e. Drape the patient using sterile procedure.

f. Inject the site with a small amount of 1% lidocaine.

g. Place in fifth intercostal space in midaxiliary line on affected side.

h. Using the needle introducer attached to a syringe, enter the skin at a 30- to 45-degree angle distal to the fourth intercoastal space, avoiding breast tissue and nipple. Guide the needle superficially above the fifth rib, avoiding the inferior structures, and into the intercostal space.

    i. Gently withdraw on the syringe while entering the pleural space. As air or fluid is aspirated, watch for improvement in vital signs. To avoid lung injury, do not evacuate the entire amount of air or fluid.

    j. Remove the syringe and insert the guide wire. In some kits the guidewire is contained in a plastic bag to detect the presence of air. Advance the guidewire through the introducer until the guide wire marker enters the hub.

    k. Keeping the guidewire in position, remove the needle introducer over the distal end of the guidewire.

    l. Advance the dilator over the guidewire and gently dilate the site.

    m. Remove the dilator, keeping the guidewire in place.

    n. Advance the pigtail catheter over the guidewire and into the pleural space. Advance until each of the side ports is intrathoracic in location. Leave 13 cm (measured from the chest wall to the hub of the catheter) of tubing extrathoracic.

    o. Attach the chest tube to an underwater drainage system.

    p. Adequately secure the chest tube.

    q. Confirm placement radiographically.

  3. Complications are the same as those seen in needle aspiration.

VI. Pneumomediastinum: This is often of little clinical importance and usually does not need to be drained. Rarely, cardiovascular compromise occurs if the air accumulation is under tension and does not decompress. Treatments include:

  A. Nitrogen washout, as described above.

  B. Needle aspiration (using technique described above for pneumothorax): Insert the needle in midline immediately subxiphoid and apply negative pressure as the needle is advanced in a cephalad direction.

  C. A mediastinal tube is rarely needed, but if necessary, it should be placed by a qualified surgeon.

VII. Pneumoperitoneum: Often this will not adversely affect the patient's clinical status, but when respiratory compromise does occur, treatment is warranted. Upward pressure on the diaphragm may compromise ventilation because of decreased lung volumes and may reduce blood return to the heart by exerting pressure on the inferior vena cava.

  A. Distinguishing the cause of a pneumoperitoneum is very important and will drastically change patient management. Pneumoperitoneum caused by a transthoracic air leak can be differentiated from pneumoperitoneum caused by bowel perforation by measuring the oxygen from a gas sample obtained from the peritoneum. Baseline gas concentration is measured and compared to gas concentration obtained from a peritoneal sample when ventilator FiO_2 is set at 1.0. If the PaO_2 from the latter sample is high, the source of the air leak is likely thoracic.

  B. Needle aspiration can be used as a temporizing measure or, in some cases, may be used to treat pneumoperitoneum. Following the general procedure for needle aspiration of pneumothorax, the needle is inserted in the midline approximately 1 cm below the umbilicus.

Negative pressure is applied while the needle is advanced through the peritoneum and air is evacuated.

   C. Peritoneal drain placement may relieve a continuous peritoneal air leak.

VIII. Pneumopericardium: Pneumopericardium occurs when air from the pleural space or mediastinum enters the pericardial sac through a defect that is often located at the reflection near the ostia of the pulmonary veins. The majority of cases occur in infants ventilated with high PIP (>32 cm H_2O), high Pāw (>17 cm H_2O), and/or long T_I (>0.7 seconds). Cardiac tamponade is a life-threatening event that may result from air leak into the pericardial sac. A symptomatic pneumopericardium should be drained immediately.

   A. Needle aspiration via the subxiphoid route may be used as a temporizing measure or to treat symptomatic pneumopericardium.

      1. Technique

         a. Prepare the subxiphoid area with an antiseptic solution.

         b. Attach a 20- or 22-gauge IV catheter to a short piece of IV tubing that is then attached via a stopcock to a syringe.

         c. Locate the subxiphoid space and insert the catheter with needle pointed at a 30- to 45-degree angle toward the infant's left shoulder.

         d. Aspirate with the syringe as the catheter is advanced.

         e. Stop advancing the catheter once air is aspirated. Remove the needle, sliding the plastic catheter into the pericardial space. Reattach the syringe and remove the remaining air, and remove the catheter, or alternatively place it to water seal if the leak is continuous.

      2. Complications of pericardiocentesis include hemopericardium and laceration of the right ventricle or left anterior descending coronary artery.

      3. The procedure can be facilitated by transillumination guidance.

   B. Pericardial tube placement and drainage may be necessary if the pericardial air reaccumulates. The pericardial tube can be managed like a chest tube, except that less negative pressures are used for suction (−5 to −10 cm H2O).

   C. Prevention of further pericardial air leak by appropriate ventilator management is very important.

Suggested Reading

Alpan G, Goder K, Glick F, et al: Pneumopericardium during continuous positive airway pressure in respiratory distress syndrome. Crit Care Med 37:511-515, 1984.

Cabatu EE, Brown EG: Thoracic transillumination: Aid in the diagnosis and treatment of pneumopericardium. Pediatrics 64:958-960, 1979.

Donn SM, Engmann C: Neonatal resuscitation: Special procedures. In Donn SM (ed): The Michigan Manual of Neonatal Intensive Care. Philadelphia, Hanley & Belfus, 2003, pp 33-41.

Donn SM, Faix RG: Delivery room resuscitation. In Spitzer AR (ed): Intensive Care of the Fetus and Neonate, St. Louis, Mosby–Year Book, 1996, pp 326-336.

Donn SM, Kuhns LR: Pediatric Transillumination, Chicago, Year Book Medical, 1983.

Douglas-Jones J, Bustamante S, Mirza M: Pneumopericardium in a newborn. J Pediatr Surg 16:75-78, 1981.

Fuhrman BP, Landrum BG, Ferrara TB, et al: Pleural drainage suing modified pigtail catheters. Crit Care Med 14:575-576,1986.

Keszler M, Donn SM, Bucciarelli RL, et al: Controlled multicenter trial of high frequency jet ventilation vs. conventional ventilation in newborns with pulmonary interstitial emphysema. J Pediatr 119:85-93,1991.

Lawless S, Orr R, Killian A, et al: New pigtail catheter for pleural drainage in pediatric patients. Crit Care Med 17:173-175, 1989.

MacDonald MG: Thoracostomy in the neonate: A blunt discussion. NeoReviews 5:e301-e306, 2004.

Madansky DL, Lawson EE, Chernick V, et al: Pneumothorax and other forms of pulmonary air leak in newborns. Am Rev Respir Dis 120:729-733, 1979.

Zak LK, Donn SM: Thoracic air leaks. In Donn SM, Faix RG (eds): Neonatal Emergencies. Mount Kisco, NY, Futura, 1991, pp 311-325.

Patent Ductus Arteriosus

67

Jonathan P. Wyllie

I. Incidence of Patent Ductus Arteriosus (PDA)
  A. Most common cardiac problem in newborns
  B. Varies inversely with gestational age (GA)
    1. Up to 20% at GA >32 weeks
    2. 20% to 40% at GA between 28 and 32 weeks
    3. 60% at GA <28 weeks
II. PDA in Fetal Circulation
  A. Derived from sixth aortic arch.
  B. May be absent in association with congenital heart disease involving severe right outflow tract obstruction (rare).
  C. Carries most of right ventricular (RV) output (50% to 60% of total cardiac output) from 6th to 7th week on; caliber equal to descending aorta.
  D. Patency is both passive (from high blood flow) and active (locally derived prostaglandin E_2 [PGE_2]).
III. Postnatal Closure
  A. Mechanisms mature after 35 weeks.
  B. Is initiated by spiral medial muscle layer starting at pulmonary end.
  C. Duct shortens and thickens with functional closure at 12 to 72 hours.
  D. Factors promoting closure:
    1. Low ductal flow ($\uparrow$ systemic + $\downarrow$ pulmonary resistance = $\uparrow$ pulmonary flow)
    2. Reduced sensitivity to PGE_2
    3. Decreased production of PGE_2
    4. Increased arterial oxygen tension
IV. Persistent Ductal Patency
  A. Isolated PDA accounts for 3.5% of congenital heart disease presenting in infancy. It occurs despite ductal constriction and has a different pathogenesis from that in the preterm infant.
  B. Preterm PDA
    1. Immature closure mechanism
    2. Decreased sensitivity to constrictors such as oxygen tension
    3. Increased sensitivity to PGE_2
    4. Other associated factors:
      a. Acidosis
      b. Severe lung disease
      c. Exogenous surfactant use

        d. Phototherapy

        e. Excessive fluid administration

        f. Lack of antenatal steroid therapy

        g. Use of frusemide/furosemide in first few days of life

V. Physiologic Effects of PDA

    A. Left-to-right shunt

        1. Exacerbation of respiratory disease

        2. Altered pulmonary mechanics

        3. Increased cardiac work load

    B. Diastolic steal

        1. Altered perfusion of brain, systemic organs

        2. Risk of necrotizing enterocolitis

VI. Clinical Effects of PDA with left-to-right shunt

    A. Increased oxygen requirement

    B. Increased ventilatory requirement

    C. Apnea

    D. Chronic lung disease

    E. Impaired weight gain

    F. Congestive heart failure

VII. Clinical Features of PDA

    A. Occurs after fall in pulmonary resistance.

    B. Onset is related to severity of lung disease and size of infant.

    C. In very low birth weight infants, the most common manifestation is seen after 4 days of age, earlier in low-birth-weight infants.

    D. Signs:

        1. Failure of respiratory distress syndrome to improve (or deterioration) at 2 to 7 days

        2. Increase in FiO_2/ventilator settings

        3. Acidosis

        4. Apnea

        5. Hyperdynamic precordium (95%)

        6. Bounding pulses (85%)

        7. Murmur (80%)

            a. Normally silent until day 4

            b. Systolic

            c. Upper left sternal border

            d. Variable

VIII. Diagnosis of PDA

    A. Chest radiograph (poor specificity)

        1. Cardiac enlargement

        2. Pulmonary engorgement (hyperemia)

        3. Absence of pulmonary explanation for deterioration

    B. ECG usually helpful unless attempting to rule out other conditions

    C. Echocardiogram

        1. Ductal patency

        2. Flow velocity/pattern

        3. Ductal diameter (>1.5 mm in first 30 hours)

        4. Left atrium (LA) volume load (LA/aortic ratio >1.5)

     5. Left ventricular end-diastolic dimension (LVEDD)/aortic ratio > 2.0
     6. LV output
     7. LV function
     8. Diastolic flow in descending aorta
     9. Diastolic flow in coeliac vessels

IX. Treatment
  A. Fluid restriction (little evidence to maintain, except for <169 mL/kg/day at day 3)
  B. Diuretics
    1. Furosemide
    2. Chlorothiazide
     a. Little evidence except in congestive cardiac failure
     b. Temporizing measure
  C. Ventilation
    1. Increase mean airway pressure (Pāw) (peak inspiratory pressure [PIP])
    2. Increase positive end-expiratory pressure (PEEP)
  D. Indomethacin
    1. Infant <2 to 3 weeks of age
    2. Reasonable renal function (serum creatinine <1.3 mg/dL)
    3. No thrombocytopenia (platelets >50,000/mm^3)
    4. No significant hyperbilirubinemia
    5. Closure in up to 79% of cases, but relapse in up to 33% of these
    6. Prophylactic treatment used unnecessarily in up to 64% of cases
    7. Dosage:
     a. 0.2 mg/kg/day × 2 to 3 doses
     b. 0.1 mg/kg/day × 6 doses
  E. Ibuprofen
    1. Fewer short-term side effects than indomethacin.
    2. No long-term advantage over indomethacin.
    3. 5% incidence of severe pulmonary hypertension if used prophylactically.
    4. Dosage: 10 mg/kg loading dose, then 5 mg/kg at 24 and 48 hours.
  F. Surgical ligation

Suggested Reading

Bracken MB (eds.): Effective Care of the Newborn Infant. Oxford, Oxford University Press, 1992, pp 281-324.

Negegme RA, O'Connor TZ, Lister G, Bracken MB: Patent ductus arteriosus. Semin Neonatol 8:425-432, 2003.

68 Neonatal Pulmonary Hemorrhage

Tonse N.K. Raju

I. Description: Neonatal pulmonary hemorrhage is a rare but severe condition characterized by massive bleeding into the lungs and airways.
   A. The clinical status deteriorates rapidly, with the associated mortality ranging from 50% to 80%.
   B. The incidence of long-term pulmonary morbidity, such as chronic lung disease (CLD), among the survivors exceeds 80%.
II. Incidence: The reported incidence figures vary, depending on the definitions used, the diligence of monitoring for pulmonary hemorrhage, and the source of the data used in the study (e.g., autopsy versus clinical).
   A. General NICU population: About 1.4% of all infants admitted to the NICU have been reported to develop pulmonary hemorrhage, more than 80% of whom are diagnosed as having respiratory distress syndrome (RDS). Such infants are also likely to have been treated with exogenous surfactant and were receiving mechanical ventilatory support at the time of the bleeding.
   B. Gestational age (GA): The incidence is inversely proportional to GA, especially between 23 and 28 weeks GA.
      1. Exogenous surfactant: Ever since exogenous surfactant therapy became the standard of care for RDS, there has been a slight but noticeable increase in the incidence of pulmonary hemorrhage. In a cohort of 14,464 very low birth weight (VLBW) infants, in the infants 25 to 26 weeks GA, the incidence of pulmonary hemorrhage incidence was 10% in 1991, increasing to 16% in 2001. In infants 27 to 28 weeks GA, the incidence was 6.5% in 1991 and 8% in 2001.
      2. In a postmarketing surveillance study of an animal-derived natural surfactant, the incidence of pulmonary hemorrhage was 6.4% among 903 infants treated with surfactant for RDS. This represents a slight increase from 3% to 4% reported in the presurfactant era.
      3. A meta-analysis study concluded that exogenous surfactants increased the risk for pulmonary hemorrhage by 47%. The risk was slightly higher with animal-derived surfactants than with synthetic preparations.

    C. At autopsy: In autopsy studies, about 80% of VLBW infants were found to have pulmonary hemorrhage.

    D. Other conditions: About 6% (range, 5% to 10%) of infants requiring extracorporeal membrane oxygenation (ECMO) were reported to develop pulmonary hemorrhage either during or after ECMO.

III. Other Antecedent Factors and Infants at Risk

    A. Prematurity, RDS, and exogenous surfactant therapy: In combination, these three risk factors are the most consistent for pulmonary hemorrhage, especially in infants <28 weeks GA (or birth weight <1000 g). The complication rate is not influenced by the type (natural or synthetic) of surfactant used or its time of administration (prophylactic, early, or rescue).

    B. Lung complications: Pulmonary interstitial emphysema (PIE) and/or pneumothorax.

    C. Infections: Bacterial, viral, or fungal infections such as *Listeria*, *Haemophilus influenzae*, and congenital cytomegalovirus were reported to be associated with pulmonary hemorrhage.

    D. General clinical status: Metabolic acidosis, especially in infants with RDS; hypothermia, hypoglycemia, and shock; and disseminated intravascular coagulation (DIC).

    E. Meconium aspiration syndrome (MAS): Infants requiring ECMO.

    F. Inherited coagulation disorders: Although rare, one must consider familial bleeding disorders, such as von Willebrand disease, especially with a family history of this disease. A report by the Centers for Disease Control and Prevention found that von Willebrand disease was the underlying condition in two of five infants dying from idiopathic pulmonary hemorrhage.

    G. Trauma: Mechanical injury to the vocal cords, trachea, or other laryngeal and oropharyngeal structures, especially from endotracheal intubation.

IV. Pathophysiology: The pulmonary effluate has very high protein content, as well as a large number of cellular elements from the blood. Thus, the hemorrhage may be a consequence of increased transcapillary pore size. A series of interrelated factors may lead to an eventual bleeding episode.

    A. Hemodynamic factors: Some experts consider pulmonary hemorrhage to be a manifestation of an exaggerated hemorrhagic pulmonary edema brought about by an acute increase in pulmonary blood flow. The latter can occur from multiple, interrelated causes: the normal postnatal drop in the pulmonary vascular resistance; improved pulmonary compliance from surfactant therapy; and normal postnatal absorption of lung fluid. These changes may lead to an acute increase in pulmonary blood flow and hemorrhagic pulmonary edema.

    B. Hematological factors: DIC secondary to sepsis can lead to abnormal coagulation and hemorrhage. Bleeding may be found at other sites, such as the gastrointestinal and renal mucous membranes and the brain. The underlying sepsis or shock could further compromise local vascular integrity, leading to an acute episode of bleeding.

V. Pathology: A wide range of pathologic appearances has been reported. In mild forms, scattered red blood cells in the intra-alveolar and intraparenchymal spaces may be the only findings, with little or no blood in the airways. In infants who die from pulmonary hemorrhage, massive amounts of frank blood may be found in the parenchyma, small and large airways, trachea, and oral cavity (Fig. 68-1).

A. Macroscopic features: The lung weight is increased, its lobar borders are obliterated, and frank blood is seen in the airways, trachea, and pleural space.

B. Microscopic features: Large islands of blood in the alveolar and parenchymal spaces may be seen. Blood may be found to occupy the lumen of larger bronchi and the trachea. Pulmonary hemorrhage is reported to be predominantly alveolar in infants treated with exogenous surfactants, whereas it is predominantly interstitial in those not treated with surfactants. Thus, surfactant therapy may alter the distribution of bleeding sites rather than causing an increase in the incidence of pulmonary hemorrhage.

C. Other changes: Reactive leucocytosis and changes of RDS and bronchopulmonary dysplasia (BPD) may be found, along with those of pneumonia and bleeding in other organs, especially the intestine, kidneys, and brain.

VI. Clinical Features: The severity and magnitude of clinical signs depend upon the magnitude of hemorrhage and the severity of the underlying condition leading to the episode. The clinical manifestations result from several interrelated pathophysiologic consequences of blood loss and hemorrhage into the lung parenchyma and airways.

A. A rapidly deteriorating pulmonary condition is the hallmark of massive pulmonary hemorrhage.

1. Hypoxia, hypercarbia, and increasing requirements of ventilatory support are seen secondary to worsening of pulmonary compliance from blood in the lung tissue.

2. Frank blood can be seen pouring out of the mouth, or in milder cases, blood-tinged tracheal and oropharyngeal effluent may be seen.

3. The blood blocks the airways, increasing resistance and further causing worsening of the already deteriorating blood gas and acid-base status.

B. Extraneous blood in the lung parenchyma increases the consumption of the administered surfactant and inhibits its function. Plasma proteins and blood also inhibit endogenous surfactant production.

C. The pulmonary deterioration almost invariably is accompanied by an acute deterioration in the systemic status; a rapid drop in blood pressure and cardiac output leads to classic signs of shock, along with severe pallor and anemia.

D. In infants who survive the acute episode, widespread pulmonary inflammation from blood in the lung tissues can lead to later complications such as pneumonia, a prolonged need for assisted ventilation, and CLD.

E. Because the clinical findings are interrelated and depend on the severity of hemorrhage, in some cases, several hours may elapse before there are signs of shock and collapse.

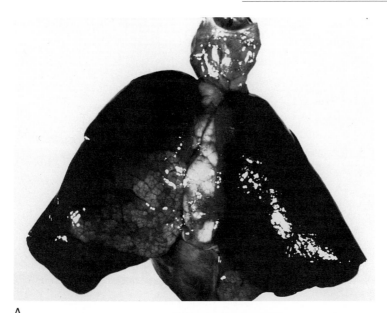

A

B

FIGURE 68-1. A, Gross appearance of the lungs of an infant who died of massive pulmonary hemorrhage. B, Microscopic findings in lung section of the same infant shows large quantities of blood in the alveolar spaces and scattered bleeding sites in the interstitial spaces. Generalized features of hyaline membrane formation and widespread inflammatory reaction are seen. In C and D, lung sections from two other cases are shown.   (*Continued*)

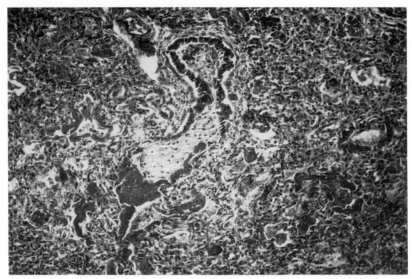

C

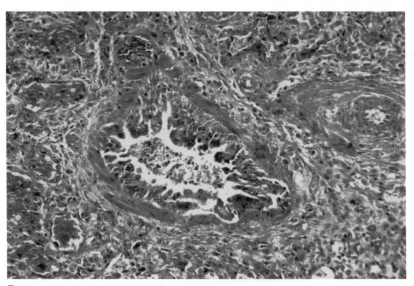

D

FIGURE 68-1 CONT'D. C, Massive pulmonary hemorrhage occurred 2 weeks prior to death. D, Infant died at 4 weeks of age from respiratory failure secondary to bronchopulmonary dysplasia; there was no clinical evidence of pulmonary hemorrhage. Scattered areas of bleeding can be identified. Both infants show varying degrees of chronic changes in the lungs.

1. Always suspect pulmonary hemorrhage in infants on assisted ventilation who appear otherwise "stable" but who gradually manifest worsening hypoxia, hypercapnia, and acidosis, requiring higher than the original ventilator settings.
2. Localized, small pulmonary hemorrhage may cause the symptoms to evolve over 6 to 8 hours; in such cases, pulmonary hemorrhage should always be high on the list of differential diagnoses.

F. In the presence of systemic shock and sudden deterioration, consider pulmonary hemorrhage even in the absence of blood or blood-tinged orotracheal effluent, because the bleeding may be interstitial.
1. A reduction in hematocrit and platelet counts may occur hours later.
2. Cardiac murmur and/or other signs of patent ductus arteriosus (PDA) may be present.

G. Other causes of left-to-right shunting and of pulmonary edema must be evaluated, such as congestive cardiac failure (ventricular septal defect, atrial septal defect, cerebral arteriovenous malformations).

VII. Investigations

A. Chest radiograph. There are no specific diagnostic features in chest radiographs.
1. Diffuse, scattered haziness, consolidation, fluffy radiodensities, and features of the underlying disease (RDS, BPD, or PIE) should suggest pulmonary hemorrhage.
2. Cardiomegaly may or may not be present, depending on the underlying cause of pulmonary hemorrhage (Figs. 68-2 and 68-3).

B. Evaluating for PDA.
1. Suspect a significant PDA in infants with pulmonary hemorrhage, even in the absence of a typical "PDA murmur," or a wide pulse pressure, heaving precordium.
2. An echocardiogram is recommended.

C. Blood tests and work-up for sepsis.
1. Blood gas and acid-base status
2. Hemoglobin and hematocrit
3. Platelet count
4. Total and differential white blood cell count
5. Bacterial culture from blood and urine should be considered
6. Viral and fungal cultures may be indicated
7. Tests for DIC (e.g., prothrombin time, partial thromboplastin time, fibrin split products) are optional

D. Search for inherited disorders of coagulation (e.g., hemophilia, von Willebrand disease).

E. For bleeding in other organs: Urinalysis to rule out major bleeding in the kidney and a cranial ultrasound examination to rule out intracranial hemorrhage are recommended, depending on other findings.

VIII. Treatment

A. General supportive care
1. Administer intensive care and antishock measures.

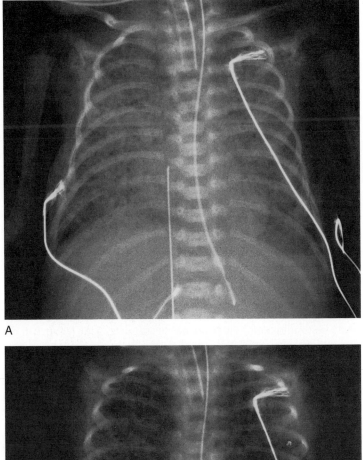

A

B

FIGURE **68-2.** Evolution of pulmonary hemorrhage in an infant with respiratory distress syndrome. Chest radiographs show typical features of severe pulmonary interstitial emphysema on the fifth day (**A**) and severe pulmonary hemorrhage on the seventh day (**B**). Heart size is normal.

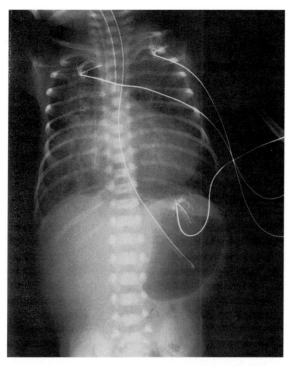

FIGURE **68-3.** Chest radiograph of a preterm infant who developed severe pulmonary hemorrhage on the sixth day secondary to a large, florid patent ductus arteriosus and signs of congestive heart failure. Pulmonary hemorrhage was accompanied by respiratory deterioration. Scattered radio-opaque densities, mostly in both lower lobes, can be seen, and there is moderate cardiomegaly.

    a. Transfuse with blood, plasma, or platelets as indicated.
    b. Correct metabolic acidosis.
    c. Administer inotropic agents to improve systemic blood pressure.
  2. Ventilatory support: With a few exceptions, most recommendations for ventilatory support have evolved based on empirical observations.
    a. Conventional ventilatory support: Increase ventilatory settings to provide a higher rate, higher PEEP, and higher Pāw.
    b. High-frequency oscillatory ventilation (HFOV) support: In a prospective observational study, it was found that 10 of 17 infants with massive pulmonary hemorrhage responded to early treatment with HFOV. All of them survived. In contrast, only one of three infants given conventional ventilatory support survived.
  3. Treat the PDA: Unless there is severe thrombocytopenia, indomethacin therapy can be used in known or suspected pulmonary hemorrhage to treat the PDA, even if had been given earlier.

    4. Treatment of infections: Antibiotics most likely to be effective against common bacterial pathogens include ampicillin (or vancomycin), along with a drug for gram-negative coverage, given until a specific etiologic agent, if any, is identified.

B. Specific treatment strategies

    1. Recombinant factor VIIa (rFVIIa): Factor rFVIIa, a vitamin K–dependent glycoprotein that is structurally similar to the plasma-derived natural factor VII, is considered a universal hemostatic agent. It acts by triggering the extrinsic coagulation cascade and forming a hemostatic seal at the site of capillary leak, providing a plug and stopping the bleeding. A dose of 80 µg/kg rFVIIa can normalize prolonged prothrombin time. This drug has been used with success in two isolated cases of neonatal pulmonary hemorrhage at doses of 50 µg/kg/dose, repeated every 3 hours for 2 to 3 days. In other studies, rFVIIa used in infants developing pulmonary hemorrhage at much higher doses also resulting in stopping pulmonary hemorrhage. More work is needed to establish the dosage and the frequency of administration, as well as to assess the consistency of response in infants with neonatal pulmonary hemorrhage.

    2. Exogenous surfactant: Exogenous surfactant improves the respiratory status in infants with pulmonary hemorrhage. The administered surfactant replenishes the endogenous surfactant pool depleted from inhibition or inactivation from blood and plasma in the alveoli.

    3. Other measures to stop pulmonary hemorrhage: Nebulized epinephrine with or without 4% cocaine has been found to temporize massive bleeding. Experience using these drugs is limited in the newborn.

IX. Outcome

  A. Mortality: Average, 50%; range, 30% to 90%.

  B. Morbidity: 50% to 75% of survivors develop CLD of varying severity.

X. Prevention

  A. Antenatal corticosteroids: Enhancing lung maturity may reduce pulmonary hemorrhage through its indirect effect on the lungs and pulmonary vascular bed.

  B. Preventing PDA: Although early administration of indomethacin and ibuprofen have shown a strong effect in reducing the incidence of significant PDA, whether such a strategy will affect pulmonary hemorrhage incidence is unclear.

  C. Monitoring for PDA and its prompt therapy: Vigilant monitoring for the signs of PDA in preterm infants treated with exogenous surfactants for RDS should be the mainstay for preventing pulmonary hemorrhage. In infants with rapid improvement in pulmonary compliance, even a minimally PDA can cause a sudden worsening of pulmonary compliance and lead to pulmonary hemorrhage.

  D. HFOV: In a large trial, the incidence of pulmonary hemorrhage was 2% (5 of 244 infants) in a group of small preterm infants treated

with HFOV, compared with 7% (17 of 254 infants) in a group
treated with conventional ventilation ($P < .02$).

Suggested Reading

Alkharfy TM: High-frequency ventilation in the management of very-low-birth-weight infants
  with pulmonary hemorrhage. Am J Perinatol 1:19-26, 2004.
Amizuka T, Shimizu , Niida Y, Ogawa Y: Surfactant therapy in neonates with respiratory failure
  due to hemorrhagic pulmonary oedema. Eur J Pediatr 162:69, 2003.
Baroutis G, Kaleyias J, Liarou T, et al: Comparison of three treatment regimens of natural
  surfactant preparations in neonatal respiratory distress syndrome. Eur J Pediatr
  62:476-480, 2003.
Centers for Disease Control and Prevention: Investigation of acute idiopathic pulmonary
  hemorrhage among infants—Massachusetts, December 2002– June 2003. MMRW Morb
  Mortal Wkly Rep 3:817, 2004.
Courtney SE, Durand DJ, Asselin M, et al: High-frequency oscillatory ventilation versus
  conventional ventilation for very-low-birth-weight infants. N Engl J Med 347:643-652, 2002.
Dufourq N, Thomson M, Adhikari M, Moodley J: Massive pulmonary hemorrhage as a cause of
  death in the neonate—A retrospective review. S Afr Med J 94:299-302, 2004.
Findlay RD, Taeusch HW, David WR, Walther FJ: Lysis of blood cells and alveolar epithelial
  toxicity by therapeutic pulmonary surfactants. Pediatr Res 37:26-30, 1995.
Goretksy MJ, Martinasek D, Warner BW: Pulmonary hemorrhage: A novel complication after
  extracorporeal life support. J Pediatr Surg 1:1276-1281, 1996.
Greisen G, Andreasen RB: Recombinant factor VIIa in preterm neonates with prolonged
  prothrombin time. Blood Coagul Fibrinolysis 14:117-120, 2003.
Kluckow M, Evans N: Ductal shunting, high pulmonary flow, and pulmonary hemorrhage.
  J Pediatr 137:68-72, 2000.
Lamboley-Gilmert G, Lacaze-Masmonteil T; Neonatologists of the Curosurf Study Group: The
  short-term outcome of a large cohort of very preterm infants treated with Poractant Alfa
  (Curosurf) for respiratory distress syndrome. A postmarketing phase IV study. Paediatr Drugs
  5:639-645, 2003.
Leibovitch L, Kenet G, Mazor K: Recombinant activated factor VII for life-threatening pulmonary
  hemorrhage after pediatric cardiac surgery. Pediatr Crit Care Med 4:444-446, 2003.
Lin TW, Su BH, Lin HC, et al: Risk factors of pulmonary hemorrhage in very-low-birthweight
  infants: A two-year retrospective study. Acta Pediatr Taiwan 45:255-258. 2004.
Long W, Corbet A, Allen A, et al: Retrospective search for bleeding diathesis among premature
  newborn infants with pulmonary hemorrhage after synthetic surfactant treatment. J Pediatr
  120:545-548, 1992.
Olomu N, Kulkarni R, Manco-Johnson M: Treatment of severe pulmonary hemorrhage with
  activated recombinant factor VII (rFVIIa) in very low birth weight infants. J Perinatol
  22:672-674, 2002.
Pandit PB, Dunn MS, Colucci EA: Surfactant therapy in neonates with respiratory deterioration
  due to pulmonary hemorrhage. Pediatrics 95:32-36, 1995.
Pappin A, Shenker N, Jack M, Redline RW: Extensive intraalveolar pulmonary hemorrhage in
  infants dying after surfactant therapy. J Pediatr 124:621-626, 1994.
Raju TNK, Langenberg P: Pulmonary hemorrhage and exogenous surfactant therapy: A meta-analysis.
  J Pediatr 123:603-610, 1993.
Rao KVS, Michalski L: Intrauterine pulmonary hemorrhage secondary to antenatal Coxsackie B-2
  infection. Pediatr Res 1:265A, 1997.
St. John EB, Carlo WA: Respiratory distress syndrome in VLBW infants: Changes in management
  and outcomes observed by the NICHD Neonatal Research Network. Semin Perinatol
  27:288-292, 2003.
Suresh GK, Soll RF: Exogenous surfactant therapy in newborn infants. Ann Acad Med Singapore
  32:335-345, 2003.
Tobias J, Berkenbosch JW, Russo P: Recombinant factor VIIa to treat bleeding after cardiac
  surgery in an infant. Pediatr Crit Care Med 41:49-51, 2003.
van Houten J, Long W, Mullett M, et al: Pulmonary hemorrhage in premature infants after
  treatment with synthetic surfactant: An autopsy evaluation. J Pediatr 120:540-544, 1992.

69 Retinopathy of Prematurity

Alistair R. Fielder

I. Introduction
  A. Retinopathy of prematurity (ROP) is a condition confined to the developing retinal vessels.
  B. ROP has acute and late phases, which are classified according to the International Classification of ROP (1984, 1987, 2005).
  C. Acute phase ROP has five stages (see Table 69-1):
    1. *Mild disease:* ROP that reaches a maximum at stage 1 or 2 and resolves fully and without visually disabling sequelae.
    2. *Severe disease:* Stage 3 is the first stage that presents a significant risk for poor visual outcome. Stages 4 and 5 (being associated with retinal detachment) always carry a dismal visual prognosis.
II. Prevention
  A. The standard of care is critical in keeping severe disease to a minimum, although it is recognized that despite meticulous neonatal care, *ROP is not entirely preventable.*
  B. The major ROP risk factor is the degree of prematurity, but many associations and complications of preterm birth have also have been implicated.
    1. Oxygen
      a. Hyperoxia, hypoxia, and fluctuations of arterial oxygen even within the normal range have all been implicated as etiologic factors.
      b. Keep arterial oxygen levels within the recommended range. Avoid fluctuations of arterial oxygen levels whenever possible.
    2. Steroids
      a. Antenatal corticosteroid administration (to induce lung maturity) has been associated with a reduced incidence of severe ROP.
      b. Postnatal steroids to treat respiratory distress syndrome may be associated with more severe ROP, but it is not known whether this is a causal relationship.
    3. Surfactant treatment does not affect ROP incidence.
    4. Light reduction. Lowering the ambient illumination of the neonatal unit does not reduce the incidence or severity of ROP.
    5. Many other risk factors have been suggested, including vitamin E deficiency, exchange transfusions, necrotizing enterocolitis, treatment for patent ductus arteriosus, and other complications of prematurity.

III. Screening
    A. Purpose: To identify severe ROP, which may require treatment and which, even if it does not, is associated with a high incidence of visually severe sequelae.
    B. Which babies should be examined?
        1. ROP incidence and severity both rise with increasing immaturity.
        2. U.S. guidelines: All babies with ≤1500 g birth weight or gestational age (GA) ≤28 weeks, as well as larger babies considered by the neonatologist, because of an unstable clinical course, to be at high risk. Such babies should have at least two examinations.
        3. U.K. guidelines: All babies ≤ 1500 g birth weight and <32 weeks GA, regardless of clinical condition.
        4. Larger babies are at risk in countries with more variable standards of neonatal care (e.g., Latin America, Eastern Europe). This emphasizes the need for locally derived protocols.
IV. Examination Protocol
    A. Principles
        1. Age at ROP onset and the rate of progression are determined mainly by postmenstrual age (PMA) rather than by neonatal events.
        2. The time available for treatment is short, within 2 to 3 days of the diagnosis of threshold ROP (usually, but not always, between 33 and 40 weeks PMA).
          a. The mean age for treatment prethreshold is 35 weeks PMA.
          b. The mean age for treatment at threshold is 37 weeks PMA.
        3. The initial examination should be between 4 and 6 weeks (U.S. guidelines) or between 6 and 7 weeks (U.K. guidelines) postnatal age.
        4. Subsequent examinations
          a. Every 2 weeks, or every week (this frequency minimizes loss to review and ensures that almost all screening is completed while the baby is in the hospital).
          b. Babies for transfer to another hospital prior to completion of the screening program. Ensure that the receiving hospital is alerted to screening requirements of the baby.
          c. Babies for discharge to home. Ensure a follow-up appointment until screening is completed.
        5. Completion of screening
          a. Vascularization that has proceeded into zone III (peripheral-most portion of the temporal retina), without ROP
          b. The development of ROP, at which point examinations are dictated by clinical criteria
        6. Screening examination
          a. To be carried out by an experienced ophthalmologist following pupillary dilatation
          b. ROP is recorded (Figure 69-1) according to the following 4 criteria:
            (1) Severity by stages: 1 to 5 and aggressive posterior ROP (AP-ROP)

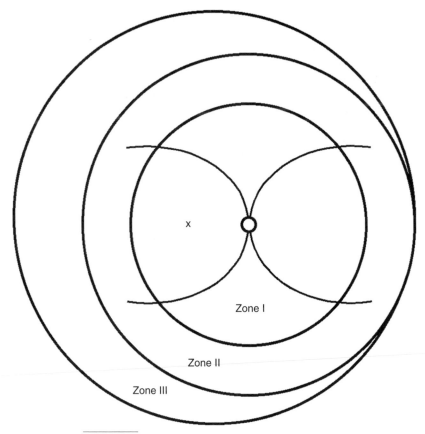

FIGURE 69-1. See text for description. X, macula fovea.

      (2) Location by zone I to III; the closer to zone I (i.e., posterior) the greater the propensity to become severe

      (3) Extent by clock hour involvement

      (4) Presence of "plus" disease (see Table 69-1)

      It is critical to record each of these criteria following every examination and to record the absence or presence of "plus" disease, even if no ROP is observed.

  V. Responsibilities and Organization

    A. Effective and efficient screening for ROP and its subsequent management require multiprofessional teamwork.

    B. National guidelines form the basis of protocols that should be developed locally and jointly by the neonatal and ophthalmic teams.

    C. Identification of babies requiring screening is the responsibility of the neonatal team.

    D. Arrangement for any postexamination follow-up required is the responsibility of the ophthalmologist.

  VI. Information for Parents

Table **69-1.** International Classification of Retinopathy of Prematurity (ROP)

A. Severity by Stage

1. *Demarcation line*
   Thin white line, lying within the plane of the retina and separating avascular from vascular retinal regions.
2. *Ridge*
   The line of stage 1 has increased in volume to extend out of the plane of the retina. Isolated vascular tufts may be seen posterior to the ridge at this stage.
3. *Ridge with extraretinal fibrovascular proliferation*
   This may:
   a. be continuous with the posterior edge of the ridge.
   b. be posterior to, but disconnected from, the ridge.
   c. extend into the vitreous.
4. *Retinal detachment—subtotal*
   Extrafoveal (4A), or involving the fovea (4B)
5. *Retinal detachment—total*
   The detached retina is funnel-shaped, which may be open or closed along all or part of its extent.
6. *Aggressive Posterior ROP (AP-ROP)*
   Commences with posterior pole vessel dilatation and tortuosity in all 4 quadrants. Deceptively featureless and does not progress from stage 1 to 3, but as a flat network of vessels at the junction between vascularized and nonvascularized retina. Typically, AP-ROP is circumferential and mostly in zone I, but also posterior zone II.

B. Location by Zone

Retinal blood vessels grow out from the optic disk in zone I toward the periphery (zone III); thus the retinal zone vascularized reflects maturity. ROP in zone I affects the most immature infant and is very likely to become severe with a poor outcome, whereas ROP located in zone III carries a very low risk for severity and adverse outcome.

C. Extent

The extent of ROP around the retinal circumference is recorded in "clock hours" 1 to 12.

D. "Plus" Disease

"Plus" disease is an indicator of ROP activity: In order of increasing severity, engorgement and tortuosity of the posterior pole retinal vessels, iris vessel engorgement, pupil rigidity, and vitreous haze. These are powerful indicators that ROP is, or will become, severe. Plus involves vessels in 2 or more quadrants. Pre-plus describes abnormalities that are insufficient for the diagnosis of plus.

    A. Mild ROP is very common, but most babies do not develop severe ROP, so conversations and literature need to convey this sense.

    B. For babies with, or close to, severe ROP who may require treatment, a personal discussion between the ophthalmologist and parents is important, and this should also involve a member of the neonatal team.

VII. Management of ROP

    A. Once ROP has been diagnosed, the baby leaves the screening program and is managed according to standard ophthalmic practice.

    B. Although most of these babies require examination every 2 weeks, more frequent examinations are indicated for babies with ROP in zone I or ROP that is close to requiring treatment.

VIII. Treatment Criteria

A. Until 2003 the indication for treatment was "threshold," the ROP stage at which the risk of blindness, if untreated, is about 50%. Threshold is defined as stage 3 ROP extending over five or more continuous, or eight or more cumulative, clock hours of the retinal circumference, with "plus" disease.

B. Acknowledging that outcome following treatment at threshold was frequently not ideal, indications for treatment have been revised and extended. The revised indications for treatment recognize two types of prethreshold diseases:
1. Type 1 prethreshold ROP (should be treated)
   a. Zone I, any ROP with "plus" disease
   b. Zone I, stage 3 ROP without "plus" disease
   c. Zone II, stage 2 or 3 with "plus" disease
2. Type 2, prethreshold ROP
   a. Zone I, stage 1 or 2 ROP without "plus" disease
   b. Zone II, stage 3 ROP without "plus" disease

Eyes should be reviewed, with treatment, if there is progression to type 1 prethreshold or to threshold ROP (i.e., to "plus" disease).

C. "Plus" disease is now the key criterion for treatment and the major difference between type 1 that requires treatment and type 2 prethreshold that does not.

D. Some eyes with type 2 prethreshold ROP will progress to threshold, which remains another criterion for treatment.

IX. Treatment Timing
A. Once type 1 or threshold ROP has been diagnosed, treatment by laser (cryotherapy is now infrequently used) should be performed within 2 to 3 days.
B. It is recognized that the window of opportunity for treatment is not precisely defined and that some eyes require intervention more urgently than others.

X. Long-Term Follow-up
A. All severe ROP requires ophthalmic follow-up, at least to 5 years of age because of the risk of reduced vision, myopia, and strabismus.
B. The follow-up of very low birth weight babies who did not develop severe ROP is less well defined, but the likelihood of developing myopia and strabismus in childhood is much higher than in their full-term counterparts.

XI. Future Directions
A. The revised classification of ROP recognizes that:
1. ROP in zone I and posterior zone II (AP-ROP), that has a poor outcome, appears deceptively innocuous.
2. "Plus" disease needs further definition, and now includes milder abnormalities pre-"Plus" disease.
B. The onset of screening can begin later in the most immature babies.
C. The revised indications for treatment require more frequent examinations when prethreshold ROP has been reached.
D. These changes need to be incorporated into national clinical guidelines.

Suggested Reading

American Academy of Pediatrics, American Association for Pediatric Ophthalmology and Strabismus, and American Academy of Ophthalmology: Screening examination of premature infants for retinopathy of prematurity. Pediatrics 108:809-811, 2001.

A Second International Committee for the Classification of Retinopathy of Prematurity: The International Classification of Retinopathy of Prematurity Revisited. Arch Ophthalmol, in press.

Early Treatment for Retinopathy of Prematurity Cooperative Group: Revised indications for the treatment of retinopathy of prematurity. Arch Ophthalmol 2003; 121:1684-1696.

Fielder AR, Quinn GE: Retinopathy of prematurity. In Taylor DSI, Hoyt CS (eds): Pediatric Ophthalmology and Strabismus, 3rd ed. Philadelphia, Elsevier, 2005, pp 506-530.

Fielder AR, Reynolds JD: Retinopathy of prematurity: Clinical aspects. Semin Neonatol 6:461-477, 2001.

Gilbert C, Fielder A, Gordillo L, et al: Characteristics of babies with severe retinopathy of prematurity in countries with low, moderate and high levels of development: Implications for screening program. Pediatrics 115:e518-e525, Epub 2005.

Higgins RD, Mendelsohn AL, DeFeo MJ: Antenatal dexamethasone and decreased severity of retinopathy of prematurity. Arch Ophthalmol 116:601-605, 1998.

Report of a joint working party. Retinopathy of Prematurity: Guidelines for screening and treatment. Royal College of Ophthalmologists and British Association of Perinatal Medicine, 1995. Early Hum Dev 46:239-258, 1996.

Reynolds JD, Dobson V, Quinn GE, et al: Evidence-based screening for retinopathy of prematurity: natural history data from CRYO-ROP and LIGHT-ROP studies. Arch Ophthalmol 120: 1470-1476, 2002.

Reynolds JD, Hardy RJ, Kennedy KA, et al: Lack of efficacy of light reduction in preventing retinopathy of prematurity. New Engl J Med 338:1572-1576, 1998.

Tin W, Wariyar U: Giving small babies oxygen: 50 years of uncertainty. Semin Neonatol 7:361-367, 2002.

Wheatley CM, Dickinson JL, Mackey DA, et al: Retinopathy of prematurity: Recent advances in our understanding. Arch Dis Child 86:696-700, 2002.

70

Neurologic Complications of Mechanical Ventilation

Jeffrey M. Perlman

I. Background
   A. The developing brain of the newborn and in particular of the premature infant requiring mechanical ventilation is at increased risk for hemorrhagic and/or ischemic injury (Table 70-1).
   B. The most frequent lesions noted are periventricular intraventricular hemorrhage (PV-IVH) and injury to white matter often referred to as periventricular leukomalacia (PVL).
   C. These lesions are most likely to occur in the premature infant with respiratory distress syndrome (RDS) requiring mechanical ventilation.
   D. The etiology of both lesions is likely multifactorial.
      1. Perturbations in cerebral blood flow (CBF) are considered to be of paramount importance.
      2. In the sick newborn infant, the cerebral circulation appears to be pressure-passive—that is, changes in CBF directly reflect similar changes in systemic blood pressure.
      3. Pressure-passive flow increases the potential for cerebral injury during periods of systemic hypotension or hypertension.
      4. The cerebral circulation is also exquisitely sensitive to changes in $PaCO_2$ and to a lesser extent pH.

TABLE 70-1. Risk Factors for Cerebral Injury in Sick Premature Infants Requiring Mechanical Ventilation

A. Cerebral
   1. Vulnerable capillary beds—e.g., germinal matrix, periventricular white matter
   2. Pressure passive cerebral circulation

B. Respiratory
   1. Respiratory distress syndrome
   2. Pneumothorax/pulmonary interstitial emphysema

C. Vascular: Perturbations in systemic hemodynamics—e.g., hypotension, hypertension, fluctuations in systemic blood pressure

D. Consequences of mechanical ventilation
   1. High mean airway pressure
   2. Hypocarbia

     5. Mechanical ventilation of the sick newborn infant can directly or indirectly affect CBF via systemic vascular or acid-base changes and thus increase the risk for cerebral injury.

II. Mechanical Ventilation and Potential Brain Injury

  A. Direct effects

    1. Infants breathing out of synchrony with the ventilator: The sick infant with RDS may exhibit beat-to-beat fluctuations in arterial blood pressure. The arterial fluctuations that affect both the systolic and diastolic components of the waveform appear to be related to the infant's own respiratory effort, which invariably is out of synchrony with the ventilator breaths. Thus, the fluctuations are increased with increasing respiratory effort and are minimized when respiratory effort is absent (Fig. 70-1). The arterial blood pressure fluctuations are associated with similar beat-to-beat fluctuations in the cerebral circulation consistent with a pressure passive state. The cerebral fluctuations, if persistent, have been associated with subsequent PV-IVH. Minimizing the fluctuation is associated with a reduction in hemorrhage. Minimize fluctuations by:

      a. Increasing ventilator support

      b. Using synchronized mechanical ventilation (e.g., assist/control ventilation)

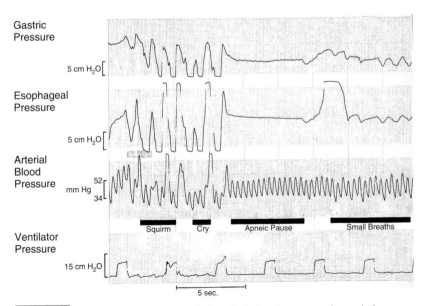

Figure 70-1. Tracing obtained from an infant depicting the temporal association between blood pressure fluctuations and gastric, esophageal, and respiratory pressure changes. Note the marked continuous fluctuations in arterial blood pressure affecting both systolic and diastolic blood pressures during "squirmlike" activity. Note also the immediate stabilization of arterial blood pressure associated with a brief variety of respiratory activities. Variability in blood pressure is again seen in association with small breaths at the end of the tracing.

    c. Sedating

    d. Using skeletal muscle paralysis (this has become less frequent in recent years given the above ventilator strategies)

  2. Impedance of venous return

    a. Increase in mean airway pressure (Pāw) may impede venous return to the heart with two consequences:

      (1) An increase in central venous pressure and, as a result, an increase in intracranial venous pressure

      (2) A decrease in cardiac output

    b. A combination of an elevated venous pressure and a concomitant decrease in cardiac output markedly increases the risk for cerebral hypoperfusion within vulnerable regions of the brain (i.e., periventricular white matter).

    c. High Pāw is often utilized with either conventional or high-frequency ventilation in the sick infant with respiratory failure.

    d. An association between the use of high-frequency ventilation and PVL has been observed.

    e. Close monitoring of the vascular system is critical in the sick infant requiring high Pāw to support respiratory function.

  3. Effects of $PaCO_2$

    a. The cerebral circulation is exquisitely sensitive to changes in $PaCO_2$ (i.e., hypocarbia decreases CBF, and hypercarbia increases CBF). This relationship appears to be intact in the sick newborn infant.

    b. Hyperventilation with a reduction in $PaCO_2$ has been utilized as a strategy to augment pulmonary blood flow. The resultant hypocarbia may significantly reduce CBF.

    c. Several studies report the association of hypocarbia and PVL as well as with subsequent neurodevelopmental defects.

    d. Conversely, hypercarbia with an increase in CBF has been associated with an increased risk for PV-IVH.

B. Indirect effects: Complications of RDS

  1. Ventilated infants with RDS are at increased risk for air leaks (i.e., pneumothorax and/or pulmonary interstitial emphysema).

  2. There is a strong association between pneumothorax and subsequent PV-IVH.

  3. The potential mechanisms that link these two conditions are likely multifactorial:

    a. An impediment of venous return

    b. A decrease in cardiac output

    c. An increase in $PaCO_2$

    d. Hemodynamic changes that accompany evacuation of pleural air

C. Other associations

  1. Sensorineural hearing loss: Term infants with pulmonary hypertension subjected to hyperventilation are at increased risk for sensorineural hearing loss. The mechanism of such injury remains unclear.

  2. Intracerebellar hemorrhage: Intracerebellar hemorrhage was noted in a series of infants who had received positive-pressure ventilation

via a face mask attached by a band across the occiput. It is presumed that the band induced occipital molding that resulted in distortion and obstruction of the major venous sinuses.

D. Potential therapeutic strategies
  1. Reduction of fluctuations in systemic hemodynamics
    a. Synchronized ventilation
    b. Sedation
    c. Paralysis
  2. Avoid systemic hypotension and/or hypertension:
    a. Consider inotropic support.
    b. Consider volume expansion.
  3. Avoid impedance of venous return by using lower Pāw (if feasible).
  4. Avoid hypocarbia:
    a. Decrease ventilator rate and/or pressure/tidal volume.
    b. Use "permissive hypercapnia" (controversial).
  5. Avoid pneumothorax:
    a. Surfactant administration for RDS
    b. Synchronized ventilation
    c. Rapid weaning, as tolerated

Suggested Reading

Fujimoto S, Togari H, Yamaguchi N, et al: Hypocarbia and cystic periventricular leukomalacia in premature infants. Arch Dis Child 71:F107-F110, 1994.

Greisen G, Munck H, Lou H: Severe hypocarbia in preterm infants and neurodevelopmental deficit. Acta Pediatr Scand 76:401-404, 1987.

Gullberg N, Winberg P, Selldén H: Changes in stroke volume cause change in cardiac output in neonates and infants when mean airway pressure is altered. Acta Anesthesiol Scand 43:999-1003, 1999.

Hendricks-Munoz KD, Walter JP: Hearing loss in infants with persistent fetal circulation. Pediatrics 81:650-656, 1988.

Hill A, Perlman JM, Volpe J: Relationship of pneumothorax to the occurrence of intraventricular hemorrhage in the premature newborn. Pediatrics 69:144-149, 1982.

Mirro R, Busija D, Green R, Leffler CB: Relationship between mean airway pressure, cardiac output and organ blood flow with normal and decreased respiratory compliance. J Pediatr 111:101-106, 1987.

Pape KE, Armstrong DL, Fitzhardinge PM: Central venous system pathology associated with mask ventilation in the very low birth weight infant. A new etiology for intracerebellar hemorrhage. Pediatrics 58:473-483, 1976.

Perlman JM, Goodman S, Kreusser KL, Volpe JJ: Reduction in intraventricular hemorrhage by elimination of fluctuating cerebral blood flow velocity in preterm infants with respiratory distress syndrome. N Engl J Med 312:1353-1357, 1985.

Perlman JM, McMenamin JB, Volpe JJ: Fluctuating cerebral blood flow velocity in respiratory distress syndrome: Relationship to subsequent development of intraventricular hemorrhage. N Engl J Med 309:204-209, 1983.

Perlman JM, Volpe JJ: Are venous circulatory changes important in the pathogenesis of hemorrhagic and/or ischemic cerebral injury? Pediatrics 80:705-711, 1987.

Pryds O, Greisen G, Lou H, Friis-Hansen B: Heterogeneity of cerebral vasoreactivity in preterm infants supported by mechanical ventilation. J Pediatr 115:638-645, 1989.

Shalak L, Perlman JM: Hemorrhagic-ischemic cerebral injury in the preterm infant: Current concepts Clin Perinatol 29:745-763, 2002.

Wiswell TE, Graziani LJ, Kornhauser MS: Effects of hypocarbia on the development of cystic periventricular leukomalacia in premature infants treated with high frequency jet ventilation. Pediatrics 98:918-924, 1996.

Other
Considerations

71

Nursing Care of the Ventilated Newborn

Kimberly LaMar

I. History: History taking assists in focusing on an area while keeping the mind open to other possibilities.
   A. Maternal, including past and existing medical conditions
   B. Family
   C. Social
   D. Delivery room
   E. Neonatal
II. Assessment: Normal physiology, pathophysiology, and embryology are key to understanding the concepts of respiratory disease in the newborn.
   A. Observation
      1. Color
         a. Generalized color, as well as central color, is determined by examining the mucous membranes.
         b. Cyanosis results from the presence of >5 g/dL unsaturated Hb in the blood.
         c. Oxyhemoglobin dissociation curve: Fetal Hb has high affinity for oxygen, leading to an association of high saturation at a lower PaO_2.
      2. Mouth and nose
         a. Secretions: Amount, color, consistency. Usually clear or white. Excessive secretions may be associated with a tracheoesophageal fistula. Coryza with thick, white secretions may be seen with respiratory synctial virus infection.
         b. Nasal flaring to decrease resistance in upper airways.
         c. Nasal stuffiness associated with maternal illicit drug use.
         d. Nasal snuffles with copious amounts of nasal drainage seen with congenital syphilis.
      3. Chest
         a. Size and shape: Normal chest size in a full-term infant is 33 ± 3 cm, or 2 cm less than the head circumference.
         b. Deviations include pigeon chest with protrusion of the sternum and funnel chest with an indented sternum. These may be seen in Marfan syndrome and neonatal rickets.
         c. An increased diameter or "barrel chest" may be seen in meconium aspiration syndrome.

   d. Symmetry of chest is assessed at the nipple line.
   e. Synchrony of chest during ventilation and chest excursions with ventilator breaths are assessed.
   f. Respirations are counted for a full minute to determine rate. Tachypnea is a rate >60 breaths/min; apnea is cessation of respirations for 20 seconds; hypopnea is shallow spontaneous respiratory effort.
   g. High-frequency ventilation is assessed by amount of chest vibration or "wiggle."
   h. Retractions are caused by baby's soft cartilage and muscle groups that pull on this cartilage in an effort to augment respiration. They may be intercostal, subcostal, sternal, suprasternal, and subxiphoid. "Seesaw" pattern of chest and abdominal breathing also may be exhibited.
   i. Work of breathing is observed as a comfortable, easy pattern or increased work of breathing when the infant is entirely involved in respiratory effort to the exclusion of all other activity.
B. Auscultation
   1. External
      a. Grunting is heard without the use of a stethoscope. It is the sound of the baby exhaling against a partially closed glottis in an attempt to prevent alveolar collapse.
      b. Air leak may be heard in very small babies or in those with higher support, as the endotracheal tube (ETT) is uncuffed. This may also be identified with graphic monitoring on the ventilator.
      c. Cry may be lusty, weak, absent, hoarse, shrill, or high-pitched as in cri du chat syndrome.
      d. Stridor is a high-pitched sound heard either at inspiration or expiration that indicates partial obstruction of the airway. It may be associated with postextubation edema, laryngomalacia, and damage to the vocal cords.
   2. Internal
      a. Assess with the warmed bell side of a neonatal stethoscope.
      b. Compare and contrast side to side of chest on the anterior chest and posterior chest.
      c. Crackles are fine, medium, or coarse and represent air or fluid moving in the small or large airways. Fine crackles originate in the dependent lobes of the lungs and are heard at the end of inspiration and may be associated with respiratory distress syndrome (RDS) or chronic lung disease (CLD). Medium crackles originate in the bronchioles and may be associated with air moving through tenacious fluid, as in pneumonia or transient tachypnea of the newborn. Coarse crackles are bubbly and are associated with fluid in the large airways and usually resolve with clearing of the airway.
      d. Rhonchi are musical and seldom heard in the newborn.

    e. Wheezes may be heard on inspiration or expiration and are louder with expiration.

    f. Rubs may be heard with inflammation of the pleura but are seldom heard in the newborn.

    g. Assess breath sounds for symmetry, diminished or absent sounds, tight sounds, and synchrony with the ventilator.

    h. It is imperative to listen to babies on high-frequency ventilation both on and off the ventilator to make a full assessment of the lungs. The time of this inspection should be coordinated to coincide with care requiring brief pauses off the ventilator.

  C. Palpation and percussion are not widely used in the newborn unless palpating for crepitus or percussing for dull sounds such as those in congenital diaphragmatic hernia.

III. Radiology: Nurses need to understand basic principles for assisting in making a quality radiographic examination and in interpreting the findings.

  A. Anything placed on the skin should be carefully considered for absolute necessity and potential for interference with imaging examinations. Such items include heat probe patches, electrodes and wires, and warming pads that can cause a "waffle" appearance on film. Keep lines and tubes from crossing the field being examined.

  B. Assist the technician in ensuring that the baby is positioned correctly in as symmetrical an alignment as possible, with the head midline and in a neutral position.

  C. Assess the reason for the examination, using a systematic approach:

    1. Soft tissue, bony structures, mediastinum, thymus

    2. Trachea, pulmonary vasculature

    3. Chest: Lungs, heart, diaphragm

    4. Abdomen: Stomach, bowel gas pattern, visible masses

    5. Lines/tubes: ETTs, umbilical catheters, peripherally inserted central catheters, chest drainage devices, nasal/orogastric tubes

IV. Monitoring

  A. Transcutaneous

    1. Allows measurement of oxygen and CO_2 levels through skin tension rather than by direct arterial sampling may have good correlation, depending on perfusion of skin.

    2. Complications include inaccurate readings, burns, and need for frequent changes, with subsequent increase in the time needed for nursing care.

  B. Pulse oximetry

    1. Emits wavelengths to a receptor that measures saturation of Hb.

    2. Monitors continuously.

    3. Accuracy depends on perfusion, body temperature, and Hb level.

    4. Used as a device to control inspired oxygen concentration with the ventilator. The procedure is still experimental in design.

    5. Knowledge of relationship between SaO_2 and PaO_2 is essential.

  C. End-tidal carbon dioxide ($ETCO_2$): To monitor $ETCO_2$, a device is attached to an ETT adapter to ensure position of the tube in the airway.

It contains filter paper sensitive to carbon dioxide, which changes color from purple to yellow if exposed to carbon dioxide (and confirms that the ETT is indeed in the trachea).

V. Pharmacotherapy: Neonatal nurses should be well versed in the drug therapies that have impact on the neonatal respiratory system. These include:
A. Sedatives
B. Analgesics
C. Muscle relaxants
D. Nitric oxide
E. Exogenous surfactants
F. Diuretics
G. Steroids
H. Vasoactive drugs
I. Bronchodilators

VI. Anticipatory Guidance: Be aware of the normal course of disease or treatments and anticipate the care required. Following are some examples.
A. RDS has a diuretic phase 48 to 72 hours after birth that generally coincides with increased compliance and improvement in condition.
B. Surfactants: Immediate increase in compliance after dosing requires less ventilator support. Failure to recognize this may result in pneumothorax.
C. CLD: As lungs develop dependency on ventilation or supplemental oxygen, the baby may have an increase in frequency and severity of desaturation spells.

VII. Documentation
A. Documentation should be timely and accurate.
B. The American Nurses Association has set standards for nurses that they must document in the medical record to communicate with other health-care providers any information concerning the patient whether in flowsheets, care plans, patient teaching, and so forth.
C. The Standards for Nursing Practice in British Columbia has set the purpose of documentation as improving communication with other nurses and care providers, promoting good nursing care in determining the effectiveness of treatments and necessary changes to the plan of care and assisting in decision making about funding for nursing research and resource management. Finally, it meets professional and legal standards for nursing measured against the standard of a reasonable and prudent nurse with similar education and experience.
D. Inclusions
1. Assessment of the patient
2. Baseline vital signs, ventilatory settings, oxygen saturation, and/or transcutaneous readings
3. Need for any nursing procedure, outcome, tolerance, and complications of procedure, if any
4. Amount, type, color, and consistency of secretions

5. Any apneic, desaturation, or bradycardic episodes not iatrogenically caused, such as associated with suctioning, positioning, tube placements

E. Abbreviations
1. Use as few as possible.
2. Use only approved abbreviations.
3. Print (not cursive writing) all abbreviations.
4. Use appropriate symbols.
5. Do not invent new symbols.
6. Clarify unknown abbreviations with the writer.

VIII. Chest Physiotherapy (CPT)/Postural Drainage (PD)
A. These procedures are of no benefit in the delivery room.
B. PD rarely is used because of concerns about the baby's lack of cerebral autoregulation.
C. CPT may include vibration, although there is no evidence to support its use.
D. There is no evidence that routine CPT assists in clearing secretions or in weaning from the ventilator. CPT has been associated with an increase in intracranial hemorrhage in the first 24 hours of life.
E. The baby's tolerance must be monitored during CPT.
F. Complications include hypoxia, bradycardia, rib fractures, and subperiosteal hemorrhage.

IX. Suctioning
A. Suctioning should never be performed on a schedule, but rather according to need per assessment, with an understanding of the disease process. Studies have shown no increase in secretions or occluded ETTs when suctioning was extended to occur once every 12 hours versus every 6 hours in babies ventilated for RDS.
B. Indicators for suctioning may include visible secretions, coarse or decreased breath sounds, decrease in saturations, acute change in blood gas results, and agitation or change in vital sounds related to the respiratory system. Turbulence on graphic monitoring may indicate airway secretions.
C. Upper airways should be suctioned gently.
D. Tracheal suctioning in the delivery room has been reserved for nonvigorous newborns or those requiring resuscitation in the immediate period after delivery regardless of the consistency of secretions or meconium.
E. ETT suctioning is performed to maintain the patency of the ETT and includes the following factors:
1. Complications include hypoxemia, bradycardia, tachycardia, atelectasis, pneumonia, lability in blood pressure and intracranial pressure, trauma to airway, sepsis, tube blockage and dislodgement, and pneumothorax.
2. Preoxygenation has been shown to result in a higher PaO_2 after suctioning, with decreased recovery time, although the effect on other outcomes such as retinopathy of prematurity, intracranial hemorrhage, and CLD is not known.

3. There are theoretical concerns regarding the use of ETT suctioning for deep suctioning; however, there is no evidence to refute deep suctioning according to a recent Cochrane review.
4. There is *no* clear evidence about how many passes should be made when suctioning, and this needs to be established each time suctioning is performed. One small study found no increase in secretion removal in two passes versus one pass.
5. Saline should be used only as a lubricant for the catheter and never instilled in the ETT. Research has shown that it does not thin secretions, nor does it mobilize secretions.
6. Head turning does not improve secretion removal and may be associated with intracranial pressure fluctuations and hemorrhage.
7. A Cochrane review found that use of a device that allows for suctioning without disconnection from the ventilator may have short-term benefits such as decreased variability in oxygenation and heart rate. The review was unable to assess the clinical relevance of these benefits or to assess other outcomes, and therefore it is unable to make any implications for practice.
8. The baby should be contained during suctioning to improve tolerance.
9. The nurse must stay at bedside and assure recovery from suctioning.

X. Transillumination (see Chapter 21)
A. This modality is used as an adjunct to clinical assessment and radiographs.
B. A diameter >1 cm may be seen around the light when placed on anterior chest or in a midaxillary line with air leaks in the chest.
C. Edema, tape, or equipment may decrease accuracy.

XI. Chest Drainage Devices
A. Be familiar with the set-up and function of drainage devices *before* they are needed, because these are emergent procedures.
B. Connections should be secured with tape.
C. Tubing is typically very heavy and should be well secured to bed to alleviate any tension on chest tubes.
D. Drainage device should be assessed for air "bubbling" in water seal chamber.
E. Chest tubes should be assessed for secretions and for movement in tube of air or secretions.
F. There is no benefit in "milking" chest tubes, and this may cause harm.
G. Fluid removed should be assessed and documented at least once per 8-hour shift unless clinical conditions call for increased monitoring.
H. Dressings should be assessed for occlusiveness, drainage under dressing, condition of the skin, and any foul odor or change in color of secretions.
I. Use a separate wall suction for clearing airway.
J. There should be an alternative set-up for emergent need or second set-up for replacement of current set-up ready at bedside. Also, an emergent means should be available at the bedside for a qualified

health-care professional to perform thoracentesis as a means to remove air quickly while performing set-up for chest tubes.

XII. Weighing

    A. Establish frequency of weighing as part of daily plan of care.

    B. At least two persons are needed to weigh a labile baby; one person may weigh a stable baby.

    C. It is preferable to disconnect ventilating devices while transferring the baby to and from scale and then reconnect the baby to ventilatory device while on scale and when returned to bed, if using a free-standing scale. If bed scale is used, ventilator usually may be left on during the weighing.

    D. Assess patient before and after weighing.

XIII. Positioning

    A. Much published data favor prone positioning for optimizing respiratory performance of the newborn.

    B. A Cochrane review of infant position during mechanical ventilation reported that prone positioning slightly improved oxygenation but may not lead to sustained improvement or be clinically relevant.

    C. When counseling parents, it is important to reinforce the American Academy of Pediatrics' position that supine positioning during sleep is preferred for care at home where there is no monitoring or 24-hour bedside care.

    D. Kangaroo care may be beneficial as an adjunct to respiratory care in ventilated babies.

        1. Kangaroo care is a form of skin-to-skin contact for preterm/small infants who are clinically stable. The infant is held in an upright position, skin-to-skin, against the mother's chest and kept warm.

        2. Assist the mother to transfer the baby to her chest before the mother sits in the chair, rather than handing the baby to the mother while she is sitting.

    E. Co-bedding of multiple birth babies

        1. Placing two infants in the same bed is still in investigation, with very limited data.

        2. Some limited anecdotal data report use in ventilated infants with improvement in respiratory status, weaning from ventilator, and no increase in spontaneous extubation. However, this practice must be approached cautiously until research is conclusive.

Suggested Reading

Balaguer A, Escribano J, Roqué M: Infant position in neonates receiving mechanical ventilation. Cochrane Database Syst Rev (2):CD003668, 2003.
http://www.nichd.nih.gov/cochrane/Balaguer/balaguer.htm

Claure N, Gerhardt T, Everett R, et al: Closed-loop controlled inspired oxygen concentration for mechanically ventilated very low birth weight infants with frequent episodes of hypoxemia. Pediatrics 5:1120-1124, 2001.

Gale G, Franck L, Lund C: Skin-to-skin (kangaroo) holding of the intubated premature infant. Neonatal Netw 12:49-57, 1993.

Hodge D: Endotracheal suctioning and the infant: A nursing care protocol to decrease complications. Neonatal Netw 9:7-15, 1991.

Lioy J, Manginello F: A comparison of prone and supine positioning in the immediate postextubation period of neonates. J Pediatr 112:982-984, 1987.

Pritchard M, Flenady V, Woodgate P: Preoxygenation for tracheal suctioning in intubated, ventilated newborn infants. Cochrane Database Syst Rev (3):CD000427, 2001. Update in: Cochrane Database Syst Rev (3):CD000464, 2001.
http://www.nichd.nih.gov/cochrane/pritchard/pritchard.htm

Raval D, Yeh T, Mora A, et al: Chest physiotherapy in preterm infants with RDS in the first 24 hours of life. J Perinatol 7:301-304, 1986.

Spence K, Gillies D, Waterworth L: Deep versus shallow suction of endotracheal tubes in ventilated neonates and young infants. Cochrane Database Syst Rev (3):CD003309, 2003.
http://www.nichd.nih.gov/cochrane/Spence2/spence.htm

Wilson G, Hughes G, Rennie J, Morley C: Evaluation of two endotracheal suction regimes in babies ventilated for respiratory distress syndrome. Neonatal Netw 11:43-45, 1992.

Woodgate P, Flenady V: Tracheal suctioning without disconnection in intubated ventilated neonates. Cochrane Database Syst Rev (2):CD003065, 2001.
http://www.nichd.nih.gov/cochrane/Woodgate2/Woodgate.htm

Wrightson D: Suctioning smarter: Answers to eight common questions about endotracheal suctioning in neonates. Neonatal Netw 18:51-55, 1999.

Yokum F: Nursing documentation, 2004. http://www.awarenessproductions.com

72

Transport of Ventilated Babies

Steven M. Donn and Molly R. Gates

I. Equipment
    A. Goals of neonatal transport
        1. Optimally, all infants requiring neonatal intensive care should be delivered at a facility capable of providing such services. Unfortunately, numerous circumstances arise that prevent this, including geographic and economic constraints and unexpected complications of labor, delivery, or the neonatal period.
        2. The next best option is maternal transport when time and circumstances permit the transfer of a mother with an identified high-risk pregnancy to a facility able to care for the baby.
        3. When neither of these options is possible, transport of a critically ill newborn must be accomplished in a manner that maximizes safety and minimizes complications for the baby. Neonatal transport must be considered an extension of the NICU, and the same philosophy of care delivered in the NICU should be delivered in the transport vehicle.
    B. Transport vehicles
        1. Ground ambulance
            a. This is the most frequently used vehicle.
            b. Provides the best access to the patient during transport.
            c. Enables the presence of the largest number of transport team members.
            d. It is easy to stop the vehicle in the event of patient deterioration and need for medical intervention.
            e. Subject to traffic delays and bad road conditions; also may be delayed by weather, although to a lesser extent than airborne vehicles.
            f. Is usually adaptable to special needs of neonatal transport.
        2. Helicopter
            a. Provides a rapid means of transport.
            b. Is not subject to traffic or road conditions, but weather conditions may preclude use.
            c. Size of vehicle may limit number of team members.
            d. Landing pad may not be adjacent to hospital, requiring extra time and possible ambulance use.
            e. Virtually no access to patient en route.

       f. Must land in event of patient deterioration.

       g. Requires special training of crew.

       h. Expensive.

   3. Fixed-wing aircraft

       a. Enables long-distance transport.

       b. Subject to weather conditions.

       c. Size of vehicle may limit number of team members.

       d. Rapid, although travel time to/from airport and hospitals must be considered.

       e. Intermediate access to the patient en route; deterioration may be problematic.

       f. There can be special problems at higher altitudes.

       g. Expensive.

   4. Combination: At times it may be advantageous to combine modes of transport, such as in the "fly-drive" method, in which the transport team and only essential emergency equipment are flown by helicopter to the referring hospital; the helicopter returns to the tertiary facility immediately, and the ambulance is dispatched with the remainder of transport equipment. This eliminates helicopter "down time" while baby is stabilized and allows for use of a more stable environment for transport of the baby.

 C. Transport incubator and related equipment

   1. Several commercial types are available.

       a. Self-contained types include virtually all necessary components as "built-ins," which may be more economical in the long run, although repairs may be costlier and may take the device out of service for a longer period of time.

       b. More basic models are available, to which specific components can be added according to the specific needs of an institution.

   2. Basic necessities

       a. The incubator must be able to maintain the baby in a thermoneutral environment; for small babies, infant servo-controlled heaters are recommended. This is especially important in winter climates that have a significantly low ambient temperature. Additional heat-conserving or heat-generating devices are necessary in colder climates.

         (1) Heat shield or thermal blanket

         (2) Exothermic chemical mattress

       b. Electronic cardiorespiratory monitor, which should function properly despite vehicle vibration or electrical interference

       c. Pulse oximeter(strongly recommended)

       d. Means of recording the temperature of the incubator and the baby

       e. Source of air and oxygen, including a blender and an analyzer, and the means to deliver increased FiO_2 to the infant

       f. Self-contained power source (battery) and the ability to be run by an external power source (e.g., wall electricity, vehicle generator)

       g. Easy accessibility to the baby (e.g., portholes, front and side doors)

    h. Means of securely anchoring the incubator within the transport vehicle

    i. All necessary resuscitative equipment, including:

      (1) Bag and masks (assorted sizes)

      (2) Laryngoscope and endotracheal tubes (assorted sizes)

      (3) Vascular access devices

      (4) Emergency medications and the means to deliver them

  3. Recommended options

    a. Transport ventilator, especially if transporting critically ill infants or transporting long distances

    b. Communications device

      (1) Vehicle radio system

      (2) Cellular telephone

    c. Vascular infusion pump(s)

    d. Blood pressure monitoring device, either invasive or noninvasive

    e. Transcutaneous $TcPO_2/PCO_2$ device or portable blood gas analyzer for long-distance transport of critically ill baby

D. Transport equipment (Tables 72-1 and 72-2): Equipment should be readily available to treat any emergency that might occur at the referring hospital or en route.

E. Transport medications (Table 72-3): Medications should be readily available, as well as the means to deliver them (e.g., syringes, diluents, catheter connectors). Medications must be secured and checked regularly for condition and expiration date.

F. Miscellaneous issues

  1. An instant camera is useful, both to give the parents a photograph of the baby and to document any unusual physical findings.

  2. All necessary documents for the medical record as well as printed information given to the parents should be prepared in advance. Keeping them together by means of a clipboard works well.

  3. Team members must protect themselves at all times.

    a. Dress appropriately for the weather.

    b. Use flame-retardant clothing for air transport.

    c. Use approved helmets for air transport.

    d. Have provisions (e.g., snacks) for long-distance transports, especially if there is a likelihood of missing meals.

    e. Always use seat belts.

    f. Maintain current knowledge of transport supplies and procedures.

  4. Packs or containers for miscellaneous transport gear should be lightweight, sturdy, well-labeled, and secure. Housing all supplies needed for a given procedure in a single compartment is useful.

II. Stabilization of the Transported Newborn

A. Basic stabilization on arrival

  1. Respiratory

    a. Assess the adequacy of gas exchange:

      (1) Clinical assessment

        (a) Breath sounds

        (b) Chest excursions

TABLE 72-1. Typical Transport Equipment

Adapters	Lubricating gel
Adhesive tape: ½″, 1″	Microbore tubing
Alcohol wipes	Nasogastric tubes: 5 Fr, 8 Fr
Antiseptic ointment	Needles: 18 G, 21 G, 25 G
Antiseptic swabs	Occlusive dressing
Blood culture bottle	Paperwork (extra)
Blood supplies	Platelet infusion set
BP transducer	Pneumothorax aspiration set
Bulb syringe	Replogle tubes: 6 Fr, 8 Fr
Butterflies: 23 G, 25 G	Saline squirts
Camera with film	Scalpel
Catheters: 22 G, 24 G	Scissors, sterile
Chest tubes: no. 10 Fr	Stopcock plugs
Connectors	Stopcocks
Cotton balls	Suction catheters: 6 Fr, 8 Fr
DeLee suction tube	Suture: 4-0 silk
$D_{10}W$: 250-mL bag	Syringes: TB, 3 cc, 5 cc, 10 cc, 20 cc, 30 cc, 60 cc
Dressings: 4 × 4, 2 × 2	T-connectors
Forceps, sterile	Tape measure, sterile
Gauze squares: see "Dressings"	Tape, plastic: ½″, 1″
Gloves, sterile	Thermometer
Glucose screening strips	Toumey syringe: 60 cc
Heimlich valves	UAC catheters
Hemostats, sterile	UAC double lumen
Labels	UAC tray
Lancets	Umbilical tape
Large-bore tubing	Waterproof adhesive tape

UAC, Umbilical artery catheter

TABLE **72-2.** Respiratory Care Transport Equipment

Blood pressure cable	Oxygen tubing (2)
Cargo netting	Adhesive solution
Chemical exothermic mattress	Magill forceps
Connectors: 15-mm (2), 22-mm (2), rubber	Nasal cannulas: newborn, premature
ECG electrode patches and leads	Sterile water-soluble lubricant
Electronic cardiorespiratory monitor	Nasal CPAP prongs, assorted sizes
Endotracheal tube adapters	Aluminum air tank
Endotracheal tubes: 2.5-mm (2), 3.0-mm (2), 3.5-mm (2), 4.0-mm (2)	Aluminum oxygen tank
Endotracheal tube stylets (2)	
Flashlight	Adhesive tape
Hood and aerosol tubing (include extra tubing)	Pulse oximeter
Infant mask	Flowmeter nipples (2)
Infant restraints	Laryngoscope blades: Miller no. 0, no.1
Manometer	Suction catheters, 6 Fr (2)
Neonatal mask	Oxygen tubing connectors (2)
PEEP valve	Air and oxygen connectors
Resuscitation bag	Hemostats and scissors
Stethoscope	Laryngoscope handle with spare batteries and bulb
Surfactant administration devices	Cotton swabs
Venturi mask	Pulse oximetry probes with elasticized wrap (2)
Wrench for medical gas "E" tanks	Adhesive remover

        (c) Skin color
        (d) Signs of distress
     (2) Laboratory assessment
        (a) Blood gas analysis
        (b) Chest radiograph
  b. Airway management
     (1) Patency (suction if necessary).
     (2) If baby is already intubated and tube position is satisfactory, secure tube adequately.

TABLE **72-3.** Typical Transport Medications

Adenosine, 3 mg/mL	Heparin
Albumin, 5%	Isoproterenol, 1 mg/5mL
Ampicillin, 250 mg	Lidocaine, 1% and 2%
Aquamephyton, 10 mg/mL	Lorazepam, 2 mg/mL
Atropine, 0.1 mg/mL	Midazolam, 1 mg/mL
Calcium gluconate, 10%	Morphine, 0.5 mg/0.5 mL
Dexamethasone, 4 mg/mL	Narcan, 0.4 mg/mL
Dextrose, 25%	Pancuronium, 1 mg/mL
Diazepam, 5 mg/mL	Phenobarbital, 30 mg and 60 mg
Digoxin, 25 µg/mL	Potassium chloride
Dobutamine	Prostaglandin E (PGE)
Dopamine, 40 mg/mL	Sodium bicarbonate, 42% (0.5 mEq/mL)
Epinephrine, 1:10,000	Sodium chloride
Furosemide, 10 mg/mL	Sterile water
Gentamicin, 10 mg/mL	Surfactant prn
Glucagon and diluent	Tham

(3) If baby is not intubated, consider elective intubation if there is any chance that this might become necessary en route. It is safer (and easier) to do this under controlled conditions at the referring hospital than in the back of an ambulance or while in flight.
   c. Place an orogastric tube (especially important for air transport).
2. Cardiac
   a. Assess tissue perfusion, treat if inadequate.
     (1) Blood pressure
     (2) Capillary refill time
     (3) Urine output
   b. Auscultation.
     (1) Murmur
     (2) Abnormal heart sounds
     (3) Abnormal rhythm
   c. Chest radiograph.
   d. If cyanotic congenital heart disease is suspected, consider starting infusion of prostaglandin E (consult with neonatologist or cardiologist before doing so).

3. Hematologic
   a. Check for sites of active bleeding.
   b. Check that all vascular connections are secure.
   c. Check hematocrit if not already done. Consider transfusion if
      hematocrit is low, baby's condition is critical, and/or duration
      of transport is anticipated to be long.
4. Metabolic
   a. Perform glucose screen. If low, check serum glucose and treat.
   b. Assure adequate glucose load during transport. Stress may
      increase consumption.
   c. Check baby's temperature and maintain thermoneutrality.
      Prewarm transport incubator before placing baby in it.
5. Vascular access
   a. It usually is best to achieve vascular access prior to departing
      the referring hospital in the event that an emergency arises
      en route.
   b. A well-placed peripheral venous line is usually sufficient.
   c. If it is difficult to secure peripheral venous access, consider
      placing an umbilical venous catheter. Confirm position
      radiographically before infusing medications (see Chapter 14).
   d. An umbilical artery catheter (see Chapter 14) generally is
      not needed for transport unless no other vascular access
      can be achieved. It is an elective procedure that can be time-
      consuming and can significantly delay departure and prolong
      transport. Many community hospitals are ill-equipped to handle
      such a complication. As a rule, this procedure is best carried out
      after the baby is admitted to the NICU.
6. Miscellaneous issues
   a. Make sure that the baby is secured within the transport
      incubator. Restraining straps should be used but must not be so
      tight as to impair thoracic excursions.
   b. Tighten all connections (e.g., endotracheal tube adapter,
      ventilator circuit, vascular catheter connections, power lines)
      before departing. Label all lines.
   c. Consider the use of infant "ear muffs" to decrease noise
      exposure during air transport.
   d. Always have spare batteries for equipment that requires them.
   e. Give the parents the opportunity to see and touch the baby
      before departing from the referring hospital.
   f. Be sure that the baby is properly identified.
   g. Collect records from the referring hospital to accompany the baby.
B. Stabilization during transport
   1. If the baby was well-stabilized in the referring hospital, little else
      should be necessary once underway.
   2. Check to be sure all of the vehicle equipment is functioning at the
      time the switch from incubator to vehicle is made.
      a. Power (generator or inverter)
      b. Gas (air and oxygen) sources
      c. Suction source

   3. Be sure the transport incubator is securely anchored and that there
      are no loose equipment or tanks that could cause a hazard en route.
   4. Monitoring of the baby during the transport should be no different
      from that which is done in the NICU.
   5. Should the baby unexpectedly deteriorate en route, it generally is
      best to stop the vehicle (this may mean landing if in a helicopter).
      It is extremely difficult to perform resuscitative procedures and draw
      and administer medications in a moving vehicle, and to do so places
      both the patient and the transport team members at risk for injury.
C. After the transport
   1. Thorough transport notes should be written in the medical record
      to document the events of the transport, as well as any treatments
      rendered, and how the baby tolerated the procedure.
   2. All supplies should be promptly replenished.
   3. Any mechanical problems (vehicle, equipment, or other) should be
      reported and corrected immediately.
   4. Give feedback to the referring physician and notify the parents that
      the baby arrived safely.
III. Special Considerations
   A. Intensive Care
      1. Although transport vehicles are designed to extend intensive care
         services to referring hospitals, they are not intensive care units.
         One of the most difficult decisions during neonatal transport is
         deciding whether a specific procedure should be performed in the
         referring hospital/transport vehicle or deferred until admission to
         the NICU. Some aspects to consider include:
         a. Urgency of the procedure in light of the patient's condition
            (i.e., elective, semielective, or emergent)
         b. Availability of experienced personnel to assist
         c. Suitability of available equipment
         d. Ability to handle a major complication if it occurs
         e. Adequacy of monitoring the patient during the procedure
      2. Some procedures that are of an elective nature should be deferred
         in view of the difficulty with which they are performed in a
         transport vehicle.
         a. Endotracheal intubation: Control of the airway in a baby with
            respiratory distress is crucial. Do not wait until the baby is in
            marked distress to intubate.
         b. Vascular access: Placement of a peripheral intravenous line *prior to*
            departure from the referring hospital is strongly advised. This is
            an extremely difficult procedure in a dimly lit, moving vehicle,
            especially if the baby is hypotensive. Placement before departure
            also enables prompt treatment of problems such as hypoglycemia.
      3. If transport to a facility providing extracorporeal membrane
         oxygenation (ECMO) is being considered, remember the following:
         a. Not all transport teams can provide inhaled nitric oxide during
            the transport. Do not delay transfer of babies with persistent
            pulmonary hypertension of the newborn (PPHN) if this is
            the case.

     b. It is presently infeasible in most instances to transport a baby on high-frequency oscillatory ventilation. If a baby cannot be safely managed temporarily by conventional or manual ventilation, transport may be ill-advised.

B. Effects of altitude
  1. Impact on respiratory status
     a. The partial pressure of oxygen decreases as altitude increases, thus the availability of oxygen to the baby decreases and alveolar hypoxia increases. The baby must work harder to achieve satisfactory gas exchange.
     b. The cabins of fixed-wing aircraft are either pressurized or non-pressurized. If nonpressurized, this effect of altitude will occur early. Pressurized cabins generally have a pressure equivalent to that at 8000 feet rather than atmospheric pressure at sea level.
     c. These parameters must be appreciated in the management of respiratory insufficiency. They underscore the need for close monitoring (i.e., pulse oximetry) as well as anticipating the need to increase support as altitude is increased.
  2. Impact on contained gases
     a. As altitude increases, and thus barometric pressure decreases, the volume of contained gases also increases.
     b. This effect must be taken into consideration in management of the baby.
       (1) Gas in the stomach and bowel will expand, potentially aggravating respiratory distress by impinging on the diaphragm. Be sure an orogastric or nasogastric tube is in place to vent the stomach.
       (2) Abnormal accumulations of gas in the chest (e.g., pulmonary interstitial emphysema, pneumomediastinum) can also expand, leading to pneumothorax. Observe closely and be ready to intervene.
     c. The effects of altitude on various treatments must also be considered.
       (1) Medications and fluids are packaged at sea level, and thus are at higher pressure at altitude. Be cautious when drawing medications from vials.
       (2) As the aircraft descends, carefully observe gravity drip infusions; external pressure may create a gradient that causes reversal of flow from the baby, with subsequent blood loss.

C. Miscellaneous effects on the baby
  1. Noise and vibration: Although these are not totally avoidable, some measures can be taken to minimize their effects.
     a. Muffle noise by using "ear muffs" or cotton inserts.
     b. Make sure that vehicle suspension is in good order.
     c. Avoid excessive speed or poorly maintained roads, if possible.
  2. Cold stress.
  3. Position infant optimally for clinical support and to maximize the caregiver's ongoing assessment.

   D. Miscellaneous effects on the transport team
     1. Motion sickness, aversion to exhaust fumes
     2. Stress.
     3. Safety issues
   E. Effects on the family
     1. Separation from the baby (especially for the mother)
     2. Economic hardship
     3. Psychosocial stress
   F. Systems issues
     1. Organized procedures must be in place and communicated to all potential participants for requesting, accepting, dispatching, and conducting neonatal transports.
     2. Periodic review of transports enables identification and correction of system problems.
     3. Contingency planning and prior consideration of unusual circumstances improves response and lessens stress.

Suggested Reading

Donn SM, Faix RG, Gates MR: Neonatal transport. Curr Prob Pediatr 15:1-63, 1985.

Donn SM, Faix RG, Gates MR: Emergency transport of the critically ill newborn. In Donn SM, Faix RG (eds): Neonatal Emergencies. Mt. Kisco, NY, Futura Publishing, 1991, pp 75-86.

Donn SM, Gates MR: Neonatal transports. In Donn SM (ed): Michigan Manual of Neonatal Intensive Care, 3rd ed. Philadelphia, Hanley & Belfus, 2003, pp 447-455.

Gates MR, Geller S, Donn SM: Neonatal transport. In Donn SM, Fisher CW (eds): Risk Management Techniques in Perinatal and Neonatal Practice. Armonk, NY, Futura Publishing, 1996, pp 563-580.

Lilly CD, Stewart M, Morley CJ: Respiratory function monitoring during neonatal emergency transport. Arch Dis Child Fetal Neonatal Ed 90:F82-F83, 2005.

73

Discharge Planning and Follow-up of the NICU Graduate

Win Tin and Unni Wariyar

I. Discharge Planning of the NICU Graduate
   A. Introduction: Hospitalization of an ill newborn is not only one of the most costly of all hospital admissions, but is also a very stressful event for the family. Discharging the neonatal intensive care unit (NICU) patient early has several advantages, including enhancement of family/infant bonding, provision of a better environment for infant development, and reduction in cost. Discharge too early, however, can impose some risk of deterioration of an infant and can lead to hospital readmissions and further stress on the family. Effective discharge planning is an important factor in making the discharge as positive and stress-free as possible.
   B. Essential features of effective discharge planning
      1. Educates parents from the early stages and forms a team of the parents and NICU care providers.
      2. Customizes planning to meet the needs of the individual infant and family.
      3. Involves multidisciplinary agencies as appropriate.
      4. Avoids duplication of services and minimizes disruption to the family.
      5. Provides good communication between the NICU and community-based primary care providers.
      6. Simplifies the care of an infant prior to discharge; does not effect major changes in infant's management immediately before discharge.
      7. Identifies unresolved medical issues and specifies arrangements for appropriate follow-up.
   C. Assessment of readiness for discharge
      1. Assessment of the infant
         a. Healthy infants can be considered ready for discharge if they:
            (1) Maintain normal temperature in an open bed or crib.
            (2) Feed well by mouth and maintain appropriate weight gain.
            (3) Do not need cardiac or respiratory monitoring.
         b. Infants with specific ongoing problems need individualized discharge plans; they should be considered ready for discharge

only when the specific needs can be provided at home by the parents, with the support of care providers in the community.

   c. Common problems among NICU graduates include chronic lung disease (CLD), dysplasia, need for home oxygen therapy, and long-term feeding problems requiring nasogastric tube feeding. Community nurse specialists and nurse practitioners play a vital role in these circumstances.

  2. Family assessment should start from the time of the admission of an infant to the NICU. Factors that will influence readiness for discharge include:

   a. Parenting skills and the willingness to take responsibility

   b. Parents' experience and understanding of routine infant care and their ability to cope with specific problems

   c. Family structure

   d. Parents' medical and psychological history

   e. Home environment

   f. Financial concerns

   g. Cultural differences and language difficulties

D. Predischarge evaluation and examination

  1. Specific evaluation and screening of NICU graduates

   a. Ophthalmologic examination

    (1) Routine retinopathy of prematurity (ROP) screening for all infants with risk factors, according to established guidelines (see Chapter 69).

    (2) Specific eye examination should be arranged for infants with congenital infections, congenital eye abnormalities, chromosomal abnormalities, and absent red reflex on routine newborn examination.

   b. Hearing screening: If universal screening is not done, hearing screening is necessary in infants with a family history of sensorineural hearing loss, neonatal meningitis or encephalitis, severe hyperbilirubinemia, congenital infection, and congenital malformation of the ear and in infants following hypoxic-ischemic injury. Prematurity per se is considered a high risk factor, and some centers also use this as a criterion.

   c. Cranial ultrasound screening for hemorrhagic and/or ischemic brain injuries in high-risk infants according to individual NICU guidelines. However, a structurally normal cranial sonogram does not rule out long-term neurodevelopmental problems, and parents need to be aware that follow-up of these infants remains the most important part of the ongoing assessment.

   d. Immunizations: Preterm infants should receive immunizations based on chronological age, using the same dosage as for term infant counterparts.

  2. Predischarge examination remains a mandatory practice and serves to ensure that good general health and growth have been maintained in an infant who is ready for discharge. It also serves as a problem-finding approach for some infants who need further evaluation (e.g., heart murmur, unstable hip). However, a normal

predischarge examination does not give complete reassurance and the parents need to be aware of this.

E. Discharge information/letter
1. Written information should be made available to the primary care providers and ideally, also to the parents.
2. All medical terminology contained in the letter should be explained to the parents and should include:
   a. Infant's particulars (name, date of birth, address, etc.)
   b. Date of admission and discharge
   c. List of important medical problems
   d. Brief clinical summary
   e. Outstanding problem(s) at the time of discharge
   f. Medications at the time of discharge
   g. Instruction on immunizations
   h. Plans for follow-up and further assessments

II. Follow-up of the NICU Graduate
A. With better understanding of neonatal pathophysiology and recent advances in medical technology, there has been an increase in long-term survival of very ill NICU graduates since the mid-1980s.
B. As this group of infants is at high risk for adverse neurodevelopmental outcomes, it is important that carefully planned follow-up is made an essential part of the NICU service provision.
C. Importance of follow-up
1. For the child:
   a. Early identification of major problems of perinatal origin (e.g., cerebral palsy, developmental delay, major hearing or visual impairment): This will facilitate any further diagnostic tests, assessment, and involvement of other appropriate professionals and agencies.
   b. Screening for other medical problems (e.g., squint, speech delay, growth failure) so that early remedial measures can be implemented.
   c. Maintenance of optimal health in order to achieve the utmost potential for growth and development.
2. For the parents/caregivers:
   a. Support of families of children with special needs: To minimize confusion and to provide consistency of care and advice, it is important that a single "lead" clinician coordinates the child's care with the help and support of other professional agencies and services.
   b. Counseling of caregivers regarding the child's problems and their relation to perinatal events, probable prognosis of the condition, appropriate investigations, and results of various assessments.
   c. Advice on immunization, medications, and diet, as well as the need for involvement of other specialists/therapists.
   d. Reassure caregivers and address concerns regarding the child's condition and progress.

3. For the professionals/institutions:
   a. Follow-up studies/programs (hospital-based or population-based) are very useful as an audit process:
     (1) To evaluate and improve the standards of neonatal intensive care.
     (2) To monitor changing patterns of prognosis (mortality and morbidity) with time.
     (3) To evaluate newer modalities of management methods and interventions when the long-term neurodevelopmental outcome will be used as primary outcome measure.
     (4) To provide reliable sources of data/information for counseling.
   b. Follow-up programs/clinics also provide training opportunities for professionals.
D. Who should be followed-up?
   1. This depends to a great extent on the resources available.
   2. The following categories of babies should be followed.
     a. Very preterm and very low birth weight infants (<32 weeks gestational age [GA] and/or <1500 g at birth). Accurately assessed GA is a better predictor than birth weight for long-term morbidity.
     b. All NICU graduates who required mechanical respiratory support
     c. Small-for-GA babies (low birth weight or head circumference more than 2 standard deviations below the mean for GA)
     d. Babies with perinatal neurologic problems such as hypoxic-ischemic encephalopathy; known ischemic and/or hemorrhagic brain injury, ventriculomegaly, microcephaly; and those with abnormal neurologic behavior (e.g., neonatal convulsion, hypotonia)
     e. Hydropic infants, from any cause
     f. Babies who had intrauterine or severe perinatal infections
     g. Babies who had metabolic derangements sush as persistent hypoglycemia and hyperbilirubinemia requiring exchange transfusion
     h. Babies with congenital abnormalities
     i. Babies exposed to toxic agents (e.g., drugs) in utero
E. Who should follow-up NICU graduates?
   1. This will vary from one unit to another, depending on structure and resources, but the follow-up team ideally should consist of:
     a. The "lead" clinician (usually a developmental pediatrician), whose role is to act as a coordinator between the family and other appropriate professionals/agencies
     b. Community liaison nurse or nurse practitioner
     c. Pediatric physiotherapist
     d. Pediatric dietician
   2. The NICU follow-up team often needs the support of and consultation with other specialties such as ophthalmology, pediatric surgery, orthopedic surgery, neurosurgery, neurology, psychology, and genetics; and with audiology, speech, language,

and occupational therapists. However, it is important that the family rely on the lead clinician to coordinate planning and facilitate communication with other professionals involved in the care of the child.

   3. Some NICU graduates may need regular follow-up at specialized clinics; (e.g., children with multiple, complex health and neurodevelopmental problems, disabling CLD, apnea requiring treatment).

F. Components of follow-up assessment

   1. Listening to the parents/caregivers and addressing their concerns is probably the most important part of follow-up.

   2. Anthropometric assessment: Weight, length, and head circumference should be regularly monitored.

   3. System review: Particularly review any health problems, including feeding and bowel habits.

   4. Assessment of vision and hearing: Some children may need further referral for detail assessment.

   5. Neurological/neurodevelopmental assessment

     a. Assessment of posture, tone, reflexes, and presence of primitive reflexes: Joint assessment may prove very useful.

     b. Assessment of gait and detailed neurologic examination in older children.

     c. Achievement of developmental milestones: It is appropriate to correct for prematurity for children who are chronologically <24 months, especially if they were born extremely preterm.

     d. Follow-up programs in some centers may include more structured developmental assessments, such as the Bayley Scales of Infant Development and Griffiths Mental Developmental Scales.

   6. Systemic examination.

   7. Review of medications (including oxygen therapy); some may need to be discontinued, whereas others may need adjustment of dosage.

   8. Check that all required immunizations have been given and all necessary screening tests have been completed.

G. How often and for how long should NICU graduates be followed?

   1. This depends on the needs of the child and family and also on the resources available. Problems such as minor cognitive and learning problems, clumsiness, or poor attention span are more common among NICU graduates than in their normal-term counterparts, and ideally NICU graduates should be followed until they are of school age, or penultimately to adulthood.

   2. Most of these children do not need follow-up regularly once their growth and development are satisfactorily progressing.

   3. Communication between the follow-up team and the community pediatrician/school is important if the child needs longer-term follow-up, mainly because of potential learning difficulties.

H. In summary, follow-up of NICU graduates is essential to facilitate better care for the child and family, to take advantage of perinatal services, and to ensure the provision of appropriate support services for these children.

Suggested Reading

Allen MC: The high risk infant. Pediatr Clin North Am 40:479-490, 1993.

Damato EG: Discharge planning from the neonatal intensive care unit. Perinatal Neonatal Nurs 5:43, 1991.

Davies PA: Follow up of low birth children. Arch Dis Child 39:794-797, 1984.

Edwards M: Discharge Planning. In Avery G, Fletcher M, MacDonald M (eds): Neonatology: Pathophysiology and Management of the Newborn. Philadelphia, JB Lippincott, 1994, pp 1349-1354.

Fielder AR, Levene MI: Screening for retinopathy of prematurity. Arch Dis Child 67:860-866, 1992.

Lefebvre F, Bard H: Early Discharge of preterm newborn infants. In Davis JA, Richards MPM, Roberton NRC (eds): Parent Baby Attachment in Premature Infants. London, Croom Helm, 1983, pp 281-287.

McCormick MC, Stuart MC, Cohen R, et al: Follow up of NICU graduates: Why, what and by whom. J Intensive Care Med 10:213-225, 1995.

Tin W, Wariyar U, Hey E: Changing prognosis for babies of less than 28 weeks' gestation in the north of England between 1983 and 1994. BMJ 314:107-111, 1997.

Wood NS, Marlow N, Costeloe K, et al: Neurologic and developmental disability after extremely preterm birth. EPICure Study Group. N Engl J Med 343:378-384. 2003.

Ethical Considerations

Initiation of Life Support at the Border of Viability

74

Daniel G. Batton and M. Jeffrey Maisels

I. Introduction: For many years, parents and caregivers have had to make a decision about whether to resuscitate an infant at the border of viability. This dilemma is not new, and there are no infallible answers to this difficult question.

II. Definitions: For a given infant, the determination of viability (or nonviability) can only be made retrospectively.
   A. Previable infants: Those born at a gestational age (GA) for which survival is currently not possible.
   B. Viable infants: Those born at a GA for which there is currently a significant survival rate (>40% to 50%).
   C. Border of viability: GA at which survival is possible but unlikely (>0% but <40% to 50%).

III. Historical Morbidity and Mortality Trends of Premature Newborns
   A. The GA representing the border of viability has declined steadily since the 1970s as survival for premature babies at all gestational ages has improved.
   B. The GA difference between previable and viable infants has continued to decrease with improved survival. At many centers this difference is now as short as 1 to 2 weeks of gestation.
   C. Surviving infants born very prematurely have significantly more long-term medical and neurodevelopmental problems than do normal term infants. However, many surviving infants, even those born at the earliest GAs, are free of significant neurosensory impairment.
   D. Current institution-specific statistics are needed to guide decisions about resuscitation.

IV. Ethical Guidelines for Making Decisions about the Resuscitation of Borderline Viable Infants
   A. The decision should represent the best interests of the infant, not the parents or caregivers.
   B. Whenever possible, the decision-making process should be deliberate. There should be sufficient time devoted to the process and parents should not feel pressured.
   C. The decision should be made jointly by parents and caregivers and should not be unilateral. If desired, the parents should be encouraged to consult others.

    D. The decision must be fully informed and all relevant data must be considered. This may require altering the process to allow time to collect more information.

    E. The process should not be arbitrary. Using an absolute GA or birth weight limit can be hazardous because these limits have changed and continue to change over time.

    F. It is important to avoid the dilemma of a self-fulfilling prophecy. If newborns at a given GA are not supported, they will all do poorly, and the results can then be used to justify nonsupport. Comparison of the institution's outcome data with national data can help to avoid this situation.

    G. Poor anticipated quality of life or impending (inevitable) death are acceptable reasons for not initiating resuscitation. However, the following facts must be recognized:

        1. These predictions have significant error rates.

        2. The perception of what is or is not an acceptable quality of life varies widely among individuals.

    H. If there is *any* uncertainty, resuscitation should be initiated, and decisions regarding subsequent care should be reevaluated frequently (see Chapter 75). Initiating resuscitation in the delivery room does not preclude subsequent withdrawal of care, and this should be emphasized in discussions with the parents.

V. Problems Involved in Decision Making

    A. It is often very difficult to make a prenatal decision not to resuscitate, because the condition of the baby (by physical examination) and the birth weight are unknown, and this information is critical in determining the prognosis. Unless a poor outcome is certain, a prenatal decision not to resuscitate could be viewed as uninformed, because not all of the relevant facts are known.

    B. Decisions made in the delivery room are, of necessity, more or less instantaneous. This means that many decisions cannot be made in a deliberate manner and that all relevant data are not available.

    C. There are no agreed-upon guidelines for how poor the prognosis must be in order to justify withholding or stopping resuscitation. The most common developmental problems of extremely premature infants who survive are learning disabilities and behavior problems. However, these issues are not usually sufficiently severe to justify a nonaggressive approach.

VI. Conclusion

The approach to borderline viable newborns should be similar to that used for older children and adults who have a comparable prognosis.

Suggested Reading

American Academy of Pediatrics: Guidelines on foregoing life-sustaining medical treatment. Pediatrics 93:532-536, 1994.

American Academy of Pediatrics: Born-Alive Infants Protection Act of 2001, Public Law No. 107-207. Pediatrics 111:680-681, 2003.

American Academy of Pediatrics: Perinatal care at the threshold of viability. Pediatrics 110:1024-1027, 2004.

American Academy of Pediatrics: Survival and long-term outcomes of infants born at 23-26 weeks. Pediatrics 113:125, 2004.

Annas G: Extremely preterm birth and parental authority to refuse treatment—the case of Sidney Miller. N Engl J of Med 351:2118-2123, 2004.

Batton DG, DeWitte DB, Espinosa R, Swails T: The impact of fetal compromise on outcome at the border of viability. Am J Obstet Gynecol 178:909-915, 1998.

Byrne PJ, Tyebkhan JM, Laing LM: Ethical decision-making and neonatal resuscitation. Semin Perinatol 18:36-41, 1994.

Lantos JD, Tyson JE, Alexander A, et al: Withholding and withdrawing life sustaining treatment in neonatal intensive care: Issues for the 1990s. Arch Dis Child 75:F218-F223, 1994.

Meadow W, Reimshisel T, Lantos J: Birth weight-specific mortality for extremely low birth weight infants vanishes by four days of life: Epidemiology and ethics in the neonatal intensive care unit. Pediatrics 97:636-643, 1996.

Peerzada J, Richardson D, Burns J: Delivery room decision-making at the threshold of viability. J Pediatr 145: 492-498, 2004.

Roy R, Aladangady N, Costeloe K, Larcher V: Decision making and modes of death in a tertiary neonatal unit. Arch Dis Child Fetal Neonatal Ed 89:F527-F530, 2004.

Shankaran S, Johnson Y, Langer J, et al: Outcome of extremely-low-birth-weight infants at highest risk: gestational age = 24 weeks, birth weight = 750 g, and 1-minute Apgar = 3. Am J Obstet Gynecol 191:1084-1091, 2004.

75 Withdrawal of Ventilatory Support

Malcolm L. Chiswick

I. Introduction
   A. Assisted ventilation, from an ethical perspective, should be viewed not as a treatment but as a temporary support measure for infants with *potentially reversible* respiratory failure. In effect, this is a *trial of life*, and the desired outcome is survival with a reasonable chance of an independent existence in later childhood.
   B. Physicians who start assisted ventilation have *a duty* to consider with the parents withdrawal of ventilatory support if it seems that the desired outcome will not be achieved.
   C. The idea that life support must be continued as long as an infant is alive and that no one has the right to terminate assisted ventilation is an extremist view that few would defend.

II. Withdrawing Ventilatory Support
   A. A robust and coherent code of practice is needed to define the circumstances that permit the withdrawal of assisted ventilation. Otherwise ad hoc ethical standards will be applied to each case and a decision will be justified only *after* it has been made.
   B. The code of practice should be derived from logical and moral concepts, based on a respect for human life that can be applied consistently across a broad range of individual circumstances. We should not have to change the rules for each infant.
   C. In practice, there are two main circumstances in which withdrawal of ventilatory support is a consideration:
      1. When it is considered that the infant has already entered the process of dying.
      2. Where the continuation of assisted ventilation might well allow the infant to survive but with a risk of severe neurodevelopmental disability.

III. The Dying Infant
   A. Physicians are not obliged to continue with treatments that serve no purpose, especially when the treatment is associated with discomfort.
   B. The problem for the physician is to decide when assisted ventilation has ceased to become a trial of life and is simply prolonging the process of dying.
   C. The infant's state is generally one of multi-organ/system failure that may include hypotension and circulatory failure, renal failure,

metabolic and electrolyte dysregulation, disseminated intravascular coagulopathy, and cardiac dysfunction against a background of poor or no respiratory drive and often an impaired level of consciousness. Specific or supportive treatments directed at these complications normally will have been offered, but without success. In effect, the decision to withdraw ventilatory support is based on *medical indications* insofar as from a medical perspective further treatment is deemed pointless.

D. Withdrawal of ventilatory support in this situation gives some control over the timing and circumstances of the death. Instead of the parents and staff presiding over an infant who is surrounded by the technological trappings of failed intensive care and who will die from cardiac standstill at an unpredictable time, a more acceptable alternative can be offered.

IV. The "Quality of Life" Decision

A. Here the judgment is that an infant might well survive as a result of continuing ventilatory support, but the quality of life is seriously called into question.

B. There are circumstances, albeit rarely, when it is ethically acceptable to withdraw assisted ventilation from an infant whose life might be saved only by further prolonged discomfiture of neonatal intensive care and in whom it is probable that substantial neurodevelopmental or physical handicap will radically limit the infant's ability to participate in human experience and will render him or her forever dependent on a caregiver for everyday living.

C. The arguments surrounding quality-of-life decisions have been well rehearsed. Reservations include the following ideas:

1. "Quality of life" is a subjective notion.
2. We can rarely be certain about the extent of any predicted handicap.
3. The infant cannot take part in the decision making.
4. No one has the right to "act like God" and to judge whether death or survival with severe handicap is the better of the two.

D. On the other hand, faced with an intolerable existence, responsible adults may exercise their right to end their own lives, and someone has to speak out on behalf of the infant.

E. The most common scenario for withdrawing ventilatory assistance on the basis of a quality-of-life decision is when an infant has bilateral gross white matter damage on a brain scan and persisting abnormal neurologic signs, including impaired level of arousal, seizures, and abnormal muscle tone. The approach to decision making will be guided by local practice. In the author's experience, a trusting relationship between the parents and a designated physician under whose care the infant was admitted, together with a consensus view among senior and experienced staff, obviate the need for involvement of an ethics committee.

F. It is rare for parents to request thoughtfully and consistently that assisted ventilation be withdrawn against medical advice. On those occasions,the physician must act in the best interests of the infant, as professionally perceived.

G. It is more common for parents to request that ventilation be *continued* against medical advice. Here, the physician's duty to the infant is to ensure that the parents understand the facts so that they are capable of acting on behalf of the infant. The author's stance is to continue to counsel the parents, but certainly not to coerce them.

V. Engaging Parents in Decision Making

A. Parents of seriously ill infants need time to make their views known. When it is clear that their infant is seriously ill, parents should be led into the discussion early rather than later.

B. Do not shoulder the burden of decision making on parents ("These are the facts; what do you want us to do?").

C. Instead, *make clear your medical view* and indicate that you are seeking the parents' support.

D. Most decisions center around infants in whom the continuation of ventilatory assistance is merely prolonging the process of dying, and it is unfair in those cases to burden parents with the complex issues surrounding quality-of-life decisions.

VI. Deceptive Signals: We need to guard against "giving up" on sick infants prematurely. Deceptive signals that may erroneously persuade care providers that continuing ventilatory support is not justified include:

A. Despair

B. Adverse appearance of infant

1. Severe malnourishment
2. Cholestatic jaundice
3. Multiple skin trauma from infusion sites ("war wounds")
4. Hydrops

C. Biased impression of prognosis based on superficial comparisons with other infants

D. Nonvisiting parents

VII. Engaging Staff in Decision Making

A. Problems arise on neonatal units where there is no proper leadership, when the staff does not work together as a team, and when there is no proper forum for discussing ethical issues. Staff may feel unable to discuss the possibility of withdrawing assisted ventilation, and instead unspoken signals occur.

1. *Standing off on clinical rounds*: Disgruntled staff turn away and show a lack of interest in discussing the infant and contributing to further management.
2. *Exaggeration of clinical signs*: An infant with pallor may be described as appearing "white as a sheet"; skin peeling may be referred to as "peeling off in layers."
3. *Therapeutic nihilism*: All suggested treatments are rejected on the basis of their side effects.
4. *Incongruous search for the expert*: Paradoxically, staff may suggest calling in an "expert" such as a nephrologist or cardiologist to advise on organ system failure.
5. *Group formation among staff*: Small groups form among the staff and discuss among themselves the apparent futility of continuing ventilatory support.

6. *"The parents don't realize how sick the infant is"*: Despite the fact that the physician discusses the infant's progress with the parents at frequent intervals, the staff insists that the parents do not understand how ill the infant is.

B. These unspoken signals reflect desperation and despair among staff who cannot communicate their feelings to the senior physician. They are cries for help. It is essential that this situation is recognized and that steps are taken to improve the organization and communication on the neonatal unit. Unless this happens, decisions about withdrawing assisted ventilation will generate a crisis each time and provoke additional suffering for parents and indeed for infants.

VIII. Care Following Withdrawal of Assisted Ventilation
   A. The concept of withdrawing assisted ventilation should not be sold to parents simply as a matter of "turning off the switch."
   B. Parents should be prepared for events and offered a choice of how they would like their infant to be cared for during and after withdrawal.
   C. A minority of parents wants simply to bid farewell to their infant, to depart from the neonatal unit and leave the details to the staff. Their wishes should be respected.
   D. At the other extreme, some parents wish to remove the endotracheal tube and intravascular lines themselves.
   E. Facilities should be made available to allow parents to remain with their infant in a secluded room immediately after withdrawal. Some will wish to bathe and dress their infant, even if death has already occurred.
   F. There are some uncomfortable facts that we must be prepared to face together with the parents.
      1. After withdrawal of assisted ventilation, parents often want to know how long it will be before their baby dies. If the indication was that the baby had "already entered the process of dying," then one can anticipate that death will occur very soon after withdrawal. This is not always the case, and parents should be made aware beforehand of the inherent uncertainty. Parents should also be advised that the baby may gasp or show other reflex activities before expiring.
      2. Normally, the action of muscle relaxants will already have been reversed before ventilation is withdrawn in order to assess spontaneous breathing activity. In the author's practice it is not necessary to stop sedatives before assisted ventilation is withdrawn. However, it is treading on a legal tightrope to introduce heavy sedation prior to withdrawal in order to facilitate death once ventilation has been withdrawn. Moreover, the use of heavy sedation *after* withdrawal in order to facilitate death probably amounts to falling from that legal tightrope. If an infant breathes vigorously and with obvious distress for a prolonged period after withdrawal of ventilatory support, the notion that he or she had "already entered the process of dying" was probably

erroneous. Retrieving this situation is challenging and illustrates how important it is to assess infants accurately and thoughtfully before making decisions, rather than being misled by deceptive signals.

3. Even more challenging is the after-care of infants in whom ventilation has been withdrawn because of quality-of-life considerations. Often, by the time agreement has been reached that ventilation should be withdrawn, the infant is no longer dependent on the ventilator and may well survive without it. In effect, the time taken for a quality-of-life decision may exceed the narrow window of opportunity to effect withdrawal of ventilation, and parents should be made aware of this in a sensitive way.

4. Withholding fluids, nutrition, and warmth during after-care is not a reasonable option for these infants. The logic behind this statement is that all infants are *expected* to breathe spontaneously and the use of assisted ventilation is an *extraordinary measure* of medical care. In contrast, all babies are *normally dependent* on a caregiver for the provision of fluid, nutrition, and warmth and therefore it is reasonable to continue to provide them.

Suggested Reading

Campbell AGM: Quality of life as a decision making criterion I. In Goldworth A, Silverman W, Stevenson DK, Young EWD (eds): Ethics and Perinatology. Oxford, Oxford University Press, 1995, pp 82-98.

Chiswick ML: Withdrawal of life support in babies: Deceptive signals. Arch Dis Child 65:1096-1097, 1990.

Delaney-Black V: Delivering bad news. In Donn SM, Fisher CW (eds): Risk Management Techniques in Perinatal and Neonatal Practice. Armonk, NY, Futura Publishing, 1996, pp 635-649.

Kraybill EN: Ethical issues in the care of extremely low birth weight infants. Semin Perinatol 22:207-215, 1998.

Kuhse H: Quality of life as a decision making criterion II. In Goldworth A, Silverman W, Stevenson DK, Young EWD (eds): Ethics and Perinatology. Oxford, Oxford University Press, 1995, pp 104-120.

Pierce SF: Neonatal intensive care decision making in the face of prognostic uncertainty. Nurs Clin North Am 33:287-297, 1998.

Roloff DW: Decisions in the care of newborn infants. In Donn SM, Faix RG (eds): Neonatal Emergencies. Mt. Kisco, NY, Futura Publishing, 1991, pp 635-643.

Weil WB Jr, Benjamin M (eds): Ethical Issues at the Outset of Life. Contemporary Issues in Fetal and Neonatal Medicine. Boston, Blackwell Scientific, 1987.

Ventilatory Case Studies

Ventilatory Case Studies

76

Jay P. Goldsmith

I. Case 1
   A. Prenatal data
      1. Mother: 24-year-old G2 P1→ 2 with intractable advanced preterm labor at 25 weeks' gestation
      2. One dose of betamethasone given 2 hours before delivery; no clinical evidence of infection
   B. Patient data
      1. Male infant, 680 g, born by spontaneous vaginal delivery, vertex presentation
      2. Apgar scores: 3 (1-minute) and 5 (5-minute)
      3. Poor lung compliance requiring high ventilatory pressures in delivery room
      4. Surfactant given at 14 minutes of age
   C. Physical findings
      1. Severe respiratory distress: Retractions, decreased air exchange, wet rales bilaterally
      2. Hypotonia
      3. Fused eyelids, poor skin integrity, visible veins
   D. Clinical course
      1. Conventional mechanical ventilation (CMV): Increasing ventilatory support up to peak inspiratory pressure (PIP) 26 cm H_2O, rate up to 60 breaths/minute, FiO_2 0.6 → 1.0. Given dopamine to support blood pressure.
      2. Increasing CO_2 retention despite increasing mean airway pressure (P̄aw)
      3. Repeat surfactant given at 6 and 12 hours of age.
   E. Chest radiographs
      1. Figure 76-1: Chest x-ray (CXR) 1 hour after birth shows severe respiratory distress syndrome (RDS) with ground-glass appearance, air bronchograms, and decreased lung volume.
      2. Figure 76-2: CXR taken at 15 hours after birth shows microradiolucencies throughout all lung fields, with areas of large bullae and hyperinflation.
   F. Laboratory values
      1. Normal complete blood cell count (CBC); C-reactive protein (CRP) <0.3
      2. Increasing hypercarbia and acidosis with increased base deficit over first 15 hours of life

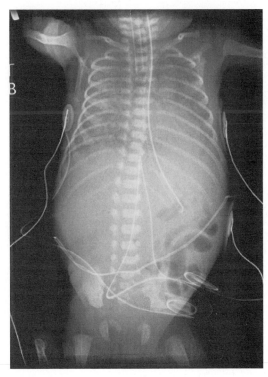

Figure 76-1. Chest radiograph 1 hour after birth showing ground-glass appearance, air bronchograms, and decreased lung volume consistent with respiratory distress syndrome.

G. Diagnosis
  1. RDS with associated pulmonary interstitial emphysema (PIE)
  2. Possible necrotizing pneumonitis (doubtful, too early)
  3. Possible lobar emphysema or cystic adenomatoid malformation of the lung (doubtful, disease process too generalized)
H. Potential therapies
  1. Ventilate with extremely short inspiratory times.
  2. Change to high-frequency ventilation (HFV): Use low-volume strategy (high-frequency oscillatory ventilation [HFOV] versus jet).
  3. Perform linear pleurotomies or scarification of lungs with creation of pnemothoracies and placement of chest tubes.
  4. Positional therapy or single lung inflation (works best with unilateral PIE)
I. Denouement
  1. Conservative therapy and HVF were unsuccessful.
  2. Patient developed pneumothoraces that were relieved with bilateral chest tubes.

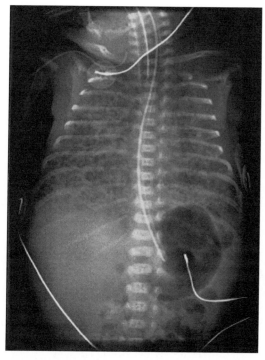

Figure 76-2. Chest radiograph 15 hours after birth showing microradiolucencies throughout all lung fields with areas of bullae and hyperinflation.

       3. Prolonged ventilatory support was necessary with the development of chronic lung disease (CLD) and grade 3 intraventricular hemorrhage (IVH).
       4. Patient discharged on oxygen at 3 months of age.
II. Case 2
    A. Prenatal data
       1. Mother: 18-year-old G2 P1 → 2
       2. Nonreassuring fetal status (meconium-stained amniotic fluid) at 41 weeks' gestation
    B. Patient data
       1. Male infant, 4670 g, born by urgent cesarean section at level II hospital
       2. Apgar scores: 1 (1-minute), 3 (5-minute), and 7 (10-minute)
       3. Intubated for meconium, ventilated in delivery room; no medications or cardiopulmonary resuscitation (CPR) given
       4. Extubated → oxyhood; pH at 1 hour of age = 7.16 → reintubated
       5. Transported to level III hospital
    C. Physical findings
       1. Large for gestational age; depressed

    2. Moderate respiratory distress: Tachypnea , 1+ retractions, rales at lung bases

    3. Duplication of right thumb

    4. Liver 4 cm below right costal margin

D. Chest radiograph (Fig. 76-3)

    1. Mild hyperinflation

    2. Patchy infiltrates consistent with meconium aspiration syndrome (MAS) or retained lung fluid

E. Laboratory values

    1. Normal CBC; normal renal and liver function panels

    2. Excellent arterial blood gases despite minimal ventilatory support ($\bar{P}aw = 7$ cm H_2O)

F. Clinical course

    1. Numerous technical problems with endotracheal tube, thought to result from plugging, displacement.

    2. Heart murmur heard on day 3 → two-dimensional echocardiogram (2D Echo) → endocardial cushion defect.

    3. Attempts to extubate from days 4 through 7 were unsuccessful.

G. Extubation failure: Differential diagnosis (Table 76-1)

H. Repeat CXR at 7 days of age (Fig. 76-4)

    1. Severe hyperinflation

    2. Volume loss in both upper lobes

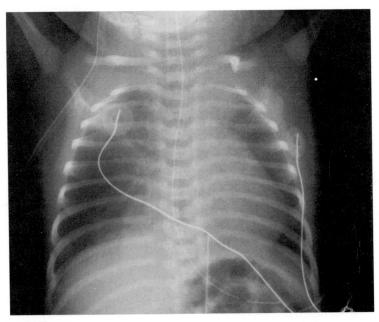

Figure 76-3. Chest radiograph on admission showing mild hyperinflation and patchy infiltrates.

TABLE **76-1.** Major Causes of Extubation Failure

Pulmonary
Primary disease not resolved
Postextubation atelectasis
Pulmonary insufficiency of prematurity
Chronic lung disease
Eventration, paralysis, or dysfunction of diaphragm
Pneumonia
Upper Airway
Edema and/or excess tracheal secretions
Subglottic stenosis
Laryngotracheomalacia
Congenital vascular ring
Necrotizing tracheobronchitis (?)
Cardiovascular
Patent ductus arteriosus
Fluid overload
Congenital heart disease with increased pulmonary flow
Central Nervous System
Apnea, hypoapnea, (extreme immaturity)
Intraventricular hemorrhage/periventricular leukomalacia
Hypoxic ischemic brain damage/seizures
Sedation
CNS infection
Miscellaneous
Unrecognized diagnosis (e.g., nerve palsy, myasthenia gravis)
Sepsis
Metabolic abnormality/severe electrolyte disturbances/alkalosis

Modified from Sinha SK, Donn SM: Weaning from assisted ventilation: Art or science? Arch Dis Child Fetal Neonatal Ed 83:F64, 2000.

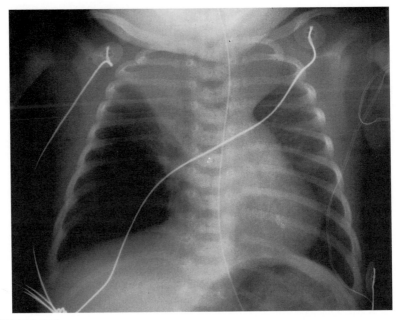

FIGURE 76-4. Chest radiograph at 7 days of age showing severe hyperinflation and bilateral upper lobe volume loss.

    I. Adjuncts to successful extubation
       1. Transition to pressure support ventilation (PSV) or nasal continuous positive airway pressure (CPAP)
       2. Methylxanthines
       3. Racemic epinephrine and/or inhalation or systemic steroids
       4. Vigorous chest physiotherapy postextubation (every 1 to 2 hours)
    J. Denouement
       1. Barium esophagoscopy, cardiac catheterization → true vascular ring with double aortic arch.
       2. Surgical division of vascular ring and ductus arteriosus ligation were accomplished without complication.
       3. Patient was successfully extubated on postoperative day 2.
  III. Case 3
    A. Prenatal data
       1. Mother: 37-year-old G4 P3 → 4 induced at 42 weeks' gestation
       2. Post dates and decreased fetal movement for 2 days
    B. Patient data
       1. Female infant, 3810 g, born vaginally, vertex presentation assisted by vacuum under epidural anesthesia
       2. Tight nuchal cord
       3. Apgar scores: 4 (1-minute), 6 (5-minute)
       4. Initial arterial blood gas at 1 hour in oxyhood ($FiO_2 = 0.4$): $pH = 7.12$, $PaCO_2 = 83$ mm Hg, $PaO_2 = 44$ mm Hg

5. Patient placed on time-cycled, pressure-limited ventilator; umbilical artery catheter placed for blood pressure and blood gas monitoring

C. Physical findings
 1. Post-term: peeling skin, decreased subcutaneous tissue, long nails
 2. Increased anterior/posterior diameter of chest, coarse inspiratory rales, tachypnea
 3. Acrocyanosis, hypotonia

D. Chest radiograph and laboratory values
 1. CXR: Fluffy lung fields, diaphragm flat, no air leaks (Fig. 76-5)
 2. White blood cell count (WBC), 27,200/mm^3 with left shift; platelets, 110,000/mm^3
 3. Normal metabolic profile

E. Clinical course
 1. Placed on antibiotics, maintenance IV fluids.
 2. Sedated.
 3. Given dopamine for hypotension.
 4. 2D Echo: Increased pulmonary vascular resistance with right-to-left shunt at foramen ovale and ductus arteriosus

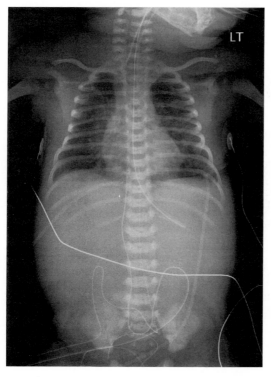

FIGURE 76-5. Chest radiograph on admission showing fluffy lung fields, flat diaphragm, and no air leaks.

5. Repeat CXR showed flattened diaphragms, interstitial fluid, small heart, no air leaks (Fig. 76-6)
6. FiO_2 increased to 1.0, ventilatory settings increased to Pāw = 16 cm H_2O. Unable to adequately oxygenate (PaO_2 <50 mm Hg).

F. Diagnosis
   1. Persistent pulmonary hypertension of the newborn (PPHN)
   2. Rule out total anomalous pulmonary venous return or other congenital heart anomaly (doubtful with normal cardiac anatomy seen on 2D Echo).

G. Potential therapies
   1. HFV
   2. Inhaled nitric oxide (iNO)
   3. Surfactant
   4. Extracorporeal membrane oxygenation (ECMO)
   5. Hyperventilation, alkalinization, paralysis (no longer favored because of side effects and availability of other options)

H. Failure of mechanical ventilation
   1. Death
   2. Inability to adequately oxygenate (unacceptably low PaO_2)
   3. Inability to adequately ventilate (unacceptably high $PaCO_2$)
   4. Toxic ventilatory settings or ventilator parameters predictive of poor outcome

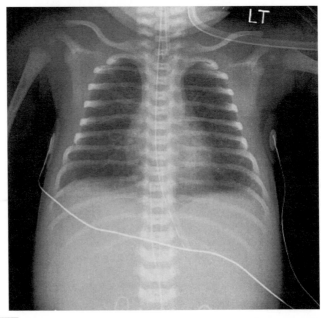

FIGURE 76-6. Chest radiograph at 24 hours showing hyperinflation, small heart, and no air leaks.

I. Predictive indices of poor outcome (term or near-term babies)
  1. Alveolar/arterial oxygen gradient (AaDO$_2$)
    a. To calculate AaDO$_2$:

$$(AaDO2) = (760 - 47) - PaCO_2 - PaO_2$$

$$760 \text{ mm Hg} = \text{atmospheric pressure}$$

$$47 \text{ mm Hg} = \text{water vapor}$$

    b. 600 to 620 mm Hg for 4 to 12 hours is predictive of high mortality.
  2. Oxygen index (OI)
    a. To calculate OI:

$$OI = \frac{100 \times (P\bar{a}w) \times (FiO_2)}{PaO_2}$$

    b. OI > 40 on 3 blood gases 30 minutes apart is predictive of high mortality.
J. Denouement
  1. Patient switched to HFV and given iNO, 20 ppm
  2. OI > 50 for 3 hours
  3. Placed on veno-venous ECMO for 140 hours
  4. Decannulated and extubated without difficulty
  5. Discharged with normal physical examination at 17 days of age
IV. Case 4
  A. Prenatal data
    1. Mother: 18-year-old G2 P1 → 2 at term
    2. Pregnancy reported as uncomplicated
  B. Patient data
    1. Female infant, 3510 g, born by precipitous vaginal delivery; vertex presentation
    2. Meconium-stained amniotic fluid
    3. Apgar scores: 7 (1-minute), 9 (5-minute)
    4. Apparent aspiration of meconium-stained amniotic fluid at delivery
  C. Initial course
    1. Oxygen by hood (FiO$_2$ = 0.4)
    2. First arterial blood gas at 30 minutes of age: pH 7.19; PaCO$_2$ = 54 mm Hg; PaO$_2$ = 29 mm Hg
    3. Intubation; placed on CMV: PIP = 20 cm H$_2$O, rate 30 = breaths/minute, constant distending pressure (CDP) = 4 cm H$_2$O
    4. Sepsis workup → antibiotics
  D. Initial CXR (Fig. 76-7)
    1. Bilateral alveolar filling
    2. Mild cardiomegaly
  E. Clinical course
    1. Patient treated for MAS, PPHN.

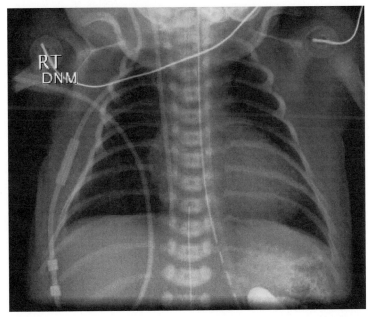

FIGURE 76-7. Initial chest radiograph showing bilateral alveolar filling and mild cardiomegaly.

    2. Required 15.5 mEq sodium bicarbonate for demonstrated metabolic acidosis over first 12 hours.
    3. Meconium fluid suctioned from trachea.
    4. Oxygen saturations fell to <60% when patient was agitated → patient paralyzed with pancuronium bromide.
    5. Increased respiratory settings on time-cycled, pressure-limited ventilator up to PIP 30 cm H_2O, FiO_2 to 1.0.

F. Further clinical testing
    1. 2D Echo (revealed normal structural heart anatomy and no right-to-left shunting)
    2. Pulmonary waveform graphic analysis (Fig. 76-8)

G. Potential therapies
    1. ECMO
    2. HFV
    3. iNO
    4. Increased settings on conventional ventilator
    5. Allow patient to wake up, normalize blood gases, and wean from ventilator rapidly using pulmonary graphics and blood gases to monitor air trapping and ventilation-perfusion (V/Q) match

H. Denouement
    1. Normal 2D Echo and pulmonary graphics revealed no PPHN and showed that patient was iatrogenically overventilated.
    2. Patient was allowed to wake up and breathe on her own.
      a. V/Q was normalized.

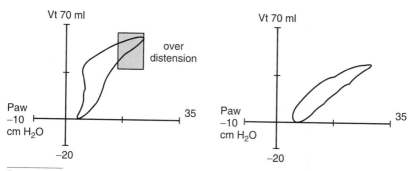

FIGURE 76-8. Pressure-volume loop demonstrating flattening of inspiratory curve ("beaking") indicative of no significant increase in lung volume despite increasing inspiratory pressure.

      b. Ventilator settings weaned quickly.
    3. Patient was extubated in next 24 hours and discharged home 6 days later.
V. Case 5
  A. Prenatal data
    1. Mother: 16-year-old G2 P1 → 3 with no prenatal care at 27 weeks' gestation
    2. Presents in active labor, complete, and ready to deliver at level I hospital
    3. Unsuspected twins
  B. Patient data
    1. Male second twin, 890 g, vertex presentation delivered by spontaneous vaginal delivery
    2. Apgar scores: 4 (1-minute), 6 (5-minute)
    3. Respiratory distress at birth
    4. Transport to level III NICU
  C. Physical findings
    1. Severe respiratory distress: Deep retractions, poor air exchange, wet rales
    2. Bruising of scalp, trunk
  D. Clinical course
    1. Intubated at 2 hours of age; exogenous surfactant given three times
    2. Poor response to CMV; switched to HFV secondary to CO_2 retention/acidosis
    3. Patent ductus arteriosus (PDA) murmur heard at 3 days; indomethacin tried, two courses → no effect; PDA ligation on day 9
    4. Unable to wean from ventilator despite adequate nutrition, blood transfusions, methylxanthines; patient requires continuous sedation/analgesia
    5. CXR at 27 days (Fig. 76-9): Areas of atelectasis alternating with cystic areas and interstitial edema consistent with early CLD
  E. Diagnosis
    1. CXR and clinical course consistent with CLD

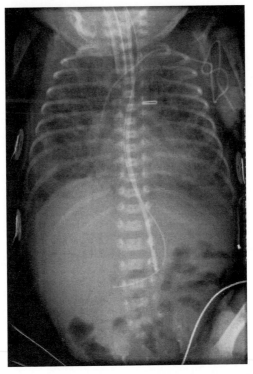

FIGURE 76-9. Chest radiograph at 27 days of age showing chronic lung disease pattern.

   2. Definition of CLD:
      a. Oxygen dependence at 28 days of age
      b. Oxygen dependence at 36 weeks postmenstrual age (PMA)
   3. Patient now 31 weeks PMA: Condition does not strictly meet definition of CLD, but CXR is suggestive of transpulmonary process.
   4. Pulmonary mechanics testing done.
F. Potential therapies
   1. Rule out other causes of ventilator dependency.
      a. Diaphragm moves bilaterally (status post-PDA ligation)
      b. Adequate methyxyanthine level
      c. CNS intact
      d. Rule out infection
   2. Goal is to extubate ASAP; may use nasal CPAP for distending pressure to prevent atelectasis/apnea.
      a. Permissive hypercapnia
      b. Bronchodilators
      c. Adequate calories with fluid restriction (120 to130 mL/kg/day) and/or diuretics

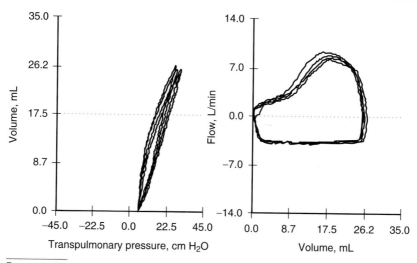

FIGURE 76-10. Pulmonary mechanics testing on synchronized intermittent mandatory ventilation demonstrating poor compliance.

      d. Corticosteroids (not recommended secondary to CNS side effects)
      e. PSV
  G. Denouement
    1. Patient is switched to volume-targeted synchronized intermittent mandatory ventilation (SIMV) with PSV at 12 cm H_2O (Fig. 76-10).
    2. Over next several days, PSV is increased, FiO_2 decreased; sedation and analgesia decreased, then discontinued.
    3. Pulmonary mechanics study is repeated (Fig. 76-11).

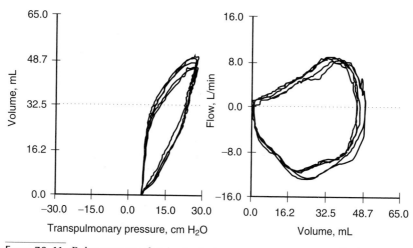

FIGURE 76-11. Pulmonary mechanics testing on pressure support ventilation only showing improved compliance.

4. SIMV is discontinued 1 week later and patient is extubated to nasal CPAP within 48 hours.
5. Patient is discharged at 76 days of age on oxygen by cannula.

Suggested Reading

Case 1

Greenough A, Dixon AK, Roberton NR: Pulmonary interstitial emphysema. Arch Dis Child 59:1046, 1984.

Keszler M, Donn SM, Bucciarelli RL, et al: Multicenter controlled trial comparing high-frequency jet ventilation and conventional mechanical ventilation in newborn infants with pulmonary interstitial emphysema. J Pediatr 119:85, 1991.

Meadow WL, Cheromcha D: Successful therapy of unilateral pulmonary emphysema: Mechanical ventilation with extremely short inspiratory times. Am J Perinatol 2:194, 1985.

Swingle HM, Eggert LD, Bucciarelli RL: New approach to management of unilateral tension pulmonary interstitial emphysema in premature infants. Pediatrics 74:354, 1984.

Case 2

Sinha SK, Donn SM: Weaning from assisted ventilation: Art or science? Arch Dis Child Fetal Neonatal Ed 83:F64, 2000.

Halliday HL: Towards earlier neonatal extubation. Lancet 355:2091, 2000.

van Son JA, Julsrud PR, Hagler DJ, et al: Imaging strategies for vascular rings. Ann Thorac Surg 57:604. 1994.

Case 3

Lewis FC, Reynolds M, Arensman RA: Extracorporeal membrane oxygenation. In Goldsmith JP, Karotkin EH (eds): Assisted Ventilation of the Neonate, 4th ed. Philadelphia, WB Saunders, 2003, pp 261-278.

Roberts JD Jr, Fineman JR, Morin FC III, et al: Inhaled nitric oxide and persistent pulmonary hypertension of the newborn. The Inhaled Nitric Oxide Study Group. N Engl J Med 336:605, 1997.

UK Collaborative ECMO Trial Group: UK Collaborative randomised trial of neonatal extracorporeal membrane oxygenation. Lancet 384:75, 1996.

Walsh MC, Stork EK: Persistent pulmonary hypertension of the newborn. Rational therapy based on pathophysiology. Clin Perinatol 28:609, 2001.

Case 4

Donn SM: Neonatal and Pediatric Pulmonary Graphics: Principles and Clinical Applications. Armonk, NY, Futura Publishing, 1998.

Nicks JJ: Graphics Monitoring in the Neonatal Intensive Care Unit. Palm Springs, CA, Bird Products, 1995.

Wood BR: Physiologic principles. In Goldsmith JP, Karotkin EH (eds): Assisted Ventilation of the Neonate, 4th ed. Philadelphia, WB Saunders, 2003, pp 15-40.

Case 5

Committee on Fetus and Newborn: Postnatal corticosteroid to treat or prevent chronic lung disease in preterm infants. Pediatrics 109:330, 2002.

Donn SM, Becker MA: Special ventilatory techniques and modalities. I: Patient triggered ventilation. In Goldsmith JP, Karotkin EH (eds): Assisted Ventilation of the Neonate, 4th ed. Philadelphia, WB Saunders, 2003, pp 203-218.

Kao, LC, Durand DJ, McCrea RC, et al: Randomized trial of long-term diuretic therapy for infants with oxygen-dependent bronchopulmonary dysplasia. J Pediatr 124:772, 1994.

Kao LC, Durand DJ, Nickerson BG: Effects of inhaled metaproterenol and atropine on the pulmonary mechanics of infants with bronchopulmonary dysplasia. Pediatr Pulmonol 6:74, 1989.

Mariani G, Cifuentes J, Carlo WA: Randomized trial of permissive hypercapnia in preterm infants. Pediatrics 104:1082, 1999.

Appendix

CONVERSION TABLE A: torr to kPa

torr	→	kPa	torr	→	kPa
20		2.7	80		10.7
25		3.3	85		11.3
30		4.0	90		12.0
35		4.7	95		12.7
40		5.3	100		13.3
45		6.0	105		14.0
50		6.7	110		14.7
55		7.3	115		15.3
60		8.0	120		16.0
65		8.7	125		16.7
70		9.3	130		17.3
75		10.0	135		18.0

Conversion Table B: kPa to torr

kPa	→	torr	kPa	→	torr
2.5		19	8.5		64
3.0		22.5	9.0		67.5
3.5		26	9.5		71
4.0		30	10.0		75
4.5		34	10.5		79
5.0		37.5	11.0		82.5
5.5		41	11.5		86.3
6.0		45	12.0		90
6.5		49	12.5		94
7.0		52.5	13.0		97.5
7.5		56	13.5		101
8.0		60	14.0		105

Index

Note: Page numbers followed by the letter f refer to figures and those followed by t refer to tables.